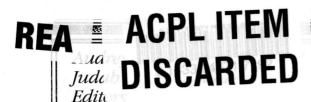

Cultural Change in Long-Term Care

Cultural Change in Long-Term Care has been co-published simultaneously as *Journal of Social Work in Long-Term Care,* Volume 2, Numbers 1/2 and 3/4 2003.

Pre-publication REVIEWS, COMMENTARIES, EVALUATIONS . . .

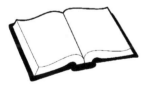

"**A** VERY IMPORTANT ADDITION to the literature about nursing homes, homes for the aged, geriatric care centers, public long-term care hospitals–all of the congregate living arrangements for functionally dependent older people. This collection illuminates the historical roots of our present-day system, and at the same time, IDENTIFIES PROBLEMS AND ISSUES THAT MUST BE FACED as the direction of long-term care is charted for the future. All of the chapters merit the attention of staff, trustees, and volunteers in our homes, and equally, the attention of other professionals, public officials, and academics who are concerned about the quality of care the homes provide."

Rose Dobrof, DSW
Brookdale Professor of Gerontology
Hunter College
City University of New York
Editor
Journal of Gerontological Social Work

The Haworth Social Work Practice Press
An Imprint of The Haworth Press, Inc.

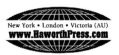

New York • London • Victoria (AU)
www.HaworthPress.com

Culture Change
in Long-Term Care

Culture Change in Long-Term Care has been co-published simultaneously as *Journal of Social Work in Long-Term Care*, Volume 2, Numbers 1/2 and 3/4 2003.

The *Journal of Social Work in Long-Term Care*™ Monographic "Separates"

Below is a list of "separates," which in serials librarianship means a special issue simultaneously published as a special journal issue or double-issue *and* as a "separate" hardbound monograph. (This is a format which we also call a "DocuSerial.")

"Separates" are published because specialized libraries or professionals may wish to purchase a specific thematic issue by itself in a format which can be separately cataloged and shelved, as opposed to purchasing the journal on an on-going basis. Faculty members may also more easily consider a "separate" for classroom adoption.

"Separates" are carefully classified separately with the major book jobbers so that the journal tie-in can be noted on new book order slips to avoid duplicate purchasing.

You may wish to visit Haworth's Website at . . .

http://www.HaworthPress.com

. . . to search our online catalog for complete tables of contents of these separates and related publications.

You may also call 1-800-HAWORTH (outside US/Canada: 607-722-5857), or Fax 1-800-895-0582 (outside US/Canada: 607-771-0012), or e-mail at:

docdelivery@haworthpress.com

Culture Change
in Long-Term Care

Audrey S. Weiner, DSW, MPH
Judah L. Ronch, PhD
Editors

Culture Change in Long-Term Care has been co-published simultaneously as *Journal of Social Work in Long-Term Care*, Volume 2, Numbers 1/2 and 3/4 2003.

The Haworth Social Work Practice Press
An Imprint of
The Haworth Press, Inc.
New York • London • Oxford

Published by

The Haworth Social Work Practice Press, 10 Alice Street, Binghamton, NY 13904-1580 USA

The Haworth Social Work Practice Press is an imprint of The Haworth Press, Inc., 10 Alice Street, Binghamton, NY 13904-1580 USA.

Culture Change in Long-Term Care has been co-published simultaneously as *Journal of Social Work in Long-Term Care,* Volume 2, Numbers (1/2)(3/4) 2002.

Cover design by Jennifer Gaska

Library of Congress Cataloging-in-Publication Data

Culture change in long-term care / [edited by] Audrey S. Weiner, Judah L. Ronch.
    p. cm.
    "Co-published simultaneously as Journal of social work in long-term care, volume 2."
    Includes bibliographical references and index.
    ISBN 0-7890-2110-2 (hard cover : alk. paper)–ISBN 0-7890-2111-0 (soft cover : alk. paper)
    1. Long-term care of the sick. I. Weiner, Audrey S. II. Ronch, Judah L. III. Journal of social work in long-term care.

RA997.C845 2003
362.1'6–dc21   2003010407

Indexing, Abstracting & Website/Internet Coverage

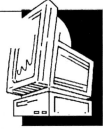

This section provides you with a list of major indexing & abstracting services. That is to say, each service began covering this periodical during the year noted in the right column. Most Websites which are listed below have indicated that they will either post, disseminate, compile, archive, cite or alert their own Website users with research-based content from this work. (This list is as current as the copyright date of this publication.)

Abstracting, Website/Indexing Coverage......... Year When Coverage Began

- *Ageline Database* **2001**

- *Alzheimer's Disease Education & Referral*
  Center (ADEAR) **2001**

- *Caredata CD: the social & community care database*
  <www.nisw.org.uk>.................................. **2001**

- *CINAHL (Cumulative Index to Nursing & Allied Health Literature),*
  in print, EBSCO, and SilverPlatter, Data-Star, and Paperchase.
  (Support materials include Subject Heading List, Database Search
  Guide, and instructional video) <www.cinahl.com> **2001**

- *CNPIEC Reference Guide: Chinese National Directory*
  of Foreign Periodicals **2001**

- *Family & Society Studies Worldwide <www.nisc.com>* **2001**

- *Guide to Social Science & Religion in Periodical Literature* **2001**

- *Social Services Abstracts <www.csa.com>*..................... **2001**

- *Social Work Abstracts* **2001**

(continued)

Special Bibliographic Notes related to special journal issues
(separates) and indexing/abstracting:

- indexing/abstracting services in this list will also cover material in any "separate" that is co-published simultaneously with Haworth's special thematic journal issue or DocuSerial. Indexing/abstracting usually covers material at the article/chapter level.
- monographic co-editions are intended for either non-subscribers or libraries which intend to purchase a second copy for their circulating collections.
- monographic co-editions are reported to all jobbers/wholesalers/approval plans. The source journal is listed as the "series" to assist the prevention of duplicate purchasing in the same manner utilized for books-in-series.
- to facilitate user/access services all indexing/abstracting services are encouraged to utilize the co-indexing entry note indicated at the bottom of the first page of each article/chapter/contribution.
- this is intended to assist a library user of any reference tool (whether print, electronic, online, or CD-ROM) to locate the monographic version if the library has purchased this version but not a subscription to the source journal.
- individual articles/chapters in any Haworth publication are also available through the Haworth Document Delivery Service (HDDS).

Culture Change in Long-Term Care

CONTENTS

SECTION 3. CASE STUDIES: IMPLEMENTING CHANGE

SECTION 4. CASE STUDIES: CULTURE CHANGE BRIEFS

SECTION 5. AN INTERNATIONAL PERSPECTIVE

SECTION 6. IS CHANGE REALISTIC?

ABOUT THE EDITORS

Audrey S. Weiner, DSW, MPH, is President and Chief Executive Officer of The Jewish Home and Hospital Lifecare System in New York, New York. She is the former Senior Vice President/Administrator and Chief Operating Officer of the Sarah Neuman Center for Healthcare & Rehabilitation and past Director of Services for Older Adults and Persons with AIDS at the Jewish Board of Family and Children's Services. An Editorial Board member of the *Jewish Social Work Forum*, published by the Wurzweiler School of Social Work at Yeshiva University, Dr. Weiner is the author or co-author of numerous articles that have appeared in the *Journal of Long-Term Care Administration*, *The Gerontologist*, *The Journal of Alzheimer's Care and Research*, *The Journal of Aging and Judaism*, and the *Journal of Applied Gerontology*. A frequent speaker in the areas of long-term care and caregiver support, she has also made numerous national and regional conference presentations. Dr. Weiner is a member of the American College of Healthcare Administration, the Gerontological Society of America, and Vice President of the World Council of Jewish Communal Services, among others.

Judah L. Ronch, PhD, is the founder and Executive Clinical Director of LifeSpan DevelopMental Systems, which for over 25 years has created numerous innovative programs of clinical service, research, staff development, systems consultation and organizational development to meet the mental health needs of the aging in various parts of the United States. Notable current activities include: culture change consultations to develop person-centered long-term care, especially for residents with dementia care in nursing homes; work with the New York State Department of Health on dementia care practices, survey and practice guidelines in Adult Care Facilities; and The EDGE program, an Internet-enabled system of tools and approaches designed to help nursing and Assisted Living facilities individualize and humanize care of residents with Alzheimer's and related dementias. He also maintains an active research program in the fields of innovative models of person-centered dementia care and culture change in long-term care. Dr. Ronch is a partner in Dementia Solutions, LLC, which hosts The EDGE online (*www.dementiasolutions.com*) and develops person-centered care approaches for a variety of long-term care settings, and is a partner in L/S Gerontology Seminars, LLC, providing staff development programs in gerontology, customer service and culture change in long-term care settings.

He is the former Executive Director of the Brookdale Center on Aging of Hunter College, the largest university based gerontology center in the Northeast, and has been on the faculties of Vassar College, The University of Miami, and Dutchess Community College.

Dr. Ronch's numerous publications include the critically acclaimed *Alzheimer's Disease: A Practical Guide for Families and Other Helpers* and *The Counseling Sourcebook: A Practical Reference on Contemporary Issues,* winner of the 1995 Catholic Press Association of the United States Book of the Year Award. He is co-editor of *Mental Wellness in Aging: Strengths Based Approaches* (with Joseph Goldfield) and *Culture Change in Long-Term Care* (with Audrey Weiner). His numerous journal articles and professional presentations include contributions in psychotherapy and counseling with the aged, care of persons with Alzheimer's Disease and related disorders, caregiver issues, staff training and service delivery issues in geriatric care. He is a popular and sought-after speaker for professional and lay audiences interested in these issues.

Foreword

Long-term care in the nursing home and kindred milieu has reached a point in its history–and in the history of our society–where new directions and innovative models are called for by all the stakeholders. Providers, residents and their families, advocates, regulators and the long-term care workforce all speak of the need for developing modern systems of caring for our dependent population that are grounded in more humanistic values and more realistic economics. We hope that this volume will provide needed expertise from multiple perspectives that will inform the diverse participants in this dialogue about how to think about the culture of long-term care and consequently, to fundamentally change it.

The prevailing wisdom in thinking about what has been termed "culture change"–a decidedly heterogeneous group of attempts to accelerate the speed and humanize the vector of institutional change, has created a shared values system that transcends the nature of any particular model. Terms like "humanistic," "person-centered," "home-like" and others have become the themes for care approaches that have as their primary mission the support and maximizing of residents' strengths (Cohen and Eisdorfer, 2001); in other words making long-term care less about care tasks and more about caring for people and the relationships between people.

We take the development of increased energy, creativity and urgency for long-term care innovation as a positive sign, though we appreciate the many barriers that still remain that thwart our attempts to achieve truly new models of care. It is not without some irony that Cohen and Eisdorfer (2001) see models for the future in earlier models of charity and compassionate care (beginning with the poorhouses of the 17th and 18th centuries) whose evolution toward medical models of care and reimbursement subordinated care of the person to care of an illness. As the articles in this collection demonstrate, some of the best attributes found in earlier years and other cultures are at the heart of

[Haworth co-indexing entry note]: "Foreword." Weiner, Audrey S., and Judah L. Ronch. Co-published simultaneously in *Journal of Social Work in Long-Term Care* (The Haworth Social Work Practice Press, an imprint of The Haworth Press, Inc.) Vol. 2, No. 3/4, 2003, pp. xix-xxi; and: *Culture Change in Long-Term Care* (ed: Audrey S. Weiner, and Judah L. Ronch) The Haworth Social Work Practice Press, an imprint of The Haworth Press, Inc., 2003, pp. xiii-xv. Single or multiple copies of this article are available for a fee from The Haworth Document Delivery Service [1-800-HAWORTH, 9:00 a.m. - 5:00 p.m. (EST). E-mail address: docdelivery@haworthpress.com].

http://www.haworthpress.com/store/product.asp?sku=J181
xiii

contemporary innovations. But the intellectual, regulatory, economic and attitudinal barriers that have arisen over time still confront innovators from all stakeholder groups as they contemplate issues of culture change for the future.

A look at our Table of Contents demonstrates, we think, both the breadth of critically important views covered in national and international perspectives as well as the expertise of our contributors. Our authors have confronted the many barriers to change on an everyday basis as they seek practical ways to bring meaning to the lives of those who live and work in long-term care.

In tackling the issue of culture change in long-term care, it is incumbent upon us to address the issue of how cultural context provides meaning to the experience of those who inhabit the institution. Perhaps the most detrimental effect of the traditional culture of long-term care, and the fact of institutional life that drives the movement for change the most, is how meaningless people's lives can become in the traditional nursing home. Any systematic attempts at culture change must therefore address the issue of teaching the requisite skills that insure cultural competency in the new order and thus add meaning to peoples' lives. This adds an additional dimension to the work of culture change, and to the traditional dialogue about cultural diversity and multi-cultural competency, by recognizing that participants in culture change programs must have the skills to manage issues of cultural diversity in the broadest sense *while* the culture is undergoing the process of change. To the extent they do not, staff will be unprepared to cope productively when inevitable clashes between the old and new cultures occur. These events represent potential opportunities to further culture change *in vivo* and strengthen the impact of formal culture programs.

We appreciate how complex and lengthy the process of culture change in long-term care will be. We also realize that each culture's "story" is perhaps best told using its own cultural and linguistic frame, and that a common language to talk about change will be developed in part as a result of this volume. These contributions are offered to the reader in the spirit of extending the dialogue about change, and with the hope that they will promote more conversations, research and practical collaborations that promote shared visions, innovative models and "cross cultural" experiences. We are proud to offer this within a collection framed by the values, knowledge and skills of the social work profession. We hope the discussion about the substance of changes and the related models, the journeys themselves and the importance of nurturing the souls of all involved in the change process is instructive.

Finally, we hope this special volume inspires dialogue and communication through letters to the editor and future articles on the subject. We thank all of the authors for their contributions and are grateful for our many new and valued colleagues. You have made our work and journey as editors more meaningful and enjoyable.

Audrey S. Weiner, DSW, MPH
Editor

Judah L. Ronch, PhD
Co-Editor

REFERENCE

Cohen, D. & Eisdorfer, C. (2001). Wanted: A new look at nursing homes in America. *Journal of Mental Health and Aging*, 7, 3, 299-300.

SECTION 1
INTRODUCTION TO CULTURE
AND VALUES IN LONG-TERM CARE

Unloving Care Revisited:
The Persistence of Culture

Bruce C. Vladeck

SUMMARY. In the almost 25 years since *Unloving Care* was written, there have been substantial changes in the characteristics of nursing homes, their residents, their staffs, and the regulatory structures in which they operate. But some of the chronic malaise that characterizes the dominant culture in many nursing homes appears to be remarkably persistent. As I argued in *Unloving Care*, significant improvements in the quality of life and quality of care in nursing homes–and as both cause and effect, in

Bruce C. Vladeck, PhD, is Senior Vice President for Policy of Mount Sinai Medical Center, and Professor of Health Policy and Geriatrics and Director of the Institute for Medicare Practice at the Mount Sinai School of Medicine. From 1993 through 1997, he was Administrator of the Health Care Financing Administration, the senior public official responsible for Medicare and Medicaid. He has been involved with nursing homes as a researcher/writer; regulator; or director/trustee since the mid-1970s.

[Haworth co-indexing entry note]: "*Unloving Care* Revisited: The Persistence of Culture." Vladeck, Bruce C. Co-published simultaneously in *Journal of Social Work in Long-Term Care* (The Haworth Social Work Practice Press, an imprint of The Haworth Press, Inc.) Vol. 2, No. 1/2, 2003, pp. 1-9; and: *Culture Change in Long-Term Care* (ed: Audrey S. Weiner, and Judah L. Ronch) The Haworth Social Work Practice Press, an imprint of The Haworth Press, Inc., 2003, pp. 1-9. Single or multiple copies of this article are available for a fee from The Haworth Document Delivery Service [1-800-HAWORTH, 9:00 a.m. - 5:00 p.m. (EST). E-mail address: docdelivery@haworthpress.com].

http://www.haworthpress.com/store/product.asp?sku=J181
10.1300/J181v2n01_01

the culture of nursing homes–will only be achieved once we have a clearer consensus on the roles we want nursing homes to play in the health care and long-term care systems. The generalized confusion in this area continues to be exacerbated by the twists and turns of public policy. *[Article copies available for a fee from The Haworth Document Delivery Service: 1-800-HAWORTH. E-mail address: <docdelivery@haworthpress.com> Website: <http://www.HaworthPress.com> © 2003 by The Haworth Press, Inc. All rights reserved.]*

KEYWORDS. Nursing homes, long-term care, public policy, regulation, culture

INTRODUCTION

Unloving Care: The Nursing Home Tragedy (Vladeck, 1980) was published in February, 1980; the manuscript had been completed in late 1978. Coming from a tradition that insists on at least the appearance of humility, I would ordinarily shy away from any evaluative comments, but in this case I think it is fair to say that *Unloving Care* remains the definitive study of nursing home policy in the United States–since it is still the only one to address this topic comprehensively. In preparation for this article, I pulled out a copy (amazingly enough, I happen to own the world's largest supply) for the first time in many years. The author pictured on the back of the hardcover's book jacket is almost unrecognizable to me: He looks extremely youthful, has a very full head of hair, and only one chin. In fact, at least in some ways, nursing homes have changed less over the last 25 years than has the author of *Unloving Care*.

Nursing home residents today are significantly older, sicker, and more likely to be demented than they were 25 years ago. They are far less likely to be restrained, either physically or chemically, and much more likely to be cared for by physicians who have had some formal training in the care of nursing home residents and–perhaps more importantly–by aides with at least some formal training. The nursing homes in which they reside are subject to a much more stringent and comprehensive regulatory regime, which is increasingly enforced, and, at least in some parts of the country, are also at substantially more risk from tort litigation.

Still, the glass may be only half full. In 1978, I wrote that

Although the overall quality of nursing homes improved substantially in the preceding decade, there were still, in the United States in 1978, nursing homes with green meat and maggots in the kitchen, narcotics in unlocked cabinets, and disconnected sprinklers in nonfire-resistant structures. The increasingly small proportion of truly horrible nursing homes may be less distressing in the aggregate, though, than the quality of life in the thousands that meet the minimal public standards of adequacy. In these, residents live out the last of their days in an enclosed society without privacy, dignity, or pleasure, subsisting on minimally palatable diets, multiple sedatives, and large doses of television–eventually dying, one suspects, at least partially of boredom. (Vladeck, 1980)

What might, perhaps somewhat grandiosely, be defined as the existential crisis in nursing home care remains essentially unchanged. Nursing homes are occupied largely by people who, if they could choose, would choose not to be there; staffed by employees of whom many will leave at the first opportunity; and financed primarily by public officials who resent every penny and feel trapped, without alternatives. Stories of patient abuse and related Congressional investigations once again fill the headlines (Pear, 2002). Under the circumstances, it is a tribute to the human spirit that as many nursing homes are as good as they are. But not enough seems to have changed over the last 25 years.

The problem really is cultural (a concept that, as applied to organizations, hardly existed 25 years ago). The confusions about role and identity described in *Unloving Care* persist, and have in some ways grown stronger. Nursing homes continue to be organized as health care facilities, although relatively little actual health care is provided there. They continue to be organized around health professional hierarchies, although relationships in nursing homes should be very different from those in other parts of the health sector. Care planning is still driven by an enumeration of residents' deficits, not their capabilities. And everyone who works or resides in a nursing home (if they are capable of rational consciousness) is conscious of the general perception that nursing homes are facilities of last resort.

These negative attributes of nursing home culture are reinforced by governmental regulation and payment mechanisms, as part of a mutually-reinforcing and mutually-symbiotic relationship between government and the nursing home industry. The negative feedback loop is very powerful. So while the quality of care in most nursing homes has undoubtedly improved significantly in the last 25 years, the forces creating or at least exacerbating our nursing home problem continue to be very powerful.

The fundamental problem with nursing homes, I argued in *Unloving Care*, was what might be called one of identity. They were neither fish nor fowl–neither full-fledged health facilities, like hospitals, nor completely residential facilities (since "merely custodial" services, to use the language of the Social

Security Act, are excluded, at least in theory, from public reimbursement programs, without which the nursing home industry in anything like its current configuration is literally inconceivable). Their patients were overwhelmingly people whose continued presence constituted a problem for some other family or facility–patients go *from* home or hospital more than they go *to* the nursing home. The nursing home "problem" therefore arose from efforts to solve hospitals' problems, or families' problems, or the problems of administrators of state mental health facilities. And almost by definition, the clients who went to nursing homes were far too frail and too limited cognitively to do very much to advocate for themselves. If they could, in many instances, they literally would not be there.

IDENTITY CONFUSION AND THE MEDICAL MODEL

Unloving Care was published at the very outset of the 1980s. By the middle of that decade, efforts to improve nursing homes and nursing home care were gathering strength in a number of different arenas. As has so often happened in the history of the evolution of nursing homes in the United States, though, policy efforts focussed on other issues altogether inadvertently reinforced the role confusion concerning nursing homes, and thus the perpetuation of a dysfunctional culture. Halfway measures seeking to improve the situation resulted in solidifying it.

In 1986, the Committee on Nursing Home Regulation of the Institute of Medicine issued its landmark report (I was honored to be among the members of that Committee) (Committee on Nursing Home Regulation, 1986). The Committee's recommendations were quite comprehensive, categorized into 45 specific areas. But the overall thrust of the report was clear: Nursing homes took care of sick people, but they were also the places where their residents (the choice of that term was itself deemed important) *lived*; quality of life was as important as quality of care; residents' rights needed to be systematically protected; and the regulation of nursing homes for the future should address such issues as air conditioning and increasing the supply of private rooms, as well as matters of medical competence. In short, the Committee emphasized the "home" part of the description more than the "nursing."

To everyone's surprise–certainly to that of most of the Committee's members–the Institute of Medicine recommendations were very soon thereafter enacted into law, almost verbatim. The Omnibus Budget Reconciliation Act (OBRA) of 1987 totally rewrote the federal rules concerning the definition, standards, regulation, and payment of nursing homes, largely along the lines recommended by the Committee. A clear path for the future development of nursing homes was thus laid out in law.

Even before a reluctant Reagan Administration could begin to implement OBRA '87, however, the Congress changed course. Only a year after OBRA's enactment, the Congress, no doubt inadvertently, largely undid much of what it had accomplished when it passed the Medicare Catastrophic Coverage Act of 1988. In an attempt to further encourage the demedicalization of nursing home care, and improve access to nursing home services, the Congress removed the requirement of a three-day prior acute hospital stay for the Medi*care* skilled nursing facility benefit, without at the same time changing the benefit itself. And the following year, when Congress repealed the major provisions of the Catastrophic Coverage Act, they kept the nursing home provisions in law. The three-day prior stay requirement was not reinstated until several years thereafter, and the requirements for receiving the benefit were otherwise unchanged.

The Medicare Skilled Nursing Facility benefit was originally titled "Extended Care," and even while the nomenclature changed, the nature of the benefit did not. It was clearly designed to provide for time-limited, recuperative or rehabilitative services arising from an acute illness, or acute exacerbation of a chronic illness, that prior to 1988 would have required an acute-care hospitalization. Thus, the benefit remained limited to 100 days during a specific "spell of illness," and was to be available only so long as the beneficiary required "skilled" services. When the requirement for the three-day prior hospitalization was lifted, the benefit itself was unchanged.

By 1988, almost everywhere in the country, Medicare paid substantially higher rates for nursing home care than did Medicaid–a differential attributable not only to Medicare's greater political popularity and financial resources, but also to the fact that Medicare patients did receive much more intensive and expensive services. So the nursing home industry responded avidly to the opportunity created by the elimination of the three day prior-stay requirement, by seeking to admit and serve patients with very different characteristics from those they had historically served. At the same time, the burgeoning HMO industry, which was to a large extent driven economically by its ability to purchase inpatient hospital and other services at marginal cost, discovered the advantages of buying putatively hospital-level services at nursing home prices. And so the "subacute" sector of the nursing home industry was born.

To this day, there is no general consensus on what "subacute" services are or who provides them (Lewin-VHI, 1995), and the evolution of subacute nursing home services has been substantially affected, generally negatively, by the Medicare Prospective Payment System for SNFs mandated in the Balanced Budget Act of 1997 and implemented in 1999 and by the continuing deterioration of HMOs' position in both private and public health insurance markets. But the very rapid growth in subacute services in the 1990s drove organizational cultures in many organizations in a direction directly opposite to that which had been laid out in the Institute of Medicine Report and OBRA '87.

Compared to the models of nursing home care promoted by the Institute of Medicine report, subacute care (to the extent that one can generalize at all about such an amorphous phenomenon) moved aggressively back towards a medical model, in which patients remained in the facility only so long as they were receiving time-limited treatment for a particular ailment, in which physicians were much more directly involved in day to day patient management–as indeed, patients' conditions were expected to change more rapidly day-to-day–and in which nurse staffing more closely resembled that of a general hospital than a traditional nursing home. Such medically intensive services (relatively speaking, at least), were not only reimbursed at a higher rate than traditional nursing home care, but they also partook of the greater social cachet attached to medical care in most communities, while avoiding the widespread stigmatization of conventional nursing home care.

Of course, even with the explosive growth in subacute care in many regions of the country in the 1990s, the vast majority of individuals residing in nursing homes on any given day continued to be more "traditional" nursing home residents, remaining in the facility for a long time while suffering from multiple, irreversible chronic conditions, generally including at least some cognitive impairment. Indeed, since very few facilities managed to convert their services entirely to subacute care, the vast majority of patients in most particular *facilities* remained those who fit the more traditional models. But the growing appeal of "subacute" status for facility operators and their professional staffs meant that those "traditional" residents were stigmatized not only relative to community-dwelling individuals, but relative *to other patients in the same buildings*.

While the growth of subacute services in nursing homes provided enormous benefits to facility proprietors, its benefits to nursing home patients or residents are much more difficult to identify. For those receiving subacute services, the only difference in their care from that which they would have received in an earlier time was that they received it in a facility with lesser technological capabilities and a more limited medical staff–and often their care required an additional inter-institutional transfer. Non-subacute nursing home residents often became second-class citizens within the facilities in which they resided. Federal policymakers were extremely aware of these issues, which is why the damage imposed on the growth of subacute services, and the companies that provided them most aggressively, by the Balanced Budget Act was far from accidental, and was quite substantial.

IDENTITY CONFUSION
AND THE GROWTH OF COMMUNITY-BASED SERVICES

At the same time that much of the nursing home industry was pursuing the chimera of subacute care, delivery systems in many communities throughout the United States were developing increasing capacity to serve in their own homes or other community settings individuals who might otherwise have been receiving nursing home services. Community-based services as an "alternative" to nursing homes had been the preferred nostrum of all reformers for a generation, and did in fact expand in the 1980s and '90s to a much greater extent than is generally recognized (Bishop, 1999). This emphasis on growth in the home and community-based sector was certainly reinforced by the continued stigmatization of nursing homes, a process that reached its ultimate apotheosis in the Supreme Court's 1999 *Olmstead* decision, which extended the Court's imprimatur to the perception of nursing homes as facilities of last resort, legally as well as clinically.

The growth in the capacity and capability of community-based care providers, and the continued public perception of the greater desirability of community-based care, in an increasingly affluent society, has meant that those admitted to nursing homes increasingly fall into two overlapping categories: frail elderly people with no family to arrange for and make possible community-based services, and those with dementias or other significant cognitive impairments, who are the clients least appropriate for community-based care. The resident population of nursing homes is thus increasingly comprised of cognitively-impaired individuals with no immediate families. The consequences for the culture of nursing homes are profound.

Everyone needs sources of satisfaction and psychic reward in their jobs, over and apart from direct compensation, and the harder and less well-paid a job is, the more important such satisfaction will be. For the nursing aides who provide the overall proportion of hands-on care in nursing homes, and the nurses who supervise them as well, there are simply fewer and fewer people to say "thank you" for the ways in which they do their jobs. Residents' family members are simply less numerous, while the ability of residents themselves to express appreciation is increasingly constrained by the residents' impairments. A difficult job is thus made all the harder.

In this regard, perhaps the most promising development in recent years affecting the quality of nursing home care, one certain to have a profound effect on nursing home culture in the years to come, is the growing recognition that individuals with even extremely significant cognitive impairments may be much more responsive to a broad range of stimuli than had previously been believed. Even the most demented patient can not only benefit, but in some ways respond to, care that is more compassionate and expert, and caregivers can thus rationally maintain expectations of some feedback associated with a job well done.

PUBLIC POLICY AND THE CULTURE OF NURSING HOMES

Recent years have seen a small number of exciting, and well-publicized, efforts to alter the culture of nursing home care in ways more consistent with the now fifteen-year old recognition of the Institute of Medicine committee that nursing homes remain, at root, fundamentally residential facilities. Several articles in this volume describe efforts that have been at least partially successful in improving the quality of life for nursing home residents (and staff) by effecting cultural change in nursing homes. But the federal government, perhaps the single most important influence on the evolution of nursing homes, and on the quality of care in nursing homes, appears to still be confused about nursing homes' role, and therefore continues to send mixed signals about the future evolution of nursing home culture.

Amidst a major publicity effort, in the Spring of 2002, the Centers for Medicare and Medicaid Services (CMS, formerly known as the Health Care Financing Administration, or HCFA), recently posted on its web site the results of quality "measurements," along eight parameters, for nursing homes in a sample of states, with the announced intention of extending the information to all states in the near future (Pear, 2000a). This approach fulfills important ideological and political objectives of the current Administration. It reflects a preference for market-driven consumer "choice" and consumer information rather than more traditional regulation as a technique for improving quality–despite the utter irrelevance of consumer behavior to the quality of nursing homes–and covers the political tracks of an Administration suspected by advocates of being prepared to weaken the regulatory enforcement mechanisms created in response to OBRA '87, but only really implemented in the late 1990s.

There are a number of technical problems with the CMS quality data, but for the purposes here the relevant point is that the quality measures being publicized by CMS mostly involve clinical dimensions of care–important issues to be sure, but issues that are more consistent with persistence of the medical model of nursing homes than more residential models. A nursing home could score well on all of CMS's measures and still be a dismal, cold place in which to live, and to work. Yet it is hard to imagine that any nursing home proprietor could ignore the priorities implicit in CMS list of measurements, even if paying close attention to those measures precluded significant positive cultural change in the facility.

In summary, despite a few notable exceptions, we seem no closer to consensus on the appropriate role of nursing homes in the health care system, and in society, than we were twenty-five years ago, and thus no closer to a clear articulation about the kind of internal cultures nursing homes ought to have. But in the process of getting nowhere, we do seem to have learned a lot along the way, and maybe the experiences of the last two and a half decades will provide the necessary background material for the next generation of significant cultural change. Sooner or later, *Unloving Care* must become obsolete.

REFERENCES

Bishop, C.E. (1999). Where are the Missing Elders? The Decline in Nursing Home Use, 1985 and 1995. 18 *Health Affairs*, July/August, 146-155.

Committee on Nursing Home Regulation, Institute of Medicine. (1986). *Improving the Quality of Care in Nursing Homes*. Washington, D.C.: National Academy Press.

Lewin-VHI, Inc. (1995). Subacute Care: Policy Synthesis and Market Area Analysis. Report prepared for the Office of the Assistant Secretary for Planning and Evaluation, Department of Health and Human Services. NTIS. November 1.

Pear, R. (2002). Unreported Abuse Found in Nursing Homes. *The New York Times*. March 3, 25:1.

Pear, R. (2002a). US Begins Issuing Data on Individual Nursing Homes' Quality of Care. *The New York Times*. April 25, Section A, 26:1.

Vladeck, B.C. (1980). *Unloving Care: The Nursing Home Tragedy*. New York: Basic Books.

Managing Organizational Culture Change: The Case of Long-Term Care

Donald E. Gibson

Sigal G. Barsade

SUMMARY. Recent research has focused on organizations as continuously confronted by forces for change. These forces may cause organizations to rethink their deeply held cultural values and beliefs in order to survive in the changing landscape. Using the long-term care industry as an exemplar, we argue that effective change requires understanding what organizational culture means, and understanding how organizational change typically occurs. Though some scholars emphasize that change is largely out of the control of organization leaders and primarily the result of evolutionary and revolutionary forces, we argue that culture change can be effectively managed. We conclude with implementation strategies for effective culture change management. *[Article copies available for a fee from The Haworth Document Delivery Service: 1-800-HAWORTH. E-mail address: <docdelivery@haworthpress.com> Website: <http://www.HaworthPress.com> © 2003 by The Haworth Press, Inc. All rights reserved.]*

Donald E. Gibson, PhD, is Associate Professor of Management, Fairfield University, Dolan School of Business.

Sigal G. Barsade, PhD, is Associate Professor, Yale School of Management.

Address correspondence to: Donald E. Gibson, PhD, Fairfield University, Dolan School of Business, North Benson Road, Fairfield, CT 06430-5195 (E-mail: dgibson@mail.fairfield.edu).

[Haworth co-indexing entry note]: "Managing Organizational Culture Change: The Case of Long-Term Care." Gibson, Donald E., and Sigal G. Barsade. Co-published simultaneously in *Journal of Social Work in Long-Term Care* (The Haworth Social Work Practice Press, an imprint of The Haworth Press, Inc.) Vol. 2, No. 1/2, 2003, pp. 11-34; and: *Culture Change in Long-Term Care* (ed: Audrey S. Weiner, and Judah L. Ronch) The Haworth Social Work Practice Press, an imprint of The Haworth Press, Inc., 2003, pp. 11-34. Single or multiple copies of this article are available for a fee from The Haworth Document Delivery Service [1-800-HAWORTH, 9:00 a.m. - 5:00 p.m. (EST). E-mail address: docdelivery@haworthpress.com].

10.1300/J181v2n01_02

KEYWORDS. Organizational culture, organizational change, long-term care

Recently, managers and management theorists alike have become concerned about understanding and implementing organizational change (Kanter, Stein, & Jick, 1992; Kotter, 1995; Nadler & Tushman, 1990; Weick & Quinn, 1999). The urgency to understand change processes is well warranted: uncertainty and instability abound in the current environment facing organizations. In examining these trends, long-term care organizations make a particularly apt exemplar; they are undergoing dramatic changes as a result of upheavals in health care specifically and the worldwide economy more generally. They are changing in response to market forces. They are changing in the nature of their relationship to residents, offering new levels of choice and freedom (Guagliardo, 2001). They are changing in their simultaneous attention to dramatically reducing costs and dramatically enhancing services. They are changing in the direction of operating larger and larger facilities, yet trying to offer more and more personalized care. Social work professionals are faced with an increasing rate and complexity of change, and how they respond to that change will determine their role in the changing health care marketplace and the degree to which they will remain a "core discipline" in long-term care organizations (Gordon, 2002). Given this setting, it is not surprising that professionals in long-term care organizations may feel like pawns in a game over which they have little control.

Drawing on current research in organizational behavior, in this article we offer a framework for conceptualizing organizational change and organizational culture and a set of themes essential to understanding how organizational change comes about and how to more effectively manage that change. Taking an "organizational behavior" perspective means that as researchers we are concerned with the social and psychological responses individuals have to their organizations. We draw on social science research to help us understand how individuals tend to act in complex organizations, and we attempt to use that understanding to increase the effectiveness of managers confronted by turbulent organizational change. The lessons we provide here are drawn from empirical studies in a variety of organizational settings, across private and not-for-profit sectors.

Using the long-term care industry as an exemplar, we first address some of the causes for change in current systems, and show why culture change is often necessary. We next define organizational culture, and outline research that has depicted culture as a means to solve organizational problems, as comprised of multiple sub-cultures, and as effective to the extent that it "fits" or is congruent with environmental forces and internal strategy and structure. We then analyze how organizational change occurs, whether as survival of the fittest, as an evolutionary, revolutionary, or a managed process, and advocate approaching it as the latter as the most effective route for managers in long-term care organizations. We then conclude with key themes in managing organizational culture change that help to ensure achievement of change goals.

OVERVIEW

Why the Concern About Change and Culture in Long-Term Care?

Organizational changes are departures from the status quo or from smooth trends (Huber & Glick, 1995). Forces for change in organizations come from two primary sources: externally, or from the organization's environment–including regulatory and market forces, changing styles and preferences, and political and legal trends–and internally, including initiatives of the organization's management, and political forces (Kanter et al., 1992). In the health care environment, external forces are often the ones emphasized: More attention is typically placed on how health care organizations are being buffeted by turbulent environmental forces rather than on how health care professionals can effect change within their organizations (Moore, 1996). As we have noted, however, environmental change and its increasing complexity is a constant, and a given. The deciding factor in whether environmental change hurts, destroys, or strengthens an organization is how managers *respond* to changes from the inside. While we will briefly address the key ways that the environment is changing for long-term care in the U.S. the primary focus of this article is an organizational behavior perspective on how to approach culture change.

There is little argument that long-term care organizations are facing a range of daunting environmental changes. As Thomas (2001) describes, underfunding of Medicare and Medicaid relative to need, along with increasing liability insurance costs and an increasing gap between those most able and those least able to pay has created a financial crisis for long-term care providers. Within long-term care facilities, there is a workforce crisis characterized by high staff turnover and absenteeism, low morale, and difficulty in recruiting skilled professionals. And there is a liability crisis looming from the conflicting trends of rising expectations of family members of what long-term care facilities should provide, admitted shortcomings in resident quality of life, and the increasing likelihood that litigation may be used to correct the discrepancy in expectations and quality.

To determine how organizations might respond to these external forces for change, we first draw a distinction between organizational structure and culture. Organizational structure refers to the formal roles and responsibilities of people within an organization, and the control and coordination mechanisms in place to ensure that the goals and mission of the organization are carried out (Katz & Kahn, 1978). The organization chart is one representation of this structure, though this chart is typically more symbolic than actual, representing an ideal vision of how people might relate to each other rather than how they actually do. Organizational culture, as we will detail in the next section, is the informal aspect of organizations. It is the value-laden glue that can bind people to each other and to the organization; it is made up of deeply held values, like respect and integrity, and held in place by behavioral norms–the often unspoken expectations for how people ought to behave (Martin, 1992).

A typical response to the complex external forces currently buffeting long-term care providers is to make structural changes–to hire different kinds of professionals to respond to business or market forces, for example, or to enlarge the organization by adding new facilities. However, there is also a call in some quarters, for a deeper response to the changing environmental landscape, a change involving culture and values. Some long-term care professionals argue that rather than reacting to external forces, long-term care organizations should fundamentally change the way they conceive of long-term care and address alternative models of long-term care. They argue that the "medical model" which has guided the thinking in long-term care for decades–characterized by large hierarchical institutions in which the frail and elderly are "placed" for ongoing clinical care–needs to be replaced with a new "person-centered" or "human habitats" or "social model" characterized by increased elder choice and personalized service (Gold, 2002; Stevens, 2001).

These kinds of changes, often termed "transformational" or "paradigmatic" change, involve much more than structural shifts; they involve changes in the underlying beliefs and values of an organization. At first blush, professionals may be tempted to assume that these deeply held cultural ideas are impossible to change. We would be the first to agree that change at the cultural level is difficult and fraught with potential barriers. At the same time, recent organizational research has suggested important ways in which professionals can understand and actually *manage* cultural change.

THEORETICAL PERSPECTIVES

Defining Organizational Culture

Organizational culture is "the glue that holds an organization together through a sharing of patterns of meaning. The culture focuses on the values, beliefs, and expectations that members come to share" (Siehl & Martin, 1984: 227). These shared values and beliefs tend to operate unconsciously and

> define in a basic 'taken-for-granted' fashion an organization's view of itself and its environment. These assumptions and beliefs are learned responses to a group's problems of survival in its external environment and its problems of internal integration. (Schein, 1991: 6)

One might think of culture as a set of layers. Representing the top layer are "artifacts," or visible aspects of an organization's culture. These are the behaviors and attributes of an organization that are apparent as soon as one walks through the door: informal versus formal dress, the presence or absence of personal objects in work spaces, the presence or absence of visible symbols characterizing the organization. These visible cultural aspects indicate and reinforce the non-visible layers that lie below.

At the second layer are norms for behavior in an organization, that is, expectations that are shared by the group about what is and is not appropriate behavior. These unspoken rules can apply to all aspects of behavior, including norms about conflict–the degree to which participants openly air their differences, or cloak them behind "politeness" norms (O'Reilly, 1989), the appropriateness of emotional expression (Hochschild, 1983; Morris & Feldman, 1996), and the degree of emphasis on professionalism (Smith & Kleinman, 1989). It is critical to note that norms develop and maintain the culture through informal rewards and sanctions; that is, behavior that is seen as appropriate to the culture is encouraged, and behavior that is seen as incongruous is punished. Norms set the boundaries for how people are expected to act in their organization, and are thus a strong form of social control (O'Reilly & Chatman, 1996). Cultural norms actually tend to be more pervasive and effective than formal control systems, such as written policies and procedures or supervisory monitoring, because of the motivation behind compliance. That is, participants conform to cultural norms because they care about the expectations of the people around them and like the certainty and stability of guidelines for behavior (O'Reilly, 1989). This is a stronger, more pervasive motivator than conforming to formal policies and procedures, because it comes from inside ("intrinsic" motivation–Deci & Ryan, 1985) rather than from external sources, such as a supervisor or policy ("extrinsic" motivation–Deci & Ryan, 1985; Herzberg, 1966).

At the third, and deepest layer, culture is constructed of values, beliefs and assumptions about how the world works. Values represent the organization's ideas about what *ought to be*. Typical organizational values may emphasize teamwork over individual autonomy, respect for individual differences, innovation and flexibility, or stability and tradition (Chatman, 1991). The value layer is the most important aspect of culture. It provides the foundation and guiding elements for the other two layers. At the same time, it is difficult to observe and gains some of its impact from the fact that it is taken for granted; employees may not even think about these values, and may not be able to put them into words, but they implicitly believe in them, and the outcomes of these values can have a dramatic impact on how the organization operates and how employees relate to it (Schein, 1991). Several empirical studies have documented links between cultural values and organizational outcomes. For example, organizational cultural values emphasizing ethical values have been shown to influence nurses' job satisfaction (Joseph & Deshpande, 1997), with differing attitudinal outcomes depending on the degree to which the culture emphasized rules, efficiency, and caring. Strong organizational cultural values have been related to innovation (O'Reilly, 1989); commitment (O'Reilly & Chatman, 1986); effectiveness and cohesion (Ouchi & Wilkins, 1985); and increased organizational performance (Kotter & Heskett, 1992); though some researchers caution that these associations are difficult to support, given the inherent complexity of accurately measuring either culture or outcomes such as performance (see critique in Martin, 1992).

Outlining these three layers helps to understand why it is difficult to change a culture. Truly changing a culture–as opposed to merely changing its superficial aspects–means changing elements of the organization at all three levels, including the deepest one, which involves employees' deeply held values and beliefs. Based on this analysis, we are not arguing that changing a culture is easy. Rather, we are arguing that organizational leaders can *manage* their cultures–they can begin by understanding why people behave the way they do, and seek to shape that behavior based on an understanding of the norms, values and beliefs. Before we present our ideas on managing cultural change, however, we emphasize three additional critical aspects of culture.

Culture emerges in an organization by solving critical organizational problems. Why do unique organizational cultures develop? Cultures emerge because they help to solve a group's basic problems, which include: (1) survival in and adaptation to forces in the external environment; and (2) coordination of its internal processes to ensure the capacity to survive in the environment and adapt to its changes (Homans, 1950; Merton, 1957; Schein, 1991). A group or organization faces an environment that provides resources and opportunities, but also presents challenges and threats. For long-term care organizations, the environment presents opportunities in the increasing demand for quality elder care; it presents threats in the limitation of resources and increasing regulation and litigation surrounding care of the elderly. As noted, some organizations are responding by increasing the homelike aspects of their facilities by allowing, for example, residents to eat and bathe whenever they want (Guagliardo, 2001). But this structural response implies a cultural one: New cultural norms must develop that encourage a value of staff flexibility, such that increasing resident control over surroundings and schedule is not perceived by the staff as a loss of control.

Cultures also solve the problem of how to organize internally–how different professional groups in the organization, for example, will deal with each other. How much autonomy will social workers, for example, be allowed in making decisions surrounding resident care? How much impact will clinical staff have in the admissions process, as opposed to marketing or finance departments? How much emphasis will there be on forming a team of professionals to manage care, versus emphasizing separate functional departments responsible for specific resident needs? These are examples of the problems long-term care organizations might face in terms of how to organize internally–how to develop rules and norms for how employees deal with each other. Internal norms thus develop to respond to unique problems facing the organization, and represent how leaders and professionals have dealt with critical issues. This is why to understand a current culture, one needs to understand aspects of its history–important leaders, important events and crises, and the solutions the organization took to address its past problems.

Organizations are comprised of multiple cultures and sub-cultures. It is important to recognize that organizations are rarely made up of one, homogenous culture, but are better thought of as multicultural. Though organizational leaders may attempt to foster a monolithic culture, subgroups within the organization–based on occupational, departmental, ethnic or other divides–inevitably generate their own expectations, means, and clear senses of priorities (Martin, 1992). Leaders may attempt to bring organizations together by emphasizing images and values of a "family," for example, but subcultures may develop which are at odds with the organization-wide culture, and may be at odds with each other. In hospitals, for example, the clinical culture of emphasizing quality care without necessarily considering costs may clash with a more cost-centered emphasis of business- and market-oriented professionals intentionally brought in to think about cost-control in their marketing, admissions, and administrative positions. The clash of sub-cultures is exemplified in this quote from a nurse in a hospital that was carrying out cost-reduction restructuring, who refers to administrators as "they":

> Well, they're trying to run it like a business now instead of a hospital. I mean they say they are caring for the community and that people matter but it really boils down to dollars and cents. That's what matters! (Blythe et al., 2001)

O'Reilly (1989) has argued that cultural norms and values may vary depending on one's location in the organization: Top managers may have guiding beliefs and visions that are quite different from the "daily" beliefs and norms held by those at lower levels in the organization. As O'Reilly (1989: 12) notes, "the former reflect top managements' beliefs about how things ought to be. The latter define how things actually are." Further, he argues that norms vary on two primary dimensions: the *intensity* or amount of approval or disapproval attached to an expectation; and the *crystallization*, or degree of consensus or consistency with which a norm or value is shared. For example, an organization could have a high degree of consensus around some shared values ("we're a family here"; "we value innovation"), but with little intensity; that is, the values are stated and talked about, but they aren't really meaningful, and don't actually shape everyday behavior. On the other hand, an organization could have a value intensely believed in by one occupational group (social workers who emphasize resident autonomy and freedom) that is at odds with the values of another group (administrative managers who emphasize efficiency and control). This is a setting with high intensity but little crystallization–a setting with a high potential for cultural conflict.

There has been much attention raised in organizational research on organizations with "strong" cultures–that is, organizations who have clear-cut values that differentiate the organization and help employees to feel actively committed (Collins & Porras, 1994). IBM, for example, is often cited as a strong culture firm that deeply values "respect for the individual," and professional codes of conduct, and these values help develop very high employee loyalty and motivation to achieve for the company. Strong cultures only exist when there is both high intensity of belief in cultural values and high consensus about what the values are (O'Reilly, 1989).

The manager seeking to manage cultural change, then, must understand the extent of the culture's value intensity and crystallization. Strong cultures may be especially difficult to change, because values are widely and deeply held. On the other hand, if there is little crystallization, the lack of agreement across levels or between occupational groups about what the central values are may also contribute to a difficult task. In this case, the leaders may have to create new organization-wide values that have not been in place before. They must recognize the multicultural aspect of organizations, but creatively seek ways to tie together their diverse sub-cultures.

There is no "perfect" culture. An unfortunate by-product of the recent interest in organizational culture by both academic and popular writers is the notion that there is one kind of strong culture that should work in all organizations. This orientation tends to foster an effort by organizations to emulate those companies with successful strong cultures and to try to adopt their values. For example, department stores have been drawn to emulating Nordstrom's emphasis on superior customer quality and service "heroics" by salespeople; airlines have tried to mimic Southwest Airlines' emphasis on low-cost, high efficiency service; and long-term care facilities may be drawn to emulate the success of the Eden model or Pioneer Network values emphasizing "person-centered" resident freedom and autonomy (see related articles in this volume).

It can be helpful to benchmark the actions of successful organizations. As in viewing successful personal role models, examining successful organizational models can introduce new ideas of how to operate and challenge the organization to achieve at a higher level. At the same time, organizational research emphasizes that the successful culture for a particular organization will not necessarily be one that another organization has adopted; rather, the successful culture will be one that "fits"–fits the organization's environmental factors, fits its long-term strategy, and fits its people. As Schein (1991: 315) notes,

> Do not assume that there is a 'correct' or 'better' culture, and do not assume that 'strong' cultures are better than weak cultures. What is correct or whether strength is good or bad depends on the match between cultural assumptions and environmental realities.

This approach, also seen in the "congruence" model (Nadler & Tushman, 1980) or the "alignment" model (Pfeffer, 1998), emphasizes that organizations will be effective to the degree that their internal components–the way tasks are coordinated, the informal ways that people deal with each other (e.g., culture), formal structure, policies and practices, and the characteristics of the organization's employees–are congruent with each other, the organization's strategy, the resources available, the organization's history, and address the threats and opportunities in the organization's environment. For example, Blythe et al. (2001) describe a restructuring process in which a hospital responded to economic threats in the healthcare environment by experimenting with changing the mix of functional backgrounds of nursing teams, adding healthcare aids and adjusting the proportion of RNs to RPNs. This structural change then caused a change in how tasks were done, given the new and different skill levels of employees now doing the work, which then led to feelings of uncertainty around roles and responsibilities. We posit that had there been an explicit, accompanying, congruent shift in values to complement this structural shift, it may well have helped to ameliorate the ensuing uncertainty and anxiety.

Types of Organizational Change

Finding a good fit between the organization's internal culture and external environment sounds like a logical imperative and one that could be resolved with analytical management tools, strategic thinking, and good intentions by organizational leadership. But this matching process is made infinitely more complicated by the fact that both the figure and ground are changing–there are continual forces, both inside and outside the organization, for alterations in the availability of resources, and the legitimacy of common ways of operating and current ways of thinking. Culture may be the social glue binding organizational members, but there are continuous forces striving to tear the glue apart. At the same time, cultures can be quite resilient: Particularly in intense and crystallized cultures there can be strong resistance to change–a strongly-held culture can prevent needed change despite substantial pressure from the external environment (Kotter & Heskitt, 1992).

Traditional models of organizational change suggest a pattern in which organizational leaders should: (1) recognize the need for change; (2) "unfreeze" the current systems by pointing out inadequacies in current practices and by breaking open the "shell of complacency and self-righteousness" inherent in the status quo way of operating (Lewin, 1997: 330); and (3) "re-freeze" the group or system at a new, more desired level of operating. The problem with this "ice cube"–unfreezing and refreezing–view of change is that it implies that a leader's task is to upset a relatively stable system, effect change, and return the system to a new, but still stable, trajectory. Newer models of change recognize that there is little stability before or after changes; that in fact change is constantly happening and is multifaceted. Also, there is no guarantee that people respond as ice cubes, being easily melted and then refrozen, thus maintaining the identical underlying atomic structure. The metaphor for organizational change is probably better seen as a moving car, as Kanter et al. (1992: 10) suggest,

> Deliberate change is a matter of grabbing hold of some aspect of the motion and steering it in a particular direction that will be perceived by key players as a new method of operating or as a reason to reorient one's rela-

tionship and responsibility to the organization itself, while creating conditions that facilitate and assist that reorientation.

Recognizing that change is constantly happening and that the ice cube model may not be a sufficient guide to scholars and managers does not, however, mean that change cannot be deliberate, planned, or managed. In order to conceptualize the change management process, we draw on scholars who have presented organizational change typologies to describe how organizational change comes about (see Kanter et al., 1992; Schein, 1991; Tushman & Romanelli, 1985). We label their approaches as survival of the fittest, evolutionary, and revolutionary models, then describe research supporting a "management of organizational culture" model–a model describing how managers can help to control this process.

Change as "survival of the fittest." The first source of change, as we have discussed, is change brought about by environmental demands. Organization theorists depict this kind of change through natural selection models, suggesting that a successful response to change is shown by organizational survival. This view asserts that there are limited resources in the environment to support a limited population of organizations. Those that adapt to the changing levels of resources and are creative in securing scarce resources will survive; those that do not respond or respond too slowly, will die out (Katz & Kahn, 1978; March & Simon, 1958; Quinn, 1981). Unfortunately, this model is not terribly helpful in recognizing how to go about the successful adaptation process. In fact, survival may be the result of organizations that are efficient and respond rapidly to change; but it may also be the result of luck, of being in the right market with the right product at the right time. Organizations may also survive because they gain institutional legitimacy–that is, stakeholders such as employees and the public may *want* certain organizations to exist, even if they are not well-suited to the current environment (Meyer & Zucker, 1989). Government agencies and programs that have outlived their objective usefulness are examples of this pattern. Finally, organizations may survive by being innovators–that is, they may seek to reshape their environment rather than merely reacting to it (Kanter et al., 1992).

Change as an evolutionary process. A second force for change comes from within the organization itself. Change may come about from the "natural" process of an organization growing and learning. Evolutionary process models emphasize that organizations tend to progress through relatively concrete "stages" as they grow and mature, and that the possibility and success of change must be viewed from the vantage point of the organization's stage of growth, with stages typically a function of age and size (Greiner, 1972;

Normann, 1977; Schein, 1991). Schein (1991) has described three major life stages for organizations, which we outline below:

Birth and early growth stages tend to be characterized by the dominance of a founder or a small founding group; communication processes and structures are informal and fast moving. This early growth stage is critical in articulating the organization's unique culture; the organization seeks to differentiate itself from other organizations, and the culture is typically strong and generates high commitment from motivated early members, who feel like they are "part of something."

Assuming the organization survives this early stage (and many do not), the organization enters a *growth or development* phase as it reaches the limit of the founder's small group and begins to emphasize professional management, more rationalized operations and more formalized procedures. At this stage, organization leaders must explicitly encourage aspects of the culture and keep the founder's values alive through intentional socialization. Otherwise, the cultural fragments as new groups enter and individuals bring in the cultures of their professions, or prior organizations, rather than the unique cultural values of the organization. Finally, in *maturity* stages, organizations expand further and foster internal stability in terms of set structures and norms, but may face stagnation in their markets and a lack of motivation to change. At this point, the "traditional" culture may become a constraint to change. Now, any proposed change to current ways of operating may meet with substantial resistance. The evolutionary model suggests that any change effort must take into account the age, size, and state of the organization's culture if it has any hope of succeeding.

Though this life cycle model of change has found support in the literature, one challenge to its dominance is the "punctuated equilibrium" model of change (Gersick, 1991; Tushman & Romanelli, 1985). This approach argues that organizations tend to progress through alternating stages of *convergence*, punctuated by *reorientation*. During convergent periods, organizations change as the life cycle model would predict, incrementally altering their structures, systems, culture, and resources to adapt to changes in the environment. These relatively long periods are characterized by stability, elaboration of current structures, and slow, small changes. Periodically, however, when organizations are confronted by exogenous "shocks" such as a substantial competitive threat, a change in the legal environment, or a change in technology, organizations may reorient themselves, a period involving a series of "rapid and discontinuous change in the organization which fundamentally alters its character and fabric," which may include key strategies, power distribution and its core cultural values (Tushman & Romanelli, 1985: 179). The punctuated equilibrium model would suggest to leaders of change that there are likely to be opportune moments for reorienting the organization, that managers may use the pressures for change that arise–often suddenly–in the environment as an opportunity to substantially change the direction and values of the organization. Apart from these tumultuous periods, however, this model would predict that change will be slow and likely to encounter strong resistance from people with an interest in preserving the status quo.

Change as a revolutionary process. A third force for change is through revolutionary forces within the organization (Kanter et al., 1992). Change from this perspective is based on shifting levels of power. Power within organizations is typically based on control of valued organizational resources, the ability to reward or punish, and the possession of critical pieces of information (Pfeffer, 1992). Revolutionary change is often the result of new people entering organizational positions with new sets of assumptions about the strategic direction of the organization or how people ought to be managed. If new people with new assumptions assume key power positions in an organization, they can foster dramatic organizational change. Leaders' understanding the levels of power held by various individuals and groups (often termed "coalitions") within an organization is essential to initiating and sustaining change efforts. Without the support of key powerful individuals in the organization, no change will result, and depending on their power, the very ability of the leader to lead may be threatened.

Change as a managed process. The previous three models suggest that from the leader's perspective, there are many aspects of the organizational setting that are "out of control." The environment makes substantial demands on organizations, and coldly rewards those that adapt and punishes those who don't. The culture is an emergent, multifaceted process that arises to solve central organizational problems, but over time becomes resistant to change and may be a constraining factor. Individuals within the organization have differing priorities and goals, and often act on their political self-interest rather than for the "good" of the organization. At the same time, we are optimistic that leaders *can* change their organizations and their cultures. In fact, the best leaders are arguably the ones who are continuously monitoring their external and internal environments so that they understand what needs to be changed and how they should go about it. Culture has the effect of reducing anxiety for group members because it provides some guidelines (informally determined, but no less concrete than more "formal" policies and procedures) for appropriate behavior (Schein, 1991). But it is also leaders who must recognize that management of the culture is an essential part of their job. As Schein (1991: 317) urges, "the unique and essential function of leadership is the manipulation of culture." Leaders and professionals need to be aware of and understand their own culture *and* the shifting trends in the environment so that they can continuously seek opportunities for change that will help to enhance fit. When a leader realizes that a cultural change is needed to adapt to changing circumstances, he or she needs to consider several critical elements in the culture change.

IMPLEMENTING CHANGE

Key Themes in Effective Organizational Culture Change

Implementing culture change involves "moving an organization to some desired future state" (Nadler, 1983: 361). This movement implies (1) understanding the current state of the organization–that is, the dominant cultural norms and underlying beliefs and values, (2) an image or vision of a desired future state–how you envision a culture that better meets needs; and (3) a transition period between these two states (Beckhard & Harris, 1977). In the current environment of long-term care, many providers are contemplating a change from the dominant medical model with its emphasis on acute care, to a patient-centered model focusing on elders' holistic well-being (Gold, 2002). The critical first step in this process is to envision specifically what that different future state would look like–how the facilities would look, what kinds of people will need to staff it, and what kind of leadership will be necessary to lead it. Without a clear vision of what the future state will look like, participants may lack the motivation to change long-held patterns, and leaders will lack guidelines to assess progress toward a different state or indeed, knowledge of whether the change has successfully taken place or not.

This does not mean to imply that managers should expect that all plans will turn out exactly as envisioned. In fact, being flexible during the change effort is critical (as we discuss below). However, having a clear direction about where one would like the organization to go (even if it changes) gives managers a better chance for "grabbing hold of some aspect of the motion and steering it in a particular direction," as Kanter et al. (1992: 10) suggest. Based on studies of organizational change in a variety of environments, the following elements are essential to successfully managing the direction of organizational change.

Leadership from the top. Effective leadership is essential to driving cultural change. Though culture change may be the result of environmental forces or political upheaval, as shown above, *managed* change implies active and intentional leadership in all aspects of the change process. To successfully manage change, leaders must create and sustain a vision of the future state; role model appropriate behaviors; manage shifting political coalitions; and manage the anxiety that naturally results from change (Nadler, 1983).

Through the use of symbols, including language, pictures, and symbolic acts, leaders must demonstrate the desirability of the potential future state, and provide a vivid image of what the future state will look and feel like. Using language, for example, to show the difference between a facility as an "institution" versus a facility as a collection of "neighborhoods" or "houses" (Gold, 2002), is critical to help participants envision what the future could look like. Even small gestures of change, such as the words used in public statements, can send potent signals during the transition time. During times of uncertainty and change, people will be acutely observing the leader's actions and words to note the seriousness and importance of change.

These changes in language, however, will be perceived as mere rhetoric if they are not also accompanied by leader behavior that accentuates and illustrates real change. The leader must recognize that he or she is a role model for participants in illustrating behaviorally what the change should look like. If the change is toward "empowerment"–that is, giving lower-level staff more decision-making and autonomy, for example, the leader must demonstrate that risk taking by empowered staff members is acceptable and that first-time failures will not be punished. Identification of the leader as a role model can be a powerful force for change. Role modeling has been shown to be an effective way to promote social and technical learning in observers (Bandura, 1977). Moreover, having role models for change also may promote a positive emotional response: Participants may be reassured by observing a leader who illustrates that change is possible, and inspired by the example (Lockwood & Kunda, 1997).

Leaders must also be attuned to the shifting power dynamics during the transition period. Leaders must marshal support for the change among key power groups, including key opinion leaders within the organization, but also key stakeholder groups, including community leaders, funding agencies, regulatory agencies, customer or client groups and families. At the same time, leaders must also build in points of stability during the transition period. Too much uncertainty about the change can promote defensive reactions, excess anxiety, and political conflict (Nadler, 1983). Providing substantial information about the change process, assuring job security where appropriate, and taking clear, consistent actions can assuage some of the natural anxiety associated with creating change.

Intentionally align structure, systems, and policies with the new culture. Organizational research consistently emphasizes that effective change and overall performance will be enhanced to the extent that the culture is consistent with organizational structure and human resource policies (Chatman, 1989;

Nadler & Tushman, 1980; Pfeffer, 1998). As noted, structure includes formal reporting relationships (who reports to whom in the organizational chart), and job descriptions (how will jobs change as a result of this change?). Human resource policies include selection and recruiting practices, performance appraisal, reward or compensation structures, and training and development. Ensuring congruence between these areas with the organization's culture is essential to creating and maintaining change. Change to a patient-centered culture, for example, will require changes to a range of HR practices. Managers will want to carefully recruit and select people who are willing and able to provide care in the new settings, using a variety of selection methods, including structured and unstructured interviews, on-the-job previews, behavioral simulations, and matching values and personality to ensure "fit" between the employee and the culture. The approach emphasizing testing to ensure fit between the employee and the firm's culture has shown that a better fit is associated with a person's future satisfaction and performance in the firm (O'Reilly et al., 1991). In line with the congruence perspective, performance appraisal and feedback processes will then need to be adjusted to reflect the new understanding of what constitutes high performance in the new culture. Where before, focus on achieving only the tasks, duties and responsibilities listed in one's job description led to successful performance, in the new setting, performance may be defined as flexibility in meeting new challenges and providing superlative elder care which includes relationships with elders, not just task completion. The reward structure will need to change to reflect more flexible job descriptions and new definitions of performance. Training will need to be re-focused to ensure that staff have the skills necessary to meet the new changes.

It is important to recognize that in some cases, the decision to create a new culture may bring about these structural and procedural changes, and in some cases, structural and procedural changes may precipitate culture change. For example, the shift from staff focusing on completing the duties as listed in a concrete, specific job description to staff focusing on taking responsibility for a range of duties that flow from their own autonomous decision-making and resident wishes requires a dramatic shift in the cultural values of an organization. Similarly, eliminating middle managerial oversight positions in favor of team-based responsibility implies a substantial change in culture, from top-down authoritarian emphasis to a bottom-up, participative structure.

Ensuring staff and stakeholder participation. It has become a cliché to argue that people believe most in those things they have a hand in creating. However, cultural change cannot succeed without involvement of many people at all levels of the organization. Without involvement, people may feel distanced from the change. Some researchers note that this can lead to employees feeling disempowered, with its associated feelings of hopelessness, alienation, victimization, loss of control, and dependency, a finding researchers have found in workers responding to change in the health care industry (Baumann & Silverman, 1998; Gibson, 1991).

However, leaders of change must also take a balanced approach to involvement. On one hand, encouraging active participation by employees in the change can help to generate excitement and motivation to change, can ensure effective communication of vision and goals, and can result in better decision-making based on input from a wider array of people. On the other hand, participation has its costs: It is time consuming, needs managers to accept a diminishment of personal control over the change process, and may contribute to a more fuzzy or ambiguous vision. Also, if not all the changes participants would like to see are actually enacted they can feel more frustrated than not participating in the first place. This is why encouraging *appropriate* participation is a balancing act. Different people may be involved in different parts of the process, including assessment and diagnosis of the current state, implementation planning, or actual execution of change. Participating in the change can range from individually offering ideas about concepts, to explicit team-building and participation used to change organizational culture (Harrison & Pietri, 1997). As Nadler (1983: 365) notes,

> Different individuals or groups may participate at different times, depending upon their skills and expertise, the information they have, and their acceptance and ownership of the change. Participation can be direct and widespread, or indirect through representatives.

There will be different levels of participation, then, depending on what different people can contribute. The key point, however, is that participation of some kind, whether direct or through representation in change teams, is essential. The participation must be real, meaningful, and participants should have a clear idea of how their ideas will be used (e.g., will go into brainstorming, but may not necessarily lead to the end product versus actually figuring out how to implement the change). If change is perceived as solely emerging from top management, implementation will be slow at best, and perhaps nonexistent.

A logical extension of the continued deep participation of organizational members in the implementation stage of change is to have this involvement continue past the "formal" change process, and proceed as part of a continuous planning toward future change. One of the most developed models of this continual participation and management of future change is Mohrman and Cummings' (1989) "self-designed change" strategy. This strategy, based on learning theory, is a way to inherently overcome many of the inertial, resistance, and structural problems that we describe above as it involves organizational members as continuously designing and implementing change (Cummings, 1995). Thus it serves as the basis of continuous improvement, which also sets the structural and psychological stage for large scale change when needed.

Criticality of communicating change. Communication is one of the most important aspects of organizational change, yet managers often underestimate how much communication is needed during change processes. Frequent, redundant and copious communication is necessary to ensure that a message, particularly a message that employees are resistant to hearing, will be transferred (Larkin & Larkin, 1994). Communication processes, both cognitive and affective, offer the vehicle through which persuasion, innovation, learning, trust, and emotional comfort occur (Laschinger & Havens, 1996; Rogers & Agarwala-Rogers, 1976), and leads to a lessening of resistance, and greater acceptance of change (Schweiger & DeNisi, 1991; Wanberg & Banas, 2000). Also, to the degree that uncertainty leads to the focus of one's emotional and cognitive resources in trying to find or process information (Bastien et al., 1995), any communication that helps to lessen this uncertainty will be helpful.

Obtain feedback and evaluate progress. It is also essential that communication about change flows in a two-way, rather than a one-way direction (Leavitt & Mueller, 1951). That is, communication needs to flow in all directions, top-down, bottom-up, and horizontally. To make this happen, managers of change must *actively* seek feedback from stakeholders in the change, rather than waiting for problems to arise that force crisis containment. The reason that feedback must actively be sought is based on theories of communication in organizational structures. Hierarchical structures shape the direction and tone of communications. As Rogers and Agarwala-Rogers (1976) note, communication in an organization, like water, tends to run downhill; those who are higher in organizational hierarchies are more likely to initiate communication flows downward to their subordinates, than the other way around. Because communicating negative feedback about organizational activities "upward" to one's superior is potentially threatening, the tendency, in organizational hierarchies, is for positive information to flow upward. As Katz and Kahn (1978: 447) note, "The upward flow of communication in organizations is not noted for spontaneous and full expression, despite attempts to institutionalize the process of feedback up the line." Rather, employees tend to send "sugar-coated" messages from lower levels to higher levels, and "the net result is highly inaccurate feedback to the top about the actual accomplishments at the bottom of an organization" (Rogers & Agarwala-Rogers, 1976: 97). It is critical, then, in the midst of organizational change, for managers to (1) minimize status differences that may attenuate accurate feedback, and (2) engage in active *listening* to the feedback being provided. Listening, though underemphasized as a component of communication, is critical to receiving and acting effectively on received feedback, particularly negative feedback that is likely to be a part of substantial change efforts (Rogers & Roethlisberger, 1991).

A common, and ironic mistake in participative change management that reflects these structural effects on communication is that once the change plan is in place, participation and feedback on how the change process is going tends to be ignored. There should be structural mechanisms built in throughout the entire implementation process to allow continuous feedback of how the technical and emotional aspects of the change are progressing, and any changes employees see needed to make the change operate more effectively. There should thus be as much participation and communication in the *implementation* of the change as in the planning of the change. Without this type of attention, the change may not work, and managers may well not understand why.

Managing the emotional response. Often forgotten in organizational change processes are the role of emotions. The concept and the reality of change is an inherently emotional one, and predictably elicits both positive and negative feelings in employees and managers alike running the gamut of positive and negative emotions (Huy, 1999; Scheck & Kinicki, 2000). Responses to dramatic cultural change may follow the typical grieving process for other life events: denial, anger, sadness and acceptance (Kubler-Ross, 1970). To truly understand and effectively guide managerial change, organizations need to manage not only the rational "facts" of change, but critically, the "feelings" around change, the need for change, and what will happen when there is no longer the status quo. In fact, sometimes employees may not be capable of really understanding the facts until they have clarified how they feel about them.

Since employee emotions will permeate the entire change process, having a clear and intentional *affective* message is important–possibly more important than the logical argumentation that typically accompanies organizational change. This is particularly important because affect can spread among organizational members in the same way that more cognitively-based rumors spread. This happens both consciously through the social sharing of emotional events among organizational members (Finkenauer & Rime, 1998; Pennebaker et al., 2001) as well as through emotional contagion, or the "catching" of other people's emotions in their work groups (Barsade, 2001). Because emotions are likely to transfer rapidly among participants, leaders need to be particularly aware of the importance of their own expressed emotions and be conscious of their followers' emotions.

During a substantial culture change, there will not be an emotional vacuum–that is, *some* type of emotion will fill the void–and managers of change should strategize as much about their affective or emotional message as they would their logical, persuasive one. They can do so intentionally by behaving in an emotionally intelligent way; that is, they should (1) pay attention to and read others' emotions, as well as pay attention to the possible effects of their own expressed emotions; (2) use emotional information to help prioritize their thinking; (3) understand emotions, particularly the progression emotions can take (fear to anger), and the existence of complex or ambivalent emotions in change participants; and (4) self-regulate their own emotions (staying open to feelings) and help to regulate the emotions of others (Mayer et al., 2000). Recent research supports the idea that leadership effectiveness, especially during change, is related at least as much to leaders' emotional intelligence as it is to their cognitive and logical/rational abilities (Palmer et al., 2001).

CONCLUSION

In this article we present the fundamentals of organizational culture and change from an organizational behavior viewpoint. In reviewing these concepts and the associated research, we are making a critical assumption: By understanding the phenomena underlying culture and change processes, managers will be better equipped to implement real and lasting change in their organizations. It is our contention that when organizational change is implemented in a well-intentioned but superficial manner, this leads to needlessly disruptive, even possibly psychologically and institutionally harmful change results (e.g., employees becoming cynical and suspicious of any future change efforts). The superficiality of most change efforts is understandable in the sense that cultural values are difficult to fully identify, let alone control or manage. The very taken-for-granted nature of cultural values makes altering them difficult and threatening–it requires surfacing what the values actually are, before change can be implemented (Garfinkel, 1967). As many have noted, it is difficult for the fish to fully appreciate and understand the water in which they swim.

Yet despite this daunting complexity, we are encouraged by the substantial research suggesting that culture change *can* be managed. The survival, evolution-adaptation, and revolutionary models of change are cautionary models: They all assume that change will happen, even if managers are resolutely standing still. They assume that change is largely out of the strategic control of organizational leaders. What the management-of-culture-change model suggests, however, is that leaders can, and must "grab hold" of the inevitable change at opportune moments, and strategically implement it.

The change process we outline requires attention to a variety of variables, including thoughtful cognitive and affective communication, rewarding behaviors, congruence between rhetoric, structures, and practices, and facilitating active involvement by a wide range of participants. This is a tall order. But if long-term care organizations–as with their counterparts in the corporate environment–wish to survive in their environments on terms that they, rather than the environment dictate, attention to cultural change and its effective implementation are essential.

Moreover, if these organizations wish to thrive in meaningful ways for elders, their families and staff, understanding the dynamics of culture change will be essential to implementing a model or amalgam of models described in this volume.

REFERENCES

Bandura, A. (1977). *Social learning theory.* Englewood Cliffs, NJ: Prentice-Hall.

Barsade, S. G. (2001). *The ripple effect: Emotional contagion in groups.* Unpublished manuscript.

Bastien, D. T., McPhee, R., & Bolton, K. (1995). A study and extended theory of organizational climate: A structural approach. *Communication Monographs, 62,* 135-151.

Baumann, A., & Silverman, B. (1998). Flattening the hierarchy: Deprofessionalization in health care. In L. Groake (Ed.), *The ethics of the new economy.* Waterloo, ON: Wilfred Laurier University Press.

Beckhard, R., & Harris, R. (1977). *Organizational transitions.* Reading, MA: Addison-Wesley.

Blythe, J., Baumann, A., & Giovannetti, P. (2001). Nurses' experiences of restructuring in three Ontario hospitals. *Journal of Nursing Scholarship, 33,* 61-68.

Chatman, J. A. (1989). Improving interactional organizational research: A model of person-organization fit. *Academy of Management Review, 14,* 333-349.

Chatman, J. A. (1991). Matching people and organizations: Selection and socialization in public accounting firms. *Administrative Science Quarterly, 36,* 459-484.

Collins, J. C., & Porras, J. I. (1994). *Built to last: Successful habits of visionary companies.* New York: HarperBusiness.

Cummings, T. G. (1995). From programmed change to self design: Learning how to change organizations. *Organizational Development Journal, 13,* 20-32.

Deci, E. L., & Ryan, R. M. (1985). *Intrinsic motivation and self-determination in human behavior.* New York: Plenum.

Finkenauer, C., & Rime, B. (1998). Keeping emotional memories secret: Health and subjective well-being when emotions are not shared. *Journal of Health Psychology, 3,* 47-58.

Garfinkel, H. (1967). *Studies in ethnomethodology.* Cambridge, UK: Polity Press.

Gersick, C. J. G. (1991). Revolutionary change theories: A multilevel exploration of the punctuated equilibrium paradigm. *Academy of Management Review, 16*(1), 10-36.

Gibson, C. H. (1991). A concept analysis of empowerment. *Journal of Advanced Nursing, 16,* 354-361.

Gold, M. F. (2002, January). Freeing the human spirit. *Provider*, 21-32.

Gordon, N. (2002). The role of social work in the nursing home admissions process: Framing the debate. *Journal of Social Work in Long-Term Care, 1*(1), 7-10.

Greiner, L. E. (1972, July-August). Evolution and revolution as organizations grow. *Harvard Business Review*, 37-46.

Guagliardo, J. (2001, July 16). Spreading a gospel of freedom. *McKnight's Long-Term Care News.*

Harrison, E. L., & Pietri, P. H. (1997). Using team building to change organizational culture. *Organization Development Journal, 15*, 71-76.

Herzberg, F. (1966). *Work and the nature of man.* Cleveland, OH: World.

Hochschild, A. R. (1983). *The managed heart: Commercialization of human feeling.* Los Angeles: University of California Press.

Homans, G. (1950). *The human group.* New York: Harcourt Brace Jovanovich.

Huber, G. P., & Glick, W. H. (Eds.). (1995). *Organizational change and redesign: Ideas and insights for improving performance.* New York: Oxford University Press.

Huy, Q. N. (1999). Emotional capability, emotional intelligence, and radical change. *Academy of Management Review, 24*(2), 325-345.

Joseph, J., & Deshpande, S. P. (1997). The impact of ethical climate on job satisfaction of nurses. *Health Care Management Review, 22*, 76-81.

Kanter, R. M., Stein, B. A., & Jick, T. D. (1992). *The challenge of organizational change.* New York: The Free Press.

Katz, D., & Kahn, R. L. (1978). *The social psychology of organizations.* New York: John Wiley & Sons.

Kotter, J. P. (1995, March-April). Why transformation efforts fail. *Harvard Business Review*, 59-67.

Kotter, J. P., & Heskett, J. L. (1992). *Corporate culture and performance.* New York: Free Press.

Kubler-Ross, E. (1970). The care of the dying: Whose job is it? *Psychiatry in Medicine, 1*, 103-107.

Larkin, T. J., & Larkin, S. (1994). *Communicating change.* New York: McGraw-Hill.

Laschinger, H. K., & Havens, D. S. (1996). Staff nurse work empowerment and perceived control over nursing practice: Conditions for work effectiveness. *Journal of Nursing Administration, 26*, 27-35.

Leavitt, H., & Mueller, R. (1951). Some effects of feedback on communication. *Human Relations, 4*, 401-410.

Lewin, K. (1997). *Resolving social conflicts & field theory in social science.* Washington, DC: American Psychological Association.

Lockwood, P., & Kunda, Z. (1997). Superstars and me: Predicting the impact of role models on the self. *Journal of Personality and Social Psychology, 73*, 91-103.

March, J., & Simon, H. (1958). *Organizations.* New York: Wiley.

Martin, J. (1992). *Cultures in organizations.* New York: Oxford University Press.

Mayer, J. D., Caruso, D. R., & Salovey, P. (2000). Emotional intelligence meets traditional standards for an intelligence. *Intelligence, 27*, 267-298.

Merton, R. K. (1957). *Social theory and social structure* (Rev. ed.). New York: Free Press.

Meyer, M. W., & Zucker, L. G. (1989). *Permanently failing organizations.* Newbury Park, CA: Sage.

Mohrman, S. & Cummings, T. G. (1989). *Self-designing organizations: Learning how to create high performance.* Reading, MA: Addison-Wesley.

Moore, J. D. J. (1996, March 25). Instill a culture of change, hospital consultants advise. *Modern Healthcare,* 52.

Morris, J. A., & Feldman, D. C. (1996). The dimensions, antecedents, and consequences of emotional labor. *Academy of Management Review, 21,* 986-1010.

Nadler, D. A. (1983). The effective management of organizational change. In M. D. Dunnette (Ed.), *Handbook of industrial and organizational psychology* (pp. 358-369). New York: John Wiley & Sons.

Nadler, D. A., & Tushman, M. L. (1980). A model for diagnosing organizational behavior. *Organizational Dynamics* (Autumn), 35-51.

Nadler, D. A., & Tushman, M. L. (1990). Beyond the charismatic leader: Leadership and organizational change. *California Management Review, 32*(2), 77-97.

Normann, R. (1977). *Management for growth.* New York: Wiley.

O'Reilly, C. (1989). Corporations, culture and commitment: Motivation and social control in organizations. *California Management Review, 31*(Summer), 9-25.

O'Reilly, C., & Chatman, J. A. (1986). Organizational commitment and psychological attachment: The effects of compliance, identification and internalization on prosocial behavior. *Journal of Applied Psychology, 71,* 492-499.

O'Reilly, C., & Chatman, J. A. (1996). Culture as social control: Corporations, cults, and commitment. In B. M. Staw & L. L. Cummings (Eds.), *Research in organizational behavior* (Vol. 18, pp. 157-200). Stamford, CT: JAI Press.

O'Reilly, C. I., Chatman, J. A., & Caldwell, D. M. (1991). People and organizational culture: A Q-sort approach to assessing person-organization fit. *Academy of Management Journal, 34,* 487-516.

Ouchi, W., & Wilkins, A. (1985). Organizational culture. *Annual Review of Sociology, 11,* 457-483.

Palmer, B., Walls, M., Burgess, Z., & Stough, C. (2001). Emotional intelligence and effective leadership. *Leadership and Organizational Development Journal, 22*(1), 5-10.

Pennebaker, J. W., Zech, E., & Rime, B. (2001). Disclosing and sharing emotion: Psychological, social, and health consequences. In M. S. Stroebe & R. O. Hansson (Eds.), *Handbook of bereavement research: Consequences, copying, and care* (pp. 517-543). Washington, DC: American Psychological Association.

Pfeffer, J. (1992). *Managing with power: Politics and influence in organizations.* Boston, MA: Harvard Business School Press.

Pfeffer, J. (1998). *The human equation: Building profits by putting people first.* Boston, MA: Harvard Business School Press.

Quinn, J. B. (1981). *Strategies for change: Logical incrementalism.* Homewood, IL: Irwin.

Rogers, C. R., & Roethlisberger, F. J. (1991, November-December). Barriers and gateways to communication. *Harvard Business Review,* 105-111.

Rogers, E. M., & Agarwala-Rogers, R. (1976). *Communication in organizations.* New York: Free Press.

Scheck, C. L., & Kinicki, A. J. (2000). Identifying the antecedents of coping with an organizational acquisition: A structural assessment. *Journal of Organizational Behavior, 21*(6), 627-648.

Schein, E. H. (1991). *Organizational culture and leadership.* San Francisco, CA: Jossey-Bass.

Schweiger, D. M., & DeNisi, A. S. (1991). Communication with employees following a merger: A longitudinal field experiment. *Academy of Management Journal, 34*, 110-135.

Siehl, C., & Martin, J. (1984). The role of symbolic management: How can managers effectively transmit organizational culture? In J. Hunt, D. Hosking, C. Schriesheim & R. Stewart (Eds.), *Leaders and managers: International perspectives on managerial behavior and leadership* (pp. 227-239). Elmsford, NY: Pergamon.

Smith, A. C. I., & Kleinman, S. (1989). Managing emotions in medical school: Student's contacts with the living and the dead. *Social Psychology Quarterly, 52*, 56-69.

Stevens, C. H. (2001, November/December). A timeless dream. *Balance,* 7-7-18.

Thomas, W. (2001). A message from Dr. Thomas. *Eden Alternative Journal, 9*(2), 6-8.

Tushman, M. L., & Romanelli, E. (1985). Organizational evolution: A metamorphosis model of convergence and reorientation. In B. M. Staw & L. L. Cummings (Eds.), *Research in organizational behavior.* Greenwich, CT: JAI.

Wanberg, C. R., & Banas, J. T. (2000). Predictors and outcomes of openness to changes in a reorganizing workplace. *Journal of Applied Psychology, 85*, 132-142.

Weick, K. E., & Quinn, R. E. (1999). Organizational change and development. *Annual Review of Psychology, 50*, 361-386.

Culture Change
in Long-Term Care Facilities:
Changing the Facility
or Changing the System?

Monsignor Charles J. Fahey

SUMMARY. This essay asserts that the long-term care system, as we know it, has grown in response to public policy initiatives in other areas. This system is lacking in clear, coherent conceptual underpinnings. If significant culture change is to occur, societal values, public policy, and provider behavior must be responsive to the clear preference of consumers for services that respect their dignity by balancing the system toward home- and community-based services and home-like residential care when needed. *[Article copies available for a fee from The Haworth Document Delivery Service: 1-800-HAWORTH. E-mail address: <docdelivery@haworthpress.com> Website: <http://www.HaworthPress.com> © 2003 by The Haworth Press, Inc. All rights reserved.]*

KEYWORDS. Culture, long-term care, Medicare, Medicaid, nursing home, public policy

Monsignor Charles J. Fahey, MSW, MDiv, is Professor Emeritus, Fordham University; Program Officer, Milbank Memorial Fund; and Senior Research Associate, Loretto Institute for the Frail Elderly.

Address correspondence to: Monsignor Charles J. Fahey, 602 Loyola Hall, Fordham University, Bronx, NY 10458 (E-mail: fahey@fordham.edu).

[Haworth co-indexing entry note]: "Culture Change in Long-Term Care Facilities: Changing the Facility or Changing the System? Fahey, Monsignor Charles J. Co-published simultaneously in *Journal of Social Work in Long-Term Care* (The Haworth Social Work Practice Press, an imprint of The Haworth Press, Inc.) Vol. 2, No. 1/2, 2003, pp. 35-51; and: *Culture Change in Long-Term Care* (ed: Audrey S. Weiner, and Judah L. Ronch) The Haworth Social Work Practice Press, an imprint of The Haworth Press, Inc., 2003, pp. 35-51. Single or multiple copies of this article are available for a fee from The Haworth Document Delivery Service [1-800-HAWORTH, 9:00 a.m. - 5:00 p.m. (EST). E-mail address: docdelivery@haworthpress.com].

10.1300/J181v2n01_03

INTRODUCTION

That which informs the behavior of the long-term care system (i.e., its culture) is a function of three interacting forces: the purchaser (demand), the provider (supply), and the regulator. In the field of long-term care, the normal interaction of supply and demand is mediated by the heavy regulatory activity of government, which is also the primary purchaser. Government controls the demand of many consumers by allowing the use of Medicare and especially Medicaid funds only in narrowly defined circumstances. This essay asserts that substantial change in facilities can occur only in the context of a change in long-term care public policy and the public's commitment to this change.

DEFINITIONS

First, we need to examine the concepts *long-term care* and *culture* as used here. In *Towards an International Consensus on Policy for Long-Term Care of the Ageing,* the World Health Organization and Milbank Memorial Fund define the first concept as follows:

> Long-term care is the system of activities undertaken by informal caregivers (family, friends, and/or neighbours) and/or professionals (health, social, and others) to ensure that a person who is not fully capable of self-care can maintain the highest possible quality of life, according to his or her individual preferences, with the greatest possible degree of independence, autonomy, participation, personal fulfillment, and human dignity. (2000, http://www.milbank.org/000712oms.pdf)

The dictionary definition of culture is

- to cultivate, i.e., that which is cultivated
- an act of developing by education, discipline, or training
- the enlightenment and refinement of taste acquired by intellectual and aesthetic training
- a particular stage of advancement in civilization or the characteristic features of such a stage or state

(*Webster's New Collegiate Dictionary*, 1951, p. 202)

ASSERTIONS

1. Significant changes in the culture of long-term care, especially in facilities, must be viewed in terms of short- and long-term possibilities.
2. The pervasiveness and structure of Medicaid will permit only marginal, albeit important, changes in the immediate future.
3. Long-range, significant changes can occur only if consumers have the power to move the long-term care field in accord with their desires.
4. Regulatory activity must better balance safety and negotiated risk.
5. Cultural change can occur only if exogenous forces can be identified and the interests of those persons providing and purchasing services are in alignment with these exogenous forces.
6. Significant cultural changes can occur only if there are changes in the broader culture and that of society including:

   - recognition of the extent of frailty and its impact on all persons;
   - valuing of the frail person;
   - willingness to share economic, psychological, and opportunity costs; and
   - community, moral, and psychological ownership of long-term care systems and facilities.

The definition of culture implies

- a definable locus;
- a deliberate cultivation; and
- refinement and civilization (i.e., an evolutionary process that contributes to the dignity of individuals and the community).

To bring about change there must be

- an understanding and delineation of the locus where change is to take place;
- an understanding of what constitutes the culture of that locus–
  - the discernable elements in the current culture and their prevalence;
  - the desirability/undesirability of these elements; and
  - the history of the prevailing culture and knowledge of how this culture is sustained;
- an agreement about what constitutes a more desirable culture–
  - specific contributors to nourishing the dignity of people; and
  - the strategies and obstacles to change.

The first step in this analysis is to clarify the scope of the effort: What culture is to be changed? Three approaches (or some combinations) that can be taken include focusing on

- the nursing home as we know it;
- the services and/or systems that purport to offer support to those who would otherwise be eligible for nursing home care; and
- the conditions that generate the need for supportive services.

DOMAINS

If there is to be a culture change in the care of the frail, there must be changes in three interlocking, overlapping domains: society, public policy, and the provision of services.

Society

American society is known for its almost pathological emphasis on independence and youth. While freedom is indeed an important value, it does not trump others such as interdependence and community. Our good life with its attendant freedoms and possibilities is a result of the inheritance from the past and many interactions with the present. We are the recipients of a congenial civic infrastructure and advances that make life richer, less painful, and even longer. Contemporaneously, we are dependent on others for the things that sustain physical life and even more importantly, for our psychological and spiritual well-being. This is true at every age.

Unfortunately, the preoccupation with independence and youth is not merely a distraction but in all too many instances is accompanied by a denial of the aging process and even a disvaluing of older people. These tendencies work against more enlightened and life-giving/sustaining approaches to a more dignified way of providing care for those in need of the help of others over an extended period of time.

Public Policy

Elderly public policy in the United States follows two distinct paths. One is premised on the assumption that old age and retirement are matters of public concern in which employed persons should share the burdens associated with nonemployment and acute illness. We have adopted social insurance models in which risk is broadly shared, and a floor for income (Social Security) and payment of needed medical services (Medicare) are assured publicly.

The other path, a concomitant welfare policy involving "means testing," provides modest income security (Supplemental Security Income) and access to needed health services for the poor (Medicaid). Unfortunately, this path dominates long-term care since such a high percentage of persons in need of long-term care services has limited means. As former Secretary of Health and Human Services Wilbur Cohen is reputed to have said, "Of one thing we can be sure, programs for the poor will be poor programs." In virtually every jurisdiction, Medicaid eligibility for and reimbursement of long-term care are modest at best. While there is some room for culture change, it is likely to be modest and without greater public outlays for a better-balanced system (i.e., more services to maintain people at home and better-staffed, more congenial physical structures).

Services: Long-Term Care Field and Long-Term Care Industry

Formal long-term care is complex and dominated by

- transactions of persons without resources to purchase needed services, largely driven by Medicaid, but also to a lesser degree by Medicare; Supplemental Security Income; Older American Act funds; veterans' benefits; and various state programs; and
- transactions of persons with private resources and Medicare who purchase services of their choice from providers
  - whose services are driven by Medicaid;
  - who are in the private, formal marketplace; and
  - who are off the books.

The Nursing Home

Why is there a need for change?

- No one likes a nursing home.
  - It is filled with sick people.
  - Most residents are close to death.
  - Many residents have limited intellectual and/or relational capacity.
- Yet for those with limited economic resources, there are few choices and likely to be fewer still in the future.
- The publicly supported system is lacking in balance.
- The system is expensive and in all probability, unsustainable
  - for the individual, family, and spouse and
  - for the Medicaid system itself.
- There is some evidence that Medicaid reimbursement in many jurisdictions is inadequate for quality services.

- While survey and certification processes have contributed to some improvement in quality, they have unintended, but nonetheless deleterious, effects as well.
- Especially in the area of direct care, there is often staffing that is inadequate in terms of numbers, education, and training. Many come from troubled circumstances.

What Is a Nursing Home, and How Did It Get To Be What It Is?

The following help to understand the nursing home as it exists today:

- The nursing home structure is dominated by the Medicaid system, which is essentially a program for sick people who are poor. These characteristics encourage a culture laden with the trappings of healthcare and medicine. Because this is a program for the sick who are poor, the economic support of the facility will be almost always assuredly minimal out of political deference to the taxpayer and other important public priorities.
- Long-term care services as they exist are largely an artifact of shifts in public policy about other modes of care and public financing. Medicaid and the availability of capital financing were major factors in the growth of nursing homes. On several occasions in recent history, policy decisions have been made to minimize the use of acute care hospitals. Each resulted in significant growth in nursing home use. Court decisions as well as economic and humane considerations brought about de-institutionalization and non-institutionalization of the mentally ill, increasing the number of persons with dementia in nursing homes.

The nursing home field grew as a result of the following factors:

- the growth of the frail elderly population, many of whom had limited resources;
- public policy designed to minimize the use of acute hospitals;
- public policy and court decisions to minimize state mental institutions;
- federal funds to build facilities; and
- Medicaid funds to pay for care (and to a lesser extent, Medicare funds).

These factors shaped and continue to shape the structure of nursing home care. Medicaid is both the primary payer of nursing home care and the regulator.

More recently, the following additional forces have come into play in shaping the culture of nursing homes:

- the growth of home- and community-based services;
- the proliferation of the private-pay assisted-living market;
- greater use of preadmission screening;
- Medicaid financing offering incentives (disincentives) to care for persons with the most intense acuity; and
- favorable Medicare and managed care reimbursement for subacute and rehab patients.

All of these factors have contributed to a stabilization of nursing home usage with a concomitant growth in the number of very sick and/or disabled residents. Nursing homes have both incentives and disincentives to admit very sick patients, even as both home care and assisted living are primary choices for those who can afford them.

In general terms, there are several types of persons in nursing homes, each with distinctive care needs such as

- very sick, multiply distressed persons, for example, ventilator-dependent patients;
- short-term rehab patients who are likely to leave the facility;
- persons, such as Alzheimer patients, whose dementia is difficult for families to manage;
- other persons who have problems with several activities of daily living because of various physical impairments; and
- the dying.

In addition to the variety of residents in nursing homes, regulation, reimbursement, staffing patterns, and the availability of competent and committed staff are other factors influencing the culture of nursing homes.

The regulatory milieu has impact on both the physical and social environments. The hospital model and the operational codes have influenced Medicaid building specifications heavily, as have medicine and the centrality of safety in regulatory approaches.

Assisted-living continuing-care residential facilities and the growth of home- and community-based services have altered the long-term care scene. The use of each evidences the preference of persons to remain at home and if that is not possible or desirable, to reside in a home-like setting.

Traditional marketplace forces are unable to bring about desired changes since nursing homes must serve the people for whom Medicaid will pay and in the mode that Medicaid requires. Virtually no nursing home can survive without Medicaid patients, and increasingly Medicaid will pay only for those who are the most frail and often difficult to manage.

Most consumers are uninformed. Often services are sought in time of crisis with few choices within the nursing home field, or in many jurisdictions, between a nursing home and other services. For example, often the decision to access long-term care is on the occasion of a hospital stay with substantial pressure upon the family or significant other to move the patient and accept whatever placement is available.

Except in the rare instance of a provider catering to an exclusively private-pay market, the provider has little incentive or margin to manage other than to minimum requirements.

OTHER INFLUENCES
IN THE CULTURE OF LONG-TERM CARE FACILITIES

Taken as a whole, the nursing home sector has characteristics of both a field and an industry. Institutional and home- and community-based providers include the publicly traded and the for-profit entities that have a dual mission of providing needed services and assuring a return for investors. A significant minority are sponsored by religious and community groups that view themselves as involved in ministry and civic responsibility. Inevitably some internal management choices, including resource allocation, are rooted in the ownership/sponsorship of the entity.

Size and geographic location are often significant factors in determining the culture of a facility, as is the existence of a unionized workforce. Each variable can exert a positive or negative impact on the overall cultural context.

Desirable cultural values include

- an atmosphere emphasizing the dignity of all who are part of the community;
- alternatives and participation in decision-making;
- a sense of mutual responsibility on the part of all community members;
- personal relationships;
- community and the promotion of the common good;
- reciprocal interactions with the broader community;
- a supportive environment;
- ethical decision-making;
- an atmosphere of caring;
- good clinical interventions;
- pleasant physical environment; and
- the opportunity for social, recreational, and spiritual engagement.

WHAT TRIGGERS THE NEED FOR LONG-TERM CARE?

Dependency and the need of assistance are at the heart of long-term care. In some instances, the dependency requires a specialized residence.

The use of the term *long-term care* itself may be both misleading and constraining. Long-term care addresses the reality of loss and how individuals, those close to them, and society as a whole deal with the loss. This loss is a sometimes gradual, sometimes dramatic loss of physiological, intellectual, and social capacity that requires substantial, costly support. This loss and accompanying need have become so pervasive that we can now characterize a period of frailty as a normal part of the human journey.

Unfortunately, long term-care carries with it considerable baggage and immediately focuses on services, often those provided in a nursing home, rather than on needs.

Frailty

It may be useful to consider frailty as the overarching concept. Frailty is not easily defined but is easily recognized. Using it as an organizing concept can better define how to address the programmatic and financial implications of long-term care. Used in this context, frailty is both a state and a process. It involves functional, social, and economic considerations. Central to the concept are the challenges of a person's relative ability to deal with activities of daily living, insults both minor and devastating, and change. Frailty is likely to be progressive with some periods of remission and will ultimately result in the need for care and finally, in death.

Frailty manifests itself in many diverse ways that ultimately often coalesce into substantial dependence. It may occur as a result of a cataclysmic physical event such as a stroke, a social event such as the loss of a significant other, or an economic event such as the loss of personal savings. In some instances, frailty occurs over time with various individual physical events and in other instances, occurs with a sudden cascading of events that can best be characterized as system degradation or failure. The common characteristic of frailty is the loss of capacity to manage without assistance.

The impact in the increase of the incidence and prevalence of frailty is both personal and social, involving the person, those significant to him or her, and society as a whole. Everyone is at multiple risk whether a potential user, a caregiver, or a payer.

Typically, increased frailty occurs in the latter part of life when one's material and social assets may be diminished and income reduced to the minimum for all but the more affluent. Simultaneously, the costs associated with pharmacological agents, new environmental arrangements, and prosthetic devices increase.

Frailty is hard to objectify. It involves endogenous and exogenous factors. Culture, value, psychological strength, and personal financial assets have an impact on a person's ability to cope with decreased physical capacity. Where one lives, the configuration of one's home, and the willingness of others to help are also significant. Whatever the cause, the frail person has difficulty dealing with the basics of life and manages to do so at economic, social, and psychological costs.

As others become involved with the frail person, there are difficult transactions to negotiate both with informal (primary) and formal helpers. For example, how long should one be able to drive, and who makes the decision? Is home care adequate in the light of the person's needs? How long should autonomy prevail over legitimate caring and the legitimate interests of the common good? Do good-willed helpers inadvertently induce need and dependency?

We may describe the etiology of frailty as stemming from various causes:

- genetics;
- trauma;
- chronic illness, both physical and emotional;
- dementia; and
- age-related loss of capacity.

The rationale for using this insight as a basis for policy helps to better understand what is to be addressed in policy: economic security, services, protective and supportive environments, and medical care.

Current policy for long-term care tends to implement care that is a step down from care for acute illness. Each intervention for current long-term care is built on a medical model with all of its trappings, but much of the problem actually lies with and calls for social, economic, and environmental approaches with medical add-ons. Unless and until the basic problem is better defined, the foundation of long-term care will be dominated by the culture of illness and disease.

In addition to the historic long-term care system that is the result of a devolution of acute medical and long-term psychiatric care, the cultural divide evidenced in virtually all developed countries between healthcare as a general public responsibility and social care as a personal and welfare function further skews the long-term care system. Western democracies, with the exception of the United States, have universal entitlements in the area of acute health care problems. However, virtually all Western democracies means-test and/or localize care of the frail.

Since care of the frail can be costly both to individuals and state governments, these payers have utilized the Willy Sutton Principle extensively (i.e., to go "where the money is"). Medicaid, a part of the compromise that also brought about Medicare, was designed for the medically indigent. Gradually it was expanded at the state level to care not only for the very sick but also for the frail. Medicare Extended Care Benefits (Part B) were intended to provide a substitute for inpatient hospital days. Over the years, Medicare Part B was expanded to meet the needs of the frail, only to be contracted for fiscal reasons.

Frailty and Persons with Handicapping Conditions

The dominant desires of persons with handicapping conditions are normalcy, activity, and participation. The Americans with Disability Act/Olmstead Decision and vibrant advocacy activity are indications of these desires, and to some extent, have moved society to foster inclusiveness, and where needed, care programs and facilities that maximize independence and consumer direction. These examples demonstrate the ability of empowered consumers to bring about cultural and systemic changes.

Frailty and the Developmentally Disabled

Analogously, various court decisions such as the Willowbrook Consent Decree and effective advocacy on the part of the Association for Retarded Citizens have changed policy. The large institutional approach has given way to smaller more home-like neighborhood settings for those in need of residential care. The medical component, no longer dictating the matrix for the care of the developmentally disabled, has become secondary. This, too, is an example of cultural and structural change resulting from strong and effective, albeit surrogate, consumer advocacy.

Frailty and the Aging

The high point of physiological capacity is during the ordinary reproductive facet of the life cycle. It is true of plants, animals, and human beings. After this period, gradual but inexorable physiological capacity declines, with death being the endpoint. It is important here to understand two points. First, many compensations can be utilized to mitigate somewhat the decline and its consequences. Second, a person's executive functions (i.e., living responsibly and ethically, developing wisdom, and making contributions to society) may increase.

Whether the incidence and prevalence of actual dependency are decreasing is yet to be settled. It is clear that many medical advances are warding off premature death, and numerous pharmacological, prosthetic, and lifestyle interventions are currently available that can mitigate the possibility of dependency but not the underlying potential for frailty, current or future.

The virtual universality in the human journey of greater or lesser frailty, with its associated costs to individuals, families, and society, makes it a matter of public concern.

Frailty Care Associated with Aging

Dealing with frailty is as complex as its etiology. Compensations, compromises, and avoidance of potential risks are part of the aging process. Early in the progression, the individual and his or her significant other engage in these strategies more or less successfully but always at a cost, often escalating. In this phase, the culture of care is largely what the culture of the individuals and their means allows or dictates. If frailty increases in intensity, the personal resource question becomes determinative. People of means continue to make choices within the context of their values and the marketplace's response to the value judgments of purchasers. Assisted-living continuing-care residential facilities and home care are interventions of choice. For those without sufficient means, the options lie within publicly subsidized programs that are largely institutional, highly regulated for safety, and intensely medicalized.

Two overlapping types of aging frailty are particularly challenging: that which involves physical cause and that which involves dementia. Often they coexist to a greater or lesser degree, but the care, at least in the extremes, is quite different. With physical frailty, there is the opportunity for greater interpersonal communication and self-direction than with dementia. Additionally, the mixture of the two is at best a challenge for the staff, as the tendency is to attend to those with little communication and self-direction capacity at the expense of the physically frail.

Chronic Conditions and Chronic Care

Virtually all older persons develop chronic (i.e., noncorrectable and persistent) conditions. In many instances, these problems do not cause a person to be dependent on others save for skilled medical practitioners who are able to prescribe and monitor life-style factors, pharmacological agents, and/or prosthetic devices. However, there are certain conditions that limit a person's capacity to manage without hands-on assistance and will ultimately be the cause of death. Chronic illness is a medical condition. Dependency may or may not be associated with it. When it is, there must be a balance between social and medical concerns, especially if the condition leads to the need for an alternate living arrangement.

End of Life Care

While all persons will die, the proximity of death, on average, increases with age and frailty. Death from disease in the developed countries has given way to various manifestations of organ deterioration. Despite our limited ability to predict with accuracy the likely time before death, even in the face of serious illness, Medicare will allow payment for hospice service only for those whose death is expected in less than six months.

Palliative care focuses on those persons whose conditions are not remediable but painful and is geared toward relieving pain and suffering rather than toward cure.

Those receiving chronic care and hospice services are likely to be the recipients of long-term care and are certainly frail. However, the converse is not correct. Many persons who are frail receive neither chronic care nor hospice service.

THOUGHTS ON REFORM

It is ironic that at a moment of relative affluence, there is little civic dialogue about a societal approach to long-term care and the culture(s) that inform it. Despite pressing problems inherent in all facets of long-term care, we are in the lull before the storm. We are missing the opportunity for structural reform.

Calls for change seem to have time and intensity elements to them, generally related to persons connected with frailty and its impact. The more immediately and intimately people are involved in frailty and long-term care, the more they see the need for reform. There are some who are keenly aware of the impending crisis but seem unable to forward an agenda or mobilize a movement that will bring systemic change. Society in general seems to suffer from mass denial, indifference, inertia, and ignorance.

Current long-term care policy is segmented, incomplete, and often occasioned by bitter exchanges among advocates for various aspects of the system. Focus tends to be upon short-term fixes to relieve the pain experienced by users and providers. There is no agreed-upon civic agenda, yet such an agenda is essential to reform a system that appears to be both unsustainable and inhumane in its current form.

Strategies toward reform and culture change must take into account immediate issues as well as longer-range concerns. Can we fashion an approach that will enable individuals to cope with the service, setting, and costs associated with dependency? Such policies must not only meet the needs of individuals but also must be sustainable in the light of other legitimate but competing societal needs.

Governments play critical roles in who gets what services, as well as in the promotion and quality of the services available.

Unless there are dramatic breakthroughs, as yet unforeseen, costs will inevitably escalate for individuals and for society as a whole. Questions must be addressed such as

- What are or should be societal expectations about the responsibility of significant others in caring for their frail partners, family members, and friends?
- Are these expectations realistic given changing social structures and personal values?
- Does government have only a residual responsibility to care for those who have no resources to alleviate their frailty?
- Should government adopt a social insurance approach that involves life-long, intergenerational sharing of and paying for risks of frailty?
- Would a policy of tax incentives for the purchase of private insurance generate a response adequate to assure that reliance on welfare-type programs would be minimal?
- Should governmental policy emphasize a consumer-directed approach in which individuals have complete control over public dollars designated to meet needs associated with frailty and dependency?
- What are preferred modes of delivery?
- Should marketplace forces determine modes of delivery exclusively, primarily, moderately, or not at all?
- What are the most effective and humane modes of public management of resources and delivery?
- What is the underlying ideology of public quality assurance?
- What is the most effective means to avoid abuse of individuals and exploitation of the system?
- What is the appropriate role of various levels of government?

The following functions are necessary in attending to both short- and long-term reform:

- clarification of the elements in the issues;
- involvement of those who
  - can contribute to understanding the issues and formulating an agenda;
  - can and want to make a difference; and
  - can influence public opinion.

Governments in their consumer protection role preside over all formal domains. In the publicly supported domain, they are purchasers and gatekeepers as well as quality regulators. In their multiple roles, governments face the conflict inherent in assuring access in quality service for those in need and restraining public expenditures.

If substantial structural and cultural changes are to occur, there must be an alignment of the interests of the following stakeholders:

- users and their families;
- providers–
  - owners and
  - management;
- hands on personnel;
- unions;
- Medicaid purchasers; and
- Medicaid regulators.

CONCLUSION: CAN CULTURE CHANGE OCCUR AND IF SO, HOW?

Some culture change can occur with any population and with modest expenditures. However, significant changes depend on the population served, the ability of the consumer to demand and choose change, and the motivation and capacity of the provider to change.

First, we must determine which persons need residential care and whether one kind of frailty-oriented facility fits all. Can a facility with mixed populations develop and sustain a culture that is suitable for all its residents? These mixed populations consist of

- persons needing complex medical care;
- those with short-term rehab needs;
- persons with physical limitations of such a nature as to require significant assistance in the activities of daily living;

- the mentally impaired with serious cognitive and interpersonal capacity deficits; and
- the dying.

While such fundamental values as dignity and community can be promoted and maintained with all these populations and within the facilities that serve them, the nature of each particular population highlights its limitations and the need for certain emphases. For example, short-stay rehab patients will relate to staff in ways that differ from that of Alzheimer residents. In turn, the Alzheimer patients will have less capacity for social interaction, autonomous decision-making, and community than will physically frail persons.

Significant culture change requires the American people to better understand that

- the lifetime risk of needing human and environmental support is high (i.e., frailty is becoming a normal part of the life journey);
- frailty affects not only the frail person but all who are significant to him or her;
- frailty is costly;
- burdens should be shared;
- the economic choices and capacities of persons through their working days are unlikely to provide adequate personal resources to meet long-term care needs; and
- through public, private, or a combination of both resources, more adequate funding must be available for decent long-term care needs.

Culture change is unlikely unless all consumers are empowered by having the resources to demand, and thereby create a supply of, supports that better enhance dignity.

Culture change is unlikely unless regulatory philosophy better balances safety and risk, and public policy better balances home- and community-based services with institutional services. In addition, public policy must better balance the medical, social, and environmental concerns within institutions.

Culture change is unlikely unless providers have adequate financial resources for quality care.

Culture change will occur only if there is a strong and coherent agreement among the principal stakeholders that frail people and those who care for them should be treated with respect.

REFERENCES

Webster's New Collegiate Dictionary. (1951, 2nd ed.). Springfield, MA: G. & C. Merriam Company Publishers, p. 202.

World Health Organization and Milbank Memorial Fund. (2000). *Towards an international consensus on policy for long-term care of the ageing.* Retrieved February 1, 2002, from http://www.milbank.org/000712oms.pdf.

The Historical Context
of "Humanistic" Culture Change
in Long-Term Care

Sheldon S. Tobin

SUMMARY. In the 1700s, there were public poor houses; in the later 1800s, more humanistic not-for-profit homes for the aged; and by the mid-1900s, less humanistic, particularly proprietary, nursing homes. The 1970s witnessed the beginning of a burgeoning literature on piece-meal programs which are beneficial for residents but often have neither produced humanistic culture change nor have persisted. Also, these cultures did not emerge from even ambitious legislated reforms. Yet, the ingredients for humanistic cultures have appeared in many publications even though they have not been incorporated into practice. This article traces the history of humanistic approaches to care and the role of government in catalyzing change. *[Article copies available for a fee from The Haworth Document Delivery Service: 1-800-HAWORTH. E-mail address: <docdelivery@haworthpress.com> Website: <http://www.HaworthPress.com> © 2003 by The Haworth Press, Inc. All rights reserved.]*

KEYWORDS. Humanistic, culture change, long-term care

Sheldon S. Tobin, PhD, is Professor Emeritus at the University of Albany-SUNY.
Address correspondence to: Sheldon S. Tobin, PhD, 5000 South East End, Chicago, IL 60615.

[Haworth co-indexing entry note]: "The Historical Context of 'Humanistic' Culture Change in Long-Term Care." Tobin, Sheldon S. Co-published simultaneously in *Journal of Social Work in Long-Term Care* (The Haworth Social Work Practice Press, an imprint of The Haworth Press, Inc.) Vol. 2, No. 1/2, 2003, pp. 53-64; and: *Culture Change in Long-Term Care* (ed: Audrey S. Weiner, and Judah L. Ronch) The Haworth Social Work Practice Press, an imprint of The Haworth Press, Inc., 2003, pp. 53-64. Single or multiple copies of this article are available for a fee from The Haworth Document Delivery Service [1-800-HAWORTH, 9:00 a.m. - 5:00 p.m. (EST). E-mail address: docdelivery@haworthpress.com].

10.1300/J181v2n01_04

INTRODUCTION

Humanistic cultures refer to environments in which all elements enhance the humanity, the essential individuality, of its inhabitants. This is a daunting challenge for nursing homes because they are a type of "total institution," which refers to living environments where residents, patients, inmates or novitiates of religious orders are handled in "batches" (Goffman, 1961). Inhabitants, that is, arise and go to bed at the same time, eat together, participate with others in organized shared activities and so forth. Whereas most total institutions handle inhabitants primarily for the purpose of resocialization, nursing homes do so for efficiency. While saving money, efficiency usually conflicts with humanistic goals. Indeed, sound fiscal management and quality of care are usually considered to be contradictory. Fottler, Smith and James (1981), for example, in an illuminating study of 43 proprietary nursing homes, demonstrated the inverse association between fiscal management and quality of care.

In the enduring attempt to maximize both efficiency and quality, many focused beneficial programs have been developed for residents such as developing reminiscence groups, staffing training programs on reality orientation, enhancing family visiting, having pets, and therapeutic touch. Yet these programs are piecemeal efforts that while humanistic in enhancing and individualizing care, do not in themselves produce a new environment, a new culture. Unless the fabric of the facility is changed in its totality, a new culture is not developed. It has been my experience, as well as the typical experience of my colleagues, that programs we have implemented have not induced pervasive change nor, unfortunately, have they tended to persist beyond our participation.

By going beyond piecemeal programs, humanistic cultures can be developed. A necessary precondition for this transformation is the belief that sound fiscal management and quality of care are not incompatible. Also persons at every level, from board members through nursing assistants, must understand that the criteria for a "good" home, as used, for example, by assessors, is insufficient. And further, all must feel that while change is never easy, transformation can be achieved. Components of humanistic cultures will be considered later in this paper whereas illustrative programs and cultures will be described later in this volume.

A cautionary comment: Over time, facilities have become increasingly proprietary and are not as innovative as those in the not-for-profit sector. Indeed, throughout this volume it will be apparent that illustrative programs and cultures are from the not-for-profit world, most faith-based. Many have subventions that help them to achieve excellence. On the other hand, I have witnessed luxurious proprietary homes that obviously charge high fees that are among the very best facilities in quality of care. As Linn, Gruel and Linn (1977) showed decades ago, the amount of dollars spent on patient care is related to outcome. Patient care necessitates staff, particularly hands-on staff. The newest report ordered by Congress and prepared by the Department of Health and Human Services, reveals: "More than 90 percent of the nation's nursing homes have too few workers to take proper care of residents" (*New York Times,* February 18, 2002, p. 1). The Bush administration will not require or advocate more staff but rather encourages better management techniques so that nursing assistants can be more productive. It is certainly difficult at times to be sanguine about the future.

The historic context for the current effort to create humanistic culture change begins with public poor houses. It took many years for long-term institutions for the chronically impaired elderly to emerge from these public poor houses of the early 1700s in America. Whereas the government poor houses sheltered the ill and impoverished, their residents essentially lived in squalor. Although not humanistic, life in these isolated and crowded places was considered to be providing a better quality of life than homelessness and possible starvation.

Later in the 1800s, religious groups developed homes for the aged. These facilities provided a haven for elderly individuals who generally did not have family members able or willing to provide a home for them. Never married women were likely to comprise a substantial proportion of the residential population. Over time, these homes for aged admitted more ill residents who had family living in the community. Concurrent with this change was the growth of the proprietary nursing home industry as the elderly population grew and as urbanization modified family relationships. The need was for family substitutes, particularly for poor, isolated and mentally ill aged. The solution was the for-profit boarding home, the precursor of the nursing home.

The Social Security Act, while providing modest financial security for elderly persons, did not permit the payment of Social Security funds to persons in public institutions. The intent of the act was to stimulate the elderly to live at home, but the effect was to displace tens of thousands of elderly persons from public institutions to privately owned, profit-making boarding homes. Time and the changing level of health of these elderly boarders led to the boarding homes adding nurses and calling themselves nursing homes. Initially, most were small and managed by a family. It was Medicare and Medicaid, like Social Security 30 years earlier that took the nursing home from a family enterprise into big business. By 1960 about four of five residents of nursing homes lived in proprietary facilities (see Cohen, 1974, for a more complete history).

As the nursing home industry grew, homes for the aged became the stimulus for humanistic care. For example, in the early 1960s (when I began my association with Drexel Home for the Aged in Chicago) staff in these facilities usually focused on, and preached, enhancing a home-like atmosphere, a "high-touch" rather than "high-tech" environment. The Drexel Home was a combination of a hotel, hospital and home; staff recognized that unless the home component was enhanced, hotel and hospital components would squeeze out the home atmosphere.

At Drexel Home in Chicago, as in other not-for-profit and usually faith-based homes for the aged, there was likely to be a wealth of programs. The Hebrew Home for the Aged in Riverdale (New York City), for example, had the eminent psychoanalyst Alvin Goldfarb (1959) as a consultant who was intimately involved in the life of the facility. Social programs at Drexel Home included cocktail hours, outdoor picnics and special holiday events. Enhancing the home by bringing in persons from the outside was ongoing. There were training programs for the diversity of students in human service, including physicians in residency programs in medicine and psychiatry. Libow (1982) reported a similar range of training programs at the Jewish Institute for Geriatric Care in New York City. Research activities were incorporated into Drexel Home under the rubric "research as program." In our double blind "memory pill" studies, for example, RNs were paid for administering the pills and also for the assessment of memory improvements. One of the evaluators later became the Director of Nursing.

Concurrently, especially in the 1970s, the proprietary nursing home industry attended to practices in the not-for-profit sector, particularly as a way to improve its image in the face of tough-minded criticism. Criticism was particularly directed at proprietary homes but not exclusively (Butler, 1975; Mendelson, 1974; Vladek, 1980). Too often the profit motive outweighed initiation of a humanistic approach, as illustrated by a vignette entitled "A Good Business" (Tobin, 1999):

> I was asked to discuss my work on institutionalization at the annual meeting of a state proprietary nursing home association. My talk, and the discussion thereafter, seemed to reflect an acceptance by the administrators of the need for family involvement. But then at lunch, a cheerful man dressed in an expensive, well-tailored suit who owned several rural nursing homes said, "Let me tell you about families. I've been in the undertaker business all my life, and what they want is for me to take over. You get them all upset if you involve them too much. I tell them I treat every resident like one of my own family, and I tell my people to tell them we are doing God's work and to let us do His work. (p. 207)

Family members, of course, can indeed be perceived as annoying and disruptive to care but their visiting is the *sine qua non* of good institutional care.

Elsewhere I (Tobin, 1995) have discussed five interventions designed to foster family involvement in institutional care: reducing apprehension and anxiety of family members; face-to-face visiting that enhances the sense of self–of residents, particularly of Alzheimer's disease victims; sharing by family members in the caring for residents; facilitating cooperation and interdependence between family members and nursing assistants; and furthering an identification with the facility as a caring community. A variety of interventions are appropriate for meeting these objectives, including family counseling, family support groups, educational programs for family members, and fundamental changes regarding institutional staff and policy (see also Gaugler, Zarit & Pearlin, 1999).

The literature on innovations, however, had been focused more on specific piecemeal programs rather than on the total environment or culture of the nursing home. When I (Tobin, 1982) reviewed articles published in *The Gerontologist* on long-term care in the 1970s, meaningful limited piecemeal programs were most in evidence. Articles reviewed encompassed family programs, coping with wandering, reality orientation, interpersonal skill training of nursing assistants, reminiscence groups and bringing visitors into the facility.

Continuing my personal odyssey, the 1970s also was the time of alternatives to institutional care that included the argument for parallel services, in community and also institutional care, rather than only alternatives. We at Drexel Home argued for community services for elderly impaired persons who could remain in the community. Our deliberations led to the development of the Council for Jewish Elderly, that now includes a variety of community services. It was apparent that for every resident of a long-term care facility there were two to three times as many elderly persons with the same level of impairments as those in nursing homes who were living in the community being cared for at home (Weissert, 1985). Soon the literature was burgeoning with research reports on the burden of caring at home, invariably by wives, daughters and daughters-in-laws. The literature, however, did not neglect piecemeal programs in facilities.

When I edited *The Gerontologist* in the mid-1980s, authors submitted a steady stream of articles on care burden, as well as on nursing homes. Popular were articles focused on the assessing of adverse effects from entering and living in nursing homes, as well as the need for autonomy of residents. Suggestions about how nursing homes could be restructured to assure autonomy, however, were too often superficial. The important dimension of care by underpaid direct service staff from lower socioeconomic groups, however, received critical attention (see, for example, Tellis-Nyak & Tellis-Nyak, 1989).

Nursing home reform was late in coming. Not unexpectedly a 1986 Institute of Medicine (IOM) study revealed how poor the quality of care had been in nursing homes. Then, using IOM's recommendations, sweeping reforms were enacted in OBRA '87 which included residents' rights, minimum nursing staffing, an interdisciplinary team approach for evaluation and care planning, measurable goals, creation of a uniform resident assessment instrument (RAI) focused on functionality and self-care, development of the minimum data set (MDS) for comprehensive care planning and outcomes, justification and monitoring of physical and chemical restraints, mandatory training and certification for all nursing assistants and a revised quality-of-care survey that was resident-centered. The enactment of this sweeping reform, however, did not lead to humanistic cultures in some nursing homes. Unannounced surveys by state health departments every 9 to 15 months focused on important but less than total aspects of nursing home milieus such as sanitation of food, hazard free environments, pressure sores, housekeeping and accident prevention. Attention, but insufficient to change the quality of care, was given to comprehensive assessment and care planning, as well as enhancement of dignity. Stated another way, compliance did not lead to humanistic cultures. Then, more recently, federal regulations in 2000 mandated a Resident Bill of Rights that emphasized preservation of resident dignity, autonomy, and choices. Included were rights to choose one's physician, participate in planning in care and treatment, and privacy with physicians and family visitors. Still, meeting of medical and nursing needs have dominated, often reducing support of individuals' choices.

The 1990s witnessed a differentiation among long-term care facilities. Continuing care retirement communities (CCRCs), assisted living and then Alzheimer's disease facilities were developed. The promise of this assortment, however, was beset with problems. CCRCs, for example, too often forced residents who entered and lived in independent living apartments to move to assisted living quarters to open up apartments for self-paying new residents. Because of the potential for abuses, New York State refused to license CCRCs. Specialized Alzheimer's disease home-like residences created another problem. Who would provide reimbursement? These facilities were considered neither housing for the physically impaired nor for the mentally ill. Essentially they became a social service for the affluent.

Spending down has plagued states throughout the country because of the heavy drain on Medicaid funds. As residents have spent down and become pauperized, states have reimbursed nursing homes from their Medicaid funds. The states have varied greatly in their reimbursements. While a review of the various formulas for reimbursement is beyond the scope of this article, an anecdote from an experience in New York State may be of interest. When a new Director of Social Services was appointed in the 1980s, an Hispanic man from New York City, he was particularly interested in developing health clinics for the poor in Hispanic neighborhoods using Medicaid funds. Because of his naivety, he was unaware that most Medicaid dollars went to nursing homes, with a heavy amount subsidizing nursing homes for residents who were formerly self-payers but now without funds. Obviously Medicaid funds for his pet project were unavailable.

Whereas, New York State provided somewhat liberal amounts to nursing homes through Medicaid, other states provided meager dollars. To be sure, some states with low Medicaid rates have innovative facilities that have been able to develop humanistic environments. Some states, however, have rates too low to facilitate these environments. Illinois, for example, did not increase funds over the years to counteract inflation and thus reimbursements did not allow for anything approaching humanistic care without heavy subsidization. To offset woeful Medicaid reimbursements, self-payers became a premium. Consequently, hospital discharge planners had difficulty placing poor and sick elderly patients. These patients often accumulated in hospital beds, euphemistically called "alternate care beds." Meanwhile, home care has also not been adequately funded, as it has been in other countries such as the Constant Attendance Allowance to family caregivers in the United Kingdom. At-home hospice care, however, has been funded through Medicare.

Returning to the 1970s and early 1980s, there were many calls for what can be considered to be "humanistic culture change." Four will be considered: enhancing control as an organizing principle (Langer & Rodin, 1976; Rodin & Langer, 1977), mobilizing aggression for therapeutic benefit (Brody et al., 1971), modifying institutional arrangements for the benefit of the mentally impaired (Edelson & Lyons, 1985), and creating environments that can reduce excess morbidity and mortality (Lieberman & Tobin, 1983; Tobin & Lieberman, 1976).

The importance of enhancing control was substantiated in the seminal study of Rodin and Langer (1977). Langer wrote in her 1987 book *Mindfulness*:

> Those in the experimental group were emphatically encouraged to make more decision for themselves. We tried to come up with decisions that mattered and at the same time would not disturb the staff. For example, these residents were asked to choose where to receive visitors: inside the home or outdoors, in their rooms, in the dining room, in the lounge, and so on. They were also told that a movie would be shown the next week on Thursday and Friday and that they should decide whether they wanted to see it and, if so, when. In addition to choices of this sort, residents in the experimental group were each given a houseplant to care for. They were to choose when and how much to water the plants, whether to put them in the window or to shield them from too much sun, and so forth. (p. 82)

Effects of these seemingly simple changes were dramatic. Three weeks after the experiment ended, residents in the experimental group participated more in activities, were happier, and were more alert. Eighteen months later, 30% of the residents in the comparison group had died but only 15% in the experimental group. Not unexpectedly, the relationship that was found between control and survival for nursing home residents mirrors our finding of how aggression and magical coping are associated with intact survivorship for those entering homes (Lieberman & Tobin, 1983; Tobin & Lieberman, 1976). Clearly, what is lethal for the very old is passivity and the lack of a sense of control, of autonomy, and of mastery. Thus, residents-to-be must not, if at all possible, be permitted to be passive and without control. In discharge planning when in the process of relocation to a nursing home, residents-to-be must be encouraged to participate in decision-making on their own behalf and even if unrealistic, to believe they are in control.

At admission, staff must determine how best to structure the new resident's institutional life to enhance control. At Drexel Home for Aged an initial treatment plan was developed based on the resident's characteristic way of coping and how the self is preserved. Over the years, we became rather creative. One example was providing the newly admitted paranoid resident with a roommate who was a "paranee," someone whose sense of self includes being critical of others. In turn, whenever a resident could be placed with a roommate who needed to nurture a more dependent partner, the marriage was made. We were not, however, always successful. Jerome Hammerman, a director of the Home, liked to tell the story of a new resident, a gentle and soft-spoken man, who timidly asked if he could talk to him for a few minutes. "Mr. Hammerman," he said, "you know you might have a nice home here, but how can you give an old man like me a man to live with. I only lived with a woman, my wife, for over 60 years."

Brody et al. (1971) found that excess disabilities could be reduced or eliminated in an institutional setting among the more aggressive residents:

> The fact remains that certain personality characteristics described with the 'aggression factor' were strongly predictive of the treatment potential of these individuals. . . . Aggressive, stubborn, nonconforming individuals elicit negative reactions from others and therefore tend to be regarded as maladjusted, difficult, and inflexible. They may be viewed as unpleasant, undisciplined children in the conscious and unconscious attitudes of the staff. They may be all these things, but our data suggest very clearly that within this aggressive behavior is a force for self-improvement. . . . It may be these 'fighters' who become management problems rather than yield to a structured environment. They, rather than

the 'adjusted' people improved when direction and means of implementation were given to help them to retrieve functions that had been important in previous years. (p. 139)

Unless the more passive elderly individuals become aggressive, even the best of therapeutic intentions and interventions may fail. Note that the factor of "aggressiveness" that was associated with therapeutic success was not simple mobilization, or nonpassivity, but rather a kind of determined nastiness that usually alienates others. Indeed, it is precisely this kind of aggressiveness that we (Lieberman & Tobin, 1983; Tobin & Lieberman, 1976) found insulates the very old from the deleterious effects of relocation stress.

Edelson and Lyons (1985) wrote that care must be provided "that is rehabilitative whenever possible, prosthetic whenever necessary, and at all times humane, identity-preserving, and ego-supporting" (p. xix). Identity-preserving is the same as preservation of the self and, of interest, is that in their next chapter, Edelson and Lyons explain how promoting mastery is the essence of ego-supporting efforts to inflate beliefs in mastery. Next, from their many years of experience at the Baycrest Geriatric Center in Toronto, Edelson and Lyons noted that "institutional arrangements that support direct care staff in establishing a supportive relationship with impaired residents focuses attention on how interdisciplinary teams work" (p. xxi). Thus individual mental health practitioners, separately or as members of teams, can best be used to structure ongoing supportive relationships between staff and individual residents. Finally, they stated: "As changes are made to meet the needs of the mentally impaired elderly, there will be resistance to change" (p. xxii). The obvious challenge to professionals is to facilitate change, but a paradox is that facilities must be assisted in changing so that they become settings where identities are not changed. Fortunately, mental health professionals are precisely those professionals who know only too well how hard it is to reduce resistance to change but, also, at the same time, know how to reduce the resistance.

An institutional orientation to enhancing residents' functioning must penetrate interactions between residents and staff at all levels. Such penetrations occur through staff's understanding of residents' behavior, but there are many barriers that must be overcome if there is to be accurate appraisals of behaviors, particularly of demented residents. Staff, like family, find it difficult to understand how seemingly pathologic processes are actually functional. Aggressiveness, nastiness, and even paranoid behaviors can, as has been shown, facilitate for adaptation to stress. Staff must learn to understand, tolerate, and even nurture verbally abusive aggressive and paranoid behaviors directed at them by residents. Obviously this is a difficult task, a task too difficult for some staff. It is also a task that is not assumed by staff in many facilities where even the most minor of deviations from ideal compliance and gratefulness are not tolerated.

We (Lieberman & Tobin, 1983) found in our four studies of relocation of the elderly, either from the community to nursing home or from state mental hospitals to long-term care facilities, that the quality of psychosocial environments predicted outcomes more than psychological attributes of residents-to-be such as assertiveness and magical mastery. To be specific, the beneficial psychosocial qualities were, first, warmth expressed in interpersonal relations between residents and staff and, also, between residents; second, activities and other forms of stimulation that are perceived and used; third, tolerance for deviancies such as aggression, drinking, wandering, complaining, and incontinence; and fourth, and lastly, individuation defined as the extent to which residents are perceived and treated as individuals in being allowed and encouraged to express individuality. It is a pattern of qualities that reflect the acceptance of aggressiveness, magical coping, mythmaking in reminiscence, and other ways for the preservation of self, that are essential for adaptation (Tobin, 1999).

These four excursions into the essentials of humanistic nursing home cultures provided the template for the direction, and even necessity, for change. To be sure, piecemeal innovative life-enhancing programs can be helpful for some residents. Yet unless the culture changes, too many residents fall by the wayside. We may have the knowledge but, apparently, the will is too often lacking. Change is never easy! Change toward a new orientation cannot be imposed but rather must come from within.

When I have discussed or argued with funding bodies for intrinsic changes toward humanistic cultures, I have usually been accused of being unrealistic. Whenever I proposed a social experiment that included meeting with boards and chief administrators, and not to simply initiate a controlled social experiment with the consent and cooperation of the Director of Nursing Services or Social Services, I was met with refusals. When, for example, in the 1990s I suggested to a funding group of the New York Department of Health that I was prepared to submit a proposal to assist nursing homes to move toward more humanistic cultures, I was told this kind of more total approach could not be authorized. Once again funds were to be used for controlled studies of rather narrow interventions. To be sure, these interventions were not without merit and certainly carried out with refined skills (by, may I add, invariably with professionals I admired and many that I had mentored). Yet, I do not believe that these innovations persisted. Still, sometimes it is all that we have and for a moment in time these piecemeal innovations may make a humanistic difference.

Without, however, changing the fabric of the milieu we persist in an archaic mode. The shame of it is that more than a quarter of a century ago we had detailed knowledge regarding those essential ingredients that make for a humanistic culture. Now articles in this volume show once again the possibilities for culture change. Moreover, they demonstrate how our optimism can be translated into reality despite the daunting challenge of life in a "total institution."

REFERENCES

Brody, E. M., Kleban, M. H., Lawton, M. P., & Silverman, H. A. (1971). Excess disabilities of mentally impaired aged: Impact of individualized treatment. *The Gerontologist, 11*, 124-133.

Butler, R. N. (1975). *Why survive when old in America?* New York: Harper & Rowe.

Cohen, E. S. (1974). An overview of long-term care facilities. In E. Brody, *A social work guide for long-term care facilities.* Rockville, MD: National Institute of Mental Health.

Edelson, J. S., & Lyons, W. (1985). *Institutional care of the mentally impaired elderly.* New York: Van Nostrand Reinhold.

Fottler, M. D., Smith, H, L., & James. W. L. (1981). Profits and patient care quality in nursing homes: Are they compatible? *The Gerontologist, 21*, 532-538.

Gaugler, J. E., Zarit, S. H., & Pearlin, L. J. (1999). Caregiving and institutionalization: Perceptions of family conflict and socioemotional support. *International Aging and Human Development, 49*, 1-25.

Goldfarb, A. I. (1959). Minor maladjustments in the aged. In S. Arieti (Ed.), *American handbook of psychiatry.* New York: Basic Books.

Goffman, E. (1961). *Asylums: Essays on the social situation of mental patients and other inmates.* New York: Doubleday.

Langer, E. J. (1989). *Mindfulness.* New York: Addison-Wesley.

Langer, E., & Rodin, J. (1976). The effects of choice and enhanced personal responsibility for the aged: A field experiment in an institutional setting. *Journal of Personality and Social Psychology, 34*, 191-198.

Lieberman, M. A., & Tobin, S. S. (1983). *The experience of old age: Stress, coping and survival.* New York: Basic Books.

Libow, L. S. (1982). Geriatric medicine and the nursing home: A mechanism for mutual excellence. *The Gerontologist*, 134-141.

Linn, M. W., Gruel, L., & Linn, B. S. (1977). Patient outcome as a measure of quality of nursing home care. *American Journal of Public Health, 67*, 337-344.

Mendelson, M. A. (1974). *Tender loving greed.* New York: Knopf.

Rodin, J., & Langer, E. (1977). Long-term effects of a control-relevant intervention with the institutionalized aged. *Journal of Personality and Social Psychology, 35*, 897-902.

Tellis-Nyak, V., & Tellis-Nyak, M. (1989). Quality of care and the burden of two cultures: When the world of the nurse's aide enters the world of the nursing home. *The Gerontologist, 29*, 307-313.

Tobin, S. S. (Ed.). (1982). *Current gerontology: Long-term care.* Washington, DC: The Gerontology Society of America.

Tobin, S. S. (1995). Fostering family involvement in nursing homes. In G. C. Smith, S. S. Tobin, E. A. Robertson-Tchabo, & P. W. Power (Eds.), *Strengthening aging families: Diversity in practice and policy.* Thousand Oaks, CA: Sage.

Tobin, S. S. (1999). *Preservation of the self in the oldest years with implications for practice.* New York: Springer.

Tobin, S. S., & Lieberman, M. A. (1976). *Last home for the aged: Critical implications of institutionalization.* San Francisco: Jossey-Bass.

Vladeck, B. C. (1980). *Unloving care: The nursing home tragedy.* New York: Basic Books.

Weissert, W. G. (1985). Estimating the long-term care population: Prevalence rates and selected characteristics. *Health Care Financing Review, 6,* 83-91.

Leading Culture Change
in Long-Term Care:
A Map for the Road Ahead

Judah L. Ronch

SUMMARY. Leaders of culture change in long-term care should have a plan to guide the entire process before they begin. This optimizes the human and financial resources devoted to ongoing culture change programs and prevents the serious mistakes that are usually visual with hindsight. An eight stage process for creating major change is presented as a basis of mapping culture change programs in long-term care that aspire to be humanistic in nature and involve all stakeholder groups in ongoing, empowering activity. *[Article copies available for a fee from The Haworth Document Delivery Service: 1-800-HAWORTH. E-mail address: <docdelivery@haworthpress.com> Website: <http://www.HaworthPress.com> © 2003 by The Haworth Press, Inc. All rights reserved.]*

KEYWORDS. Culture change, Kotter, planning, nursing home, humanistic care

Judah L. Ronch, PhD, is Executive Clinical Director of LifeSpan DevelopMental Systems, Poughkeepsie, NY and writes about, does research on and consults to long-term care organizations about culture change.

Address correspondence to: Judah L. Ronch, PhD, LifeSpan DevelopMental System, 7 Fox Street, Suite 103, Poughkeepsie, NY 12601 (E-mail: jronch@aol.com).

[Haworth co-indexing entry note]: "Leading Culture Change in Long-Term Care: A Map for the Road Ahead." Ronch, Judah L. Co-published simultaneously in *Journal of Social Work in Long-Term Care* (The Haworth Social Work Practice Press, an imprint of The Haworth Press, Inc.) Vol. 2, No. 1/2, 2003, pp. 65-80; and: *Culture Change in Long-Term Care* (ed: Audrey S. Weiner, and Judah L. Ronch) The Haworth Social Work Practice Press, an imprint of The Haworth Press, Inc., 2003, pp. 65-80. Single or multiple copies of this article are available for a fee from The Haworth Document Delivery Service [1-800-HAWORTH, 9:00 a.m. - 5:00 p.m. (EST). E-mail address: docdelivery@haworthpress.com].

10.1300/J181v2n01_05

INTRODUCTION

As one considers culture change in a long-term care setting, it is important to think about the core values that will define the ideal culture of the future. Equally critical, however, is the question of how the facility will proceed from the culture of today toward the vision of the future that embodies those values. Every social institution has a culture that is always evolving. The primary task of culture change agents is therefore to assume responsibility for identifying and managing the particular direction in which the culture will move. The change leader(s) must also simultaneously lead the process that defines and articulates the values of the new culture so that people's behavior, especially their relationships, will reflect and support the desired cultural values. In the case of the long-term care setting, that leadership involves envisioning how care processes will change for the better in the future.

The growing number of visionary models that have invigorated efforts at long-term care reform, such as the ones included in this volume, all share a desire to improve the quality of life for residents and staff of long-term care institutions by doing nothing less than changing the nature of the relationships in them. This change is truly radical; it aims to redefine the nature of how people interact in these communities from a procedure-based culture to a process-based one. Since people experience how much they are valued according to the ways others treat them, a culture change program directed at improving "quality of life" has a chance of success only if the relationships people have with each other in nursing homes are rooted in an ethic that values each participant as an equal (Buber, 1970). Such a culture will have at the moral core of its care practices the fundamental importance of processes rather than procedures.

The role of leading culture change is quite complex and requires that the leaders go beyond merely voicing the need for change or publicly articulating the particular values that they wish to see realized in the changed culture. The leader of culture change must envision and plan for the entire process of change so that it is global, comprehensive and sustainable. As organizational culture is always changing, so the process of qualitative change may have an identifiable kickoff ceremony but should also have no conclusion. Leaders of culture change in a long-term care setting should therefore prepare for an ongoing and complex process with an open-ended series of stages characterized by personal and organizational growth.

No matter which model of culture change a facility selects or develops, a map to guide the process of change is essential. Absent a map for change, or by using a "borrowed" one that guided the "model" facility, a long-term care institution seeking lasting culture change is vulnerable to many unforeseen problems that are likely to thwart both the momentum and direction of the change process. For a myriad of reasons one is at risk of discovering much too far down the road that the external model which looked attractive initially lacks a truly good fit for a facility. One might, alternatively, decide to proceed without any map and try to evolve the altered culture organically. This approach is vulnerable to many institutional and personal resistances that will skew or confuse the chosen direction for change and thereby compromising the desired system of values expected to be at the heart of the new culture. Going forward without a plan also makes sustaining the cultural evolution especially difficult because "any road you take will look good if you have no idea where you are going." This strategy makes it likely that stakeholder enthusiasm for change will collapse as participants become confused and demoralized after yet another in a series of false starts (the "flavor of the month" phenomenon).

The strategy of those who set out to change institutional culture without a plan is reflected in the words of former NY Yankee great (and Everyman's philosopher) Yogi Berra, who advised: "When you come to a fork in the road, take it." Among the many deterrents to change that befall travelers who take Yogi's advice is that they experience (again a Yogi-ism) "Déjà vu all over again" when they repeatedly encounter the same obstacles on their endless and demoralizing journey toward that genuinely desired but elusive goal called culture change.

Despite the many problems and frustrations to be encountered in leading culture change, this volume presumes that many readers will be encouraged to take risks inspired by vision and passion for meaningful change toward a more humanistic community of care. This discussion provides one map to guide facilities as they attempt to create a culture of care where "quality of life" and "quality of care" (Kane, 2001) have optimal clinical, fiscal, and regulatory synergy.

A PLAN FOR CHANGE

At the risk of elaborating on the obvious, it bears repeating that an organization seeking to change its culture needs a plan to guide its activities. A plan for change is necessary if for no other reason that changing institutional culture is a costly process that taps into scarce organizational resources of time, energy, personnel, good will and money. Because of that, and the fluid business environment of the 1980s and '90s, the topic of culture change has received a great deal of attention in the business world. Perhaps surprising is the fact that the pivotal issues that affect culture change in the corporate world echo those that hold the key to meaningful changes in the culture of health care. Among the most easily understood and best organized discussions of leading change in corporate culture is *Leading Change* (Kotter, 1996). It provides a practical and intuitively sensible map, i.e., the "how," to guide an organization's efforts in achieving the "what" reflected in the thinking of leading advocates for long-term care change (see for example Goffman, 1961; Vladek, 1980; Bowker, 1982; Kane, 1996; Lustbader, 1991, 2001; Thomas, 1994, 1999; Barkan, 1999; Fagan, Williams and Burger, 1997; Stone, 2000).

Given that hindsight is more acute than foresight, Kotter's (1996) plan for leading change provides a way to avoid the common and costly mistakes that emerge with blinding clarity after the fact. These are:

- Allowing too much complacency
- Failing to create a sufficiently powerful guiding coalition
- Underestimating the power of vision
- Undercommunicating the vision by a factor of 10 (or 100, or even 1,000)
- Permitting obstacles to block the new vision
- Failing to create short-term wins
- Declaring victory too soon
- Neglecting to anchor changes firmly in the corporate culture

Knowing the entire plan for organizational change in advance is particularly important in preventing these errors, says Kotter, because there are few charismatic leaders in any endeavor who can initiate and successfully carry out the process of culture change simply by force of personality and uncommon leadership skills. His eight-step plan for leading change is designed to prevent the most common errors that doom so many well-intentioned organizational change efforts.

Given the scarcity of charismatic change leaders in nursing homes who can carry the entire effort single-handedly, most culture change will result from a lengthy process of collaboration between stakeholder teams that include staff, residents, family members, administrators, the community and, ultimately, regulators. Culture change is difficult to achieve quickly even when all stakeholder groups and resources are aligned with a shared vision of what the new culture will look like. A significant but often overlooked reality that may slow the pace of culture change is that there are actually many "cultures" at work within an institution (staff, unions, families, administration, regulators). These variables create the multiple levels of experience that are the contexts for relationships and values assumptions that guide each individual's behavior as they work and interact with each other. Culture change is, therefore, a process that must recognize and factor in the multiple sources of cultural influence at work in the environment and the friction points between each. As they come into contact, they are likely to create disharmony (see Levine, this volume) and resistance to change in the affected individuals until and unless each level of the multi-cultural agenda is aired and integrated into the vision of an enhanced, mutually humanizing institutional culture.

The leader's job is to begin the process, and select colleagues with whom to develop a plan for leading the organization toward a new culture that fully realizes the values at the heart of the organization's mission. Because this typically cannot be done single-handedly, a team (see below) of committed individuals is needed who want culture change so much that they are prepared to contribute the extra time and effort needed to make it happen. The team, and ultimately the entire workforce, will initially experience a transition toward greater empowerment as they assume responsibility for culture change.

Regardless of which model a facility chooses to be the guiding example for the culture change effort, the issue of "empowerment" *will be a sine qua non* of humanistic values system. Leadership cannot unilaterally empower people without perpetuating the same hierarchic culture that they are seeking to change by developing a humanistic setting. It is important to emphasize that the processes that comprise Kotter's (1996) model create the conditions whereby all stakeholders are empowered by the very nature of their experience. Because they are instrumental in the process of change, and because the new culture is a visible outcome of their work and creativity, they are empowered. In other words, *empowered people are one of the significant outcomes of culture change* that aims for increased humanization. Empowerment is not something that can be bestowed on people during the culture change. Leaders who desire a more empowered citizenry have the responsibility to create the conditions that encourage and reward empowered participation by all the inhabitants of the community as they actualize their strengths and talents in service of the vision to be achieved.

THE EIGHT STEPS OF CREATING MAJOR CULTURE CHANGE

Kotter's Eight-Step process of creating major change (Kotter, 1996), summarized in Figure 1, provide the necessary building blocks for creating major change. (Space limitations preclude a more detailed discussion of Kotter's model, but it is highly recommended that leaders consult it prior to launching any culture change program.) Each of these steps takes time, and Kotter remarks that the major reason that major culture change fails is that leaders don't allow sufficient time to achieve each step before moving on to the next one. Given the institutional inertia, scarcity of resources and how entrenched the prevailing (and arguably obsolete) medical model is in contemporary long-term

FIGURE 1. The Eight-Stage Process of Creating Major Change

1.	Establishing a sense of urgency
2.	Creating the guiding coalition
3.	Developing a vision and strategy
4.	Communicating the change vision
5.	Empowering broad-based action
6.	Generating short-term wins
7.	Consolidating gains and producing more change
8.	Anchoring new approaches in the culture

care institutions, leading change toward a more humanistic care culture will definitely require patience, fortitude, and, as this article urges, a plan.

This (or any other plan) should be the centerpiece of the planning process and used as the "official map" of the leadership team. The initial orientation of the leadership team to the culture change program should include a thorough review of the Eight Steps and the goals of each step should be reviewed prior to commencing work on it and at the end of activities at each one. A thorough review of goals accomplished at each step will also provide a common focus and measures of achievement for the team and stakeholders.

Step 1. Establishing a Sense of Urgency

The energy for a successful culture change program must emanate from the institutional leadership that chose to initiate the process. Stakeholders will be less likely to rally around a culture change program if the leader's passion for change is not clearly and repeatedly in evidence. One of the elements of culture change which is the most difficult to sustain is the energy that drives the process and attracts partisans to the cause of organizational change in the face of the unknown.

If the institutional leadership fails to communicate the intensity of its passion for change to the leaders of the change process, an adequate *sense of urgency* will be missing. So, for example in one facility, the administrator perceived a gap between the institution's mission and the quality of life that all stakeholders experienced on an everyday basis which made her uncomfortable enough to recruit a team of managers whom she invited to lead culture change with her. Until that administrator spoke passionately about how she felt, the managers were reluctant to agree publicly that culture change was necessary.

Establishing and clearly communicating a sense of urgency encourages people to think in new ways and provides a countervailing force to peoples' natural tendency to return to their comfort zones as the status quo is upset during culture change. No matter how dedicated people say they are to the *idea* of culture change, their commitment will undergo repeated tests as the *process* of culture change unfolds. In nursing homes, comfort zones are influenced by power, relationships, the institutional "territory" people control, and the formal and informal influence various stakeholders exert. Resistance to change may intensify when one adds to the process all the other organizational dynamics that perpetuated the old culture and its values, procedures and practices that people are reluctant to abandon. From this perspective, it is possible to see that resistance to change is not always oppositionalism and that "resistors" may have (unrecognized) competing commitments, such as between their true commitment to change and their fear of loss of power and influence (Kegan and Lahey, 2001). Kotter (1996) predicts that most everyone, even the most outspoken and dedicated culture change advocate, may at some point experience anxiety about how change really might affect them and do something to return to the familiar comfort and safety of the old ways.

It is the sense of urgency that motivates the extra effort and willingness to take the risks inherent in culture change and acts as a countervailing force when people feel the need to seek the safety of old, familiar ways. They have to be reminded that to avoid the sacrifices involved in creating change, i.e., to go back to the ways of old, is to court danger. The temporary professional and personal discomfort that accompany culture change must come to be seen as preferable to the chronic discomfort of organizational stasis and, worse yet, loss of business and reputation.

The leader's job is to keep the sense of urgency ever-present without creating a sense of panic. There are a number of ways to raise the urgency level. Among these are to:

- create a sense of crisis by avoiding the usual quick fixes applied to significant problems, or by identifying market forces or regulations that dictate culture change;
- setting high customer satisfaction targets that can't be reached by the usual approaches to care;
- mandating regular meetings between staff and dissatisfied residents, families and other stakeholders;
- using consultants to "deliver the bad news" and facilitate more honest dialogue at management meetings;
- eliminating the "happy talk" (only accentuating the positive to avoid dealing with fundamental problems) and communicating openly about what is creating the sense of urgency in the organization's senior leader(s);

- bombarding employees with information about future opportunities in the field and the organization's inability to capitalize on these, and;
- identifying the gap between peoples' passion for their work and their current satisfaction with their own and the institution's performance levels.

The last option is the one used as the culture change process went forward in the facility mentioned earlier in this section. By initiating the culture change process with a series of stakeholder focus groups, the administrator found that staff and residents shared her view that the fit between care and mission really needed improvement. This process, and the opinions about how much the care at the facility needed to become more sensitive to residents' expressed needs, were strong motivators for change. Once stakeholders found that they shared similar opinions about the need for changes in the culture, the internal momentum for culture change was found.

Step 2. Creating the Guiding Coalition

Since most nursing homes lack a larger than life, extremely charismatic individual whose entire responsibility is to lead culture change, and because culture change needs broad-based stakeholder support to succeed, it is necessary to form a coalition of people with the (formal and informal) power and influence sufficient to lead change. This *guiding coalition* should include residents, members of the Board of Directors and/or trustees, staff at all levels inclusive of representatives of any unions in the facility, and family members. They must all have the titles, expertise, reputations, relationships and capacity for leadership that will inform and lead the process of change. Their work as team members must unambiguously illustrate those relationships desired in the new culture; they must also have real power to lead change. That is, to be seen as the real leaders of change by the other stakeholders they must have the credibility and power needed to make change.

Organizations desirous of culture change have to make a serious commitment to teaching the kind of teamwork skills and interpersonal relationships that teams will have to manifest in the future. This is an especially critical step for culture change in nursing homes if they are to move beyond the hierarchic, procedure driven communication style currently in place that is at the heart of the medical model governing institutional care. These teams will differ from the traditional care planning, performance improvement and similar teams that do the "think work" in traditional nursing home culture as regards both process and leadership. These members will all have equal status and responsibility for planning and leading change without regard to the political clout or social status of their normal work assignment. So the opinions of the nursing assistant and dietary aide on the committee, for example, will be heard with the same respect and credibility as is usually given to the licensed personnel who are traditionally looked to for answers due to their perceived "greater expertise" in the technical matters of health care. Likewise, any member of the guiding coalition with the skills and passion for change who the other coalition members regard as a natural leader can function as one no matter their job title or rank in the organization.

The guiding coalition will need time to practice the new ways of being actual teammates and accepting the mantle of leadership that is at variance with the old culture. It takes a good deal of time and practice to unlearn the many old habits they were taught when they were originally trained to be "good employees" in the old culture. When they are competent in the new model of teamwork, they will become a visible lesson for other stakeholders to make use of as they learn the nature of what teamwork will be in the new culture.

A telling example of how difficult it can be to make the transition to "new culture" teamwork in a nursing home happened at a meeting of a culture change leadership committee that had been at work for almost three years. They identified as one of their biggest barriers toward moving ahead with the change agenda their lack of certainty that they had "permission from the CEO" to make more than token changes in the facility culture. Their hesitancy appeared to arise primarily from their not having rid themselves of the hierarchic, "top-down" ways of the old culture in how they saw the committee's role and operational mandates, and their having failed to appreciate the trust placed in them by the CEO. Although the CEO had supported their activity and suggestions for changes in many aspects of institution's culture over the past years, many of the leadership team members described themselves as feeling not adequately empowered to change the culture. This is a good example of how empowerment must be felt by change leaders if they are to work effectively with senior leaders to carry out a culture change program.

Building a guiding coalition for change involves three essential steps: finding the right people with high influence, strong position power, broad expertise and high credibility with leadership and management skills; creating trust through planned team-building events (formal and informal opportunities to participate in joint activities), and; developing a common goal that is sensible to the head and appealing to the heart. Only teams with the right combination of power, trust and an abundance of needed information have a chance to succeed. Coalition members should not be individuals with personnel problems that you could ignore in the old culture. "Old problems" like these will impede culture change unless it is determined that their problems in the old culture were the result of their having embodied the values of the new culture before "its time."

Step 3. Developing a Vision and Strategy

This step involves creating a vision to help direct the change effort and developing strategies to achieve that vision. The guiding coalition must maintain its focus on what it wants to realize in the new culture despite the current barriers to change in the present. The resulting creative tension (Senge, 1995) will motivate the guiding coalition and ultimately other stakeholders to generate creative solutions to the problems encountered along the road of culture change. A good vision enables change efforts to overcome the natural resistance mentioned in Step 1 by being hopeful and motivating peoples' aspirations to be at their best (Eron and Lund, 1996), and juxtaposes the sacrifices needed with benefits to be gained by making them. A good vision is especially valuable when attempting to engage workers with fewer resources (e.g., pay, power, prestige) who will be asked to learn new skills and behaviors. The vision helps these staff by pointing out what benefits and personal satisfactions they will gain as a result of culture change and contrasts how these are superior to those available at present if no change takes place (Kotter, 1996).

A compelling vision statement will not emerge from one meeting. Good ones evolve over time as various stakeholders work on refashioning it as the realities of culture change become evident and inform the collective vision. A vision is an "imaginable image of the future" that is "desirable, feasible, focused, flexible, and is conveyable in five minutes or less" (Kotter, 1996, p. 81). Visions add clarity, increase enthusiasm, enhance communication and strengthen commitment (Senge, 1995), and because they do all those things they create a virtuous cycle of reinforcement that strengthens the culture change program. A vision statement successfully used to inspire current culture change programs at one New York facility says:

> St. Cabrini Nursing Home/Cabrini Center for Nursing and Rehabilitation will (each) be a community of residents and employees who live and work together in an atmosphere of respect and love, allowing members of the community to reach their greatest potential and experience joy. (see Nichols, this volume)

Northeast Health in Troy, NY has a clear vision statement that guides its current activities and future plans: "To provide a high-quality, accessible continuum of healthcare, supportive housing and community services" (*www.nehealth.com*).

Step 4. Communicating the Change Vision

A successful culture change process will involve planning an ongoing and multifaceted strategy to communicate the new vision. This effectively means planning an internal public relations strategy (in addition to an external one) as part of the culture change process. One "kickoff" event, general staff meeting or a series of festive events at which the culture change program is presented to stakeholders is insufficient by itself to keep the change vision in the forefront for as long as it takes to be fully understood. For the same reason, there should be no ceremony to mark the end of the culture change program since it must be ongoing if it is to be effective.

Kotter (1996) recommends using a combination of means to communicate the vision, such as meetings *not* about culture change per se, newsletters, posters, media releases, memos, formal and informal interaction, and leadership by example. Perhaps the most effective way to communicate the vision is to have the guiding coalition model the behavior expected of people in the new culture. This method of communicating the vision is especially useful since people are most apt to internalize cultural rules of behavior when they are immersed in them and repeatedly observe them at work in the context of everyday interactions. This is the way we initially learn the culture of the families in which we grew up and remains the easiest, most direct mode of demonstrating how "it is done here."

Effective communication of the vision is improved if the mission is stated simply and free of jargon, is reinforced by metaphor, analogy and especially when examples are publicly recognized and celebrated. The communication with the greatest impact, however, is when the vision is modeled by the behavior of the VIPs of the institution. If leadership by example is absent, the change vision will be lost in the confusion about what is really meant. For example, if the leadership of a culture change program has at the heart of its vision statement that staff and residents will reach their fullest potential as people but rejects their input about how policies and procedures could be changed to advance the new culture (see Step 7, below), the vision will become ineffective.

Step 5. Empowering Broad-Based Action

Bearing in mind that you cannot truly empower people, this step targets the obstacles that prevented people from attaining their own empowerment in the old culture. This step is the one most likely to be the occasion when culture change leaders confront their own anxieties about changing systems or organizational structures which they hold dear but that do not support the change vision.

Key among the structures that will need attention for change in the nursing home are the policy and procedure manuals, staffing patterns, and other ways of doing things that are hallmarks of the traditional culture, those that discourage risk-taking and trying non-traditional ideas, activities and actions. One measure of how empowered people have become because of the culture change program will be how comfortable they are with risk-taking and how creative their suggestions are for improving the practice of care in the facility.

Huy (2001) suggests that middle managers can be key players in radical culture change. Far from being obsolete in a new culture, they can be real assets as leaders, mentors and models. Look for those who are positive critics (they suggest alternate solutions rather than just saying that an idea won't work), people with informal power, i.e., the ones who lead "communities of practice" (Wenger, 1998), individuals who have adapted well to major change at work or in their personal lives, and people with emotional intelligence (Goleman, 1995) who can talk about their feelings and respond supportively to the feelings of those around them. The last trait is a most valuable one since change is stressful. The more emotional intelligence an organization's managers have, the easier it will be to ride out the change. Look also for early volunteers and "positive deviants" (Sternin and Choo, 2000), stakeholders who succeed by engaging environmental resources that the majority does not see or views as not useful.

The ability to identify and engage these resources from among the organization's stakeholders will influence the success your leadership has in identifying those people who can be trusted to take broad-based action in the service of the culture change. It is always preferable to find the potential change agents deep within your organization, develop their skills, and to give them the platform and resources to stimulate the actions that eliminate the obstacles to change.

Step 6. Generating Short-Term Wins

The guiding coalition should plan in advance how the organization will celebrate visible improvements in performance, or "wins," and create a repertoire of celebratory events to be an intrinsic part of the culture change process. Recognizing and rewarding those who made the wins possible maintains attention on how achievements are made which demonstrate the values of the new culture. Each of the two Cabrini facilities, whose vision statement was provided above, conducts a monthly "Values in Action" award ceremony that recognizes special instances of staff behavior that personify their mission and values in caring for residents. They have also introduced a "mission moments" award to celebrate the spontaneous "little things" (like giving the resident a choice of which soap to use during a bath) that staff do to make residents feel special as they provide routine care.

Short-term wins are visible, unambiguous and clearly related to the culture change effort. Recognizing and celebrating short-term wins require advance planning and a system of rewards that people can look forward to as a way of having their creativity honored and for their having grasped what the business of culture change is about. A facility will reach the "tipping point" (Gladwell, 2000; see review in this volume) in culture change more readily if there is a plan to generate and recognize wins and the people who made them happen.

Step 7. Consolidating Gains and Producing More Change

The foundation of this stage consists of all the accomplishments of the previous six stages that have brought visible change to the institutional culture. With visible accomplishments already in place, this stage therefore provides an opportunity to use the increased credibility the change leadership has achieved thus far. The work of earlier stages to change all the systems (policies, procedures, staffing patterns, use of physical space and material resources, for example) should by now fit the vision of the new culture. The organization should have hired and promoted people who can implement the desired culture change, and have created a steadily developing cadre of indigenous staff who are enthusiastic about the changes in the culture of care.

If the organization has reached this stage and finds that the number of culture change leaders has diminished, or that the change leaders are still talking to the same group that were around the table the day the program began, the process has probably gone ahead too rapidly; an honest internal appraisal must follow. By this point in the change process, there should be an ongoing procedure to reinvigorate the change process with new projects, new change agents, and a host of innovative applications of the new culture to facility life. Contrary to popular myth, one does not necessarily have to have flattened the organization by this stage to be on the right track (see discussion of the role of middle managers in Step 5, above). There should however be a clear idea of which middle managers are pivotal to success. "Top down" and "bottom up" change vectors should be visible.

Step 8. Anchoring New Approaches in the New Culture

At this final step, there should be a perception among all stakeholders that better outcomes for residents, staff and families have been achieved, and data to support this perception. Staff activity should be more productive, there should be better and broader based leadership, and management should be more effective. All policies and procedures, as pertain to clinical care and human resources functions, should be clearly connected to organizational success. For example, job descriptions, employee orientation, in-service education, and performance evaluations should by now all reflect the values of the new culture, specify how they are manifested in desired behavior (toward residents, families and to each other) in the setting, and how well staff have performed their roles *vis à vis* the expectations of the new culture.

It is vitally important that the care practices and staff evaluations tie together by using the same language or the culture change process will lose momentum and believability from a lack of recognition and reward for the desired behaviors. Success of the facility should be framed in terms how well it has fulfilled its mission as a result of the new culture, and reflect how staff helped in this achievement. The cultural priorities of the institution need to be reflected in the metrics used to evaluate staff, management and administration (Katzenbach, 2000). A planned program of staff development and resident and family life education may be a beneficial way to teach the requisite skills for living well in the new culture.

Finally, a plan to ensure leadership development and succession must be a part of the culture change program. Though this point may appear to be too remote from the starting point, the legacy of change leadership will fade quickly if there is no culturally competent, visionary leadership trained to perpetuate the new ways. Culture change in nursing homes confronts daily an overwhelming series of historical and inertial obstacles that can daunt even the most committed change agent. True culture change may take more years than any one leader is able to devote to an institution, and meaningful change has to survive changes in institutional leadership.

CONCLUSION

In essence, the message is "know what lies ahead before you start out." As culture change becomes a more frequent activity in long-term care, the models we create will surely become more diverse and customized for the realities of each facility. It is difficult to import "best practices" as a whole without importing the "best practitioners" (the staff) as well if you wish to achieve the same results (Brown and Duguid, 2000). Therefore, it seems likely that culture change programs will draw inspiration from the successful stories told by sister institutions, but each will have a unique identity despite common inspiration. Each setting must choose its own path, but must know where it wants to go. Remember, if you don't know where you're going, any road looks good.

REFERENCES

Barkan, B. (1999). *Pioneering efforts in the nursing home reform movement.* Presented at the annual meeting of the American Society on Aging, Orlando, Florida.

Brown, J.S., and Duguid, P. (2000). *The social life of information.* Boston: Harvard Business School Press.

Bowker, L. (1982). *Humanizing institutions for the aging.* Lexington, MA: Lexington Books.

Eron, J., and Lund, T. (1996). *Narrative solutions in brief therapy.* New York: The Guilford Press.

Buber, M. (1970). *I and thou.* New York: Charles Scribner and Sons.

Fagan, R., Williams, C. and Burger, S. (1997). *Meeting of the pioneers in nursing home culture change: Final Report.* Lifespan of Greater Rochester.

Gladwell, M. (2000). *The tipping point: How little things make a big difference.* Boston: Little, Brown and Co.

Goffman, E. (1961). *Assylums: Essays on the social situation of mental patients and other inmates.* Garden City: Anchor Books.

Goleman, D. (1995). *Emotional intelligence.* New York: Bantam Books.

Huy, Q.N. (2001). In praise of middle managers. *Harvard Business Review,* September; 72-79.

Kane, E. (1996). Transforming care institutions for the frail elderly: Out of one there shall be m of any. *Generations,* 19; 4.

Kane, R. (2001). Long-term care and a good quality of life: Bringing them closer together. *The Gerontologist, 41,* 3, 293-304.

Katzenbzch, J. (2000). *Peak performance: Aligning the hearts and minds of your employees.* Cambridge: Harvard Business School Press.

Kegan, R. and Lahey, L. (2001). The real reason people won't change. *Harvard Business Review,* November; 85-92.

Kotter, J. (1996). *Leading change.* Cambridge: Harvard University Press.

Levine, C. (2003). Family caregivers, health care professionals and policy makers: The diverse cultures of long-term care. *Journal of Social Work in Long-Term Care, 2*(1/2), p. 111-123.

Lustbader, W. (1991). *Counting on kindness: The dilemmas of dependency.* New York: The Free Press.

Lustbader, W. (2001). The Pioneer challenge: A radical change in the culture of nursing homes. In L. Noelker and Harel, Z. (Ed.) *Linking quality of long-term care and quality of life.* New York: Springer Publishing Company; 185-203.

Senge, P. (1995). *The fifth discipline: The art and practice of the learning organization.* New York: Currency Doubleday.

Sternin, J. and Choo, R. (2000). The power of positive deviancy. *Harvard Business Review,* January-February; p.14-15.

Stone, R. (2000). *Long-term care for the elderly with disabilities: Current policy, emerging trends, and implications for the twenty-first century.* New York: Millbank Memorial Fund.

Thomas, W. (1994). *The Eden Alternative: Nature, hope and nursing homes.* Columbia, MO: University of Missouri.

Thomas, W. (1999). *The Eden Alternative handbook: The art of building human habitats.* Summer Hill Company.

Vladek, B. (1980). *Unloving care: The nursing home tragedy.* New York: Basic Books.

Wenger, E. (1998). *Communities of practice.* New York: Cambridge University Press.

Achieving Organizational Change
Within the Context of Cultural Competence

Laura Martin
Bette R. Bonder

SUMMARY. Cultural competence has become more topical as the United States has become more diverse. Conceptualizing culture as constantly emerging in interaction, practitioners can enhance their skills through an inquiry-centered approach to clients. Using ethnographic inquiry, and building skills as culture brokers, social workers can work toward mutual cultural accommodation. This process of mutual adaptation, based on carefully obtained and interpreted information about the other's vantage, has the potential to enhance client outcomes and encourage organizational change based on mutual respect. *[Article copies available for a fee from The Haworth Document Delivery Service: 1-800-HAWORTH. E-mail address: <docdelivery@haworthpress.com> Website: <http://www.HaworthPress.com> © 2003 by The Haworth Press, Inc. All rights reserved.]*

KEYWORDS. Culture broker, diversity, ethnography

Laura Martin, PhD, is Associate Dean of Arts and Sciences and Professor of Anthropology, Modern Languages, and Health Sciences at Cleveland State University.

Bette R. Bonder, PhD, OTR/L, FAOTA, is Professor of Health Sciences and Psychology and Interim Chair, Health Sciences, at Cleveland State University.

Address correspondence to: Laura Martin, PhD, Cleveland State University, 2121 Euclid Avenue, Cleveland OH 44115-2214 (E-mail: l.martin@csuohio.edu).

[Haworth co-indexing entry note]: "Achieving Organizational Change Within the Context of Cultural Competence." Martin, Laura, and Bette R. Bonder. Co-published simultaneously in *Journal of Social Work in Long-Term Care* (The Haworth Social Work Practice Press, an imprint of The Haworth Press, Inc.) Vol. 2, No. 1/2, 2003, pp. 81-94; and: *Culture Change in Long-Term Care* (ed: Audrey S. Weiner, and Judah L. Ronch) The Haworth Social Work Practice Press, an imprint of The Haworth Press, Inc., 2003, pp. 81-94. Single or multiple copies of this article are available for a fee from The Haworth Document Delivery Service [1-800-HAWORTH, 9:00 a.m. - 5:00 p.m. (EST). E-mail address: docdelivery@haworthpress.com].

10.1300/J181v2n01_06

INTRODUCTION

As the United States becomes more culturally diverse, integrating cultural skills throughout practitioner organizations and workplaces becomes a more urgent concern (New Waves, 1993; Sleek, 1998). In long-term care settings, both clients and staff represent an increasingly wide array of ethnic and racial groups, requiring thoughtful assessment of the impact of these identities on programmatic decisions and care for individuals. However, the nature of cultural factors in care settings goes well beyond the usually identified features of ethnicity, religion, or language to include such sources of identification as profession, age cohort, sexual orientation, and so on. The cultural dimensions of situations of care inevitably also include even the professional and organizational cultures by which practitioners themselves self-identify (Hong et al., 2000). "Sensitivity" to cultural factors in such settings as nursing homes, home health, and community agencies affects not only direct care of clients, but also the nature of interdisciplinary interaction among team members and the manner in which organizational culture can be modified. Planned cultural change, as is contemplated by many health care institutions, requires for its success a clear sense of the existing cultural context. It also requires the sensitive anticipation of the inevitable clash of values that occur as a result of the dynamic and individual nature of culture change and an appreciation for the reality that, at any individual moment in the process of change, old values and new ones will co-exist and produce conflict. Our approach to these issues, we believe, offers a framework for conceptualizing cultural competence that can guide staff in managing institutional culture change programs. It provides the skills necessary to observe carefully and manage thoughtfully the issues that arise as institutional change occurs.

This essay develops a theoretical perspective on culture, cultural competence, and culture change that takes into account the individual, dynamic, and multilayered nature of culture. Our approach emphasizes the emergent quality of culture and identity as revealed in specific interactions, an understanding of culture that we term *culture emergent* (Bonder, Martin & Miracle, 2001; Bonder, Martin & Miracle, 2002). Using this conceptualization as our foundation, we have identified (1) a methodology based on *ethnographic inquiry* from which to extract the skills necessary for dealing with cultural factors in health care settings; (2) a perception of practitioners as *culture brokers*, or actors for change; and (3) a process that we call *mutual cultural accommodation* that can be mobilized to effect organizational culture change to infuse respect for individual and cultural factors throughout organizations. In what follows, we take up each of these considerations in turn.

DEFINING CULTURE

Definitions of culture are many and varied (cf., Brown, 1998; Hahn, 1995; Loveland, 1999). In pragmatic terms in practice, culture can best be thought of as a creative and dynamic process centered on the individual, rather than as a static mental model "shared" with or coterminous with a particular group. Culture is acquired through observation, life experiences, and direct instruction from a variety of sources. Multiple cultural influences are experienced by each individual in a complex society such as the United States. However, culture is only one aspect of an individual's identity, which also includes aspects of biology and personality, intertwined into a complex and multifaceted whole. Even selection of a health care profession has been shown to be related to personality factors (Spokane, 1992).

Cultural identity and other manifestations of culture emerge largely through discourse among individuals in a group, expressed in moment-by-moment interactions (cf., Urban, 1991). In each interaction, individuals select elements of their complex identities for display and attend to specific elements displayed by others. Most individuals, most of the time, interact primarily with people who share many of their values, experiences, and attributes. In this way, they jointly create groups with cultural similarities, and culture is thus transformed into a group phenomenon, emerging from many small unplanned sequences of behavior that converge to form large-scale patterns that separate one group from another. These self-defining groups may then create stated or unstated positions on the relationships of group members to the larger world and on the issues or problems that threaten or confront the group. These positions, or *worldviews*, reflect widely held common values about persons, groups, and institutions different from their own.

At the same time, in each interaction, along with their individuality and these culturally-grounded elements, participants also bring with them an immediately personal perspective–a particular *vantage* (c.f., Hill & MacLaurey, 1995). In our usage, vantage reflects a number of specific elements in the interactional moment, from the physical setting of the interaction itself to the mental assumptions, immediate interests, and focus of each participant. When we visit a client's home, for example, our vantage may cause us to attend only to some features of the environment, partly based on what we expect to see in a "normal" home and partly based on the purpose of our visit. We have witnessed many examples of students in unfamiliar household surroundings who simply fail to perceive certain crucial features, such as household shrines or evidences of traditional food-making.

All participants in an interaction are operating within their individual vantage, some aspects of which are be conditioned by cultural expectations. At the same time, they are operating within the larger contexts of the various cultural groups to which they belong or with which they interact. For example, they may be identified by profession or client class, may belong to a variety of organizations and communities, and may reflect personal and group histories of prior interaction. An important element in the organization of health care professions is the enculturation of students as professionals. Faculty teach not only content, but attitudes and modes of behavior that fit specific professional cultural expectations–everything from beliefs about health and healing to values about appropriate professional dress. Similarly, when staff are newly hired to work in particular agencies, the cultural values of the agency are part of the orientation, both formal and informal. Standards for inter-professional communication, even who eats in the lunchroom, are conveyed in the first few weeks of work in a new setting. Each emerging or instructing professional has his or her own cultural affiliation and personality, but each also interacts in ways that reflect commonly agreed upon standards for the display of professional affiliation and values. Therefore, any interaction is in some sense a cross-cultural interaction and will proceed more successfully if its participants have an awareness of the possible cultural factors that may influence it, or are at least alert to the possibility that such factors may exist.

Every individual, while able to exercise rather wide freedom in the degree of adaptation she or he exhibits in novel situations, usually acts more or less unconsciously from the basis of deeply held values and beliefs about the world that come largely from the cultural background within which early training and experience are developed. Everyone–not just "diverse" people or "minorities"–has culture. Everyone is a cultural actor, including practitioners and providers in interaction with clients or patients. Everyone responds both to personal factors as well as to cultural ones. Everyone is subject to unconscious expression of underlying assumptions, values, and beliefs about the world. Sometimes, a person may even hold conflicting assumptions, values, and beliefs, thus complicating how he or she interacts.

For example, a woman of Indian descent may subscribe to the cultural value that adult children, particularly daughters, are responsible for care of their aging parents. At the same time, the woman may be a doctorally educated, U.S. born professional who also believes that women have the right to hold challenging, high-level, professional positions. Thus, the woman may be faced with a serious conflict when an elderly parent becomes disabled and the choices for care are either a nursing home or the daughter as a personal care provider. A grasp of the complexity of such factors can contribute both to effective client care and to effective construction of organizational culture so that it responds more productively to cultural difference. These are typically the aspects of health contexts where "cultural competence" is thought to have its importance.

Our use of the term *culture emergent* is intended to capture the complexity of culture in a definition that emphasizes its dynamism and interactivity. The term incorporates both personal and communal components of culture. Further, it conveys the concept that the individual is a cultural actor, with multifaceted attributes that form multiple cultural identities, and with multiple goals that may sometimes conflict. These attributes, identities, and goals are differentially displayed, depending on the immediate circumstances of interaction and the perceived attributes, identities, and goals of the other participants. The focus on emergence–the constant creation and expression of culture by individuals through interaction with other individuals–allows an understanding of culture that more clearly delineates the way in which it is a factor in institutional settings and suggests a method for probing more closely the role of culture in health care interactions.

CULTURAL COMPETENCE

While much has been written about the need for cultural competence or the process for becoming culturally competent, most approaches fall into one of two categories. First, there is the *fact-centered approach* (DiversityRx, 1997), characterized by efforts to learn about specific cultures. What do Asians believe about family? How do Hispanics decide to seek health care? What is the preferred greeting style of African-Americans? This approach provides a starting place for interaction with individuals, but has significant limitations as a serious way to understand cultural patterns. Because labels such as "Hispanic" or "Asian" in and of themselves mask considerable diversity (Mexican-American, Salvadoran, or Puerto Rican? Chinese, Vietnamese, or Japanese?), it is difficult to learn enough facts about the particular group from which a specific individual comes. And even if one could learn facts about the specific group of origin of that individual, that person's life experiences and personality will not be reflected in mere facts or simple generalizations. Consider that an individual who self-identifies as Mexican-American might have arrived in the United States two years ago or two generations ago, might display a generally extroverted or introverted personality style, might come from an impoverished single-parent home or from an affluent extended family. People are not collections of cultural facts, but complex bundles of cultural and individual influences that shape identity.

An equally well-known approach to learning about cultural diversity is the *attitude-centered* one. In this approach the goal is to create a positive mind-set about culture. Practitioners are encouraged to examine their beliefs, to recognize negative stereotypes they may have, and to adopt a more positive outlook about those who appear different. However, research is equivocal about whether attitudes can actually be changed, and, if they can, whether changed attitudes lead to behavior change (Pruegger & Rogers, 1994). Good intentions alone cannot assure that practitioners undertake culturally aware interventions.

We have found that a more helpful and pragmatic approach to cultural competence is one that emphasizes observation and inquiry, that challenges assumptions by focusing on the individual's role in creating and manifesting culture, and that values the reconciliation of the individual and the communal. This inquiry-centered approach does not define specific cultural groups and then try to locate individuals within them. Rather, it inquires of the individual what aspects of his or her cultural influences are being emphasized in a specific setting or situation. The skills and attributes this approach requires are those basic to *ethnography*, a methodology relied upon by field workers in many disciplines and by good cultural observers everywhere. These skills and attributes include curiosity, the capacity to see pattern, the ability to tolerate ambiguity and multiple explanations, and, principally, the ability to ask questions and attend carefully to the answers.

In a nursing home, this inquiry-centered approach would be characterized by the care provider's careful questioning of the client. The provider might begin by asking the client about preferred forms of greeting–first name or last name? handshake or bow?–and notice whether the client engages directly or indirectly with the questions, making eye contact or averting the gaze, eventually following up with questions about the client's life experiences, beliefs, values, and wishes. Knowing the client's self-identified ethnic background provides a starting point for multiple questions about how that ethnicity was enacted for the individual in his or her early life and how those early cultural influences have been altered by subsequent experience. If a provider has learned facts or generalizations relevant to this cultural group, she or he can then compare them against this individual's responses. Thus, a social worker interviewing a client of Asian background would not automatically assume that the cultural value of reticence to reveal personal information characterizes the individual. Instead, the social worker would pose a series of questions, motivated by active and open curiosity, to gain insight into that particular person's attitudes toward self-revelation.

So, for example, the social worker, on meeting the client, might start by introducing himself as he prefers to be addressed, and asking the client how she prefers be addressed. He might observe whether the client exchanges greetings by shaking hands, by bowing, by smiling, or by some other means, and whether or not she looks in his eyes while greeting. He might then explain his purpose to the client, describe the kinds of questions he will be asking and the reasons for those questions, and ask permission to proceed. During the first few questions, he would observe closely to see whether she shows any signs of discomfort with the topic (fidgeting, moving away, altering eye-gaze, for example), and perhaps inquire gently to confirm his observations. He might, for instance, explain the particular relevance of a topic that seems to be sensitive for the client and ask about the client's feelings about answering questions about it. With such explanation, delivered with an empathic demeanor that helps the client realize that he understands that such questions might be uncomfortable, he may be more successful in enlisting the client's assistance. Or, sensing that the client is avoiding his gaze, he might suspend any assumption that this behavior indicates reluctance or an intention to mislead, and change his own gaze patterns to see whether the client becomes more comfortable. A series of such exchanges will give him a sense of her level of comfort with a variety of topics, and with self-disclosure in general.

Cultural competence, in this approach, is intrinsic to the definition of professional competence, rather than an add-on required by especially "diverse" communities. It assumes that every community is diverse, by virtue of the complex interaction of cultural and personal factors. Professional competence in all healing or service professions increasingly involves a client-centered orientation toward helping others (Law, 1998), based on a sound evaluation of the client's context, needs, and goals. Such an evaluation traditionally includes attention to the client's social situation, personal background, community setting, family history, and physical and psychosocial skills and goals. It is entirely consistent with the inquiry-centered approach to cultural competence that is suggested here, and positions cultural competence as a matter of the effective deployment of the skills toward which one is already predisposed by one's professional culture. For example, in a situation where a social worker is helping a family decide about nursing home placement for an elder in the family, the social worker has been educated to recognize that family members may have differing levels of acceptance of the role of informal caregiver, and of the acceptability of having a parent in a nursing home. Our premise is that the social worker can be most helpful if he or she recognizes that some of the family members' attitudes may be based in cultural, as well as personal, factors. Naturally, inquiry into such matters must be accompanied by receptivity to the information obtained and the ability to suspend judgmental reactions while assessing what is in the best interests of the client.

Generally, exposure to human variation, if non-threatening, evokes the humanizing responses of curiosity, caring, and attention. Since these attributes are always features of good care, it is important to promote them. Our observation is that organizations, work teams, and supervisors can encourage a respectful climate governed by the idea that cultural variation is an inevitable aspect of human interaction. They can foster the expectation that "people who work with people" will naturally be curious and open to that variation. Such people may even be the most likely to take pleasure in observing and understanding people's culture differences, so the climate can define itself as one of opportunities to learn and share as well. We believe that individuals will be more likely to exhibit curiosity and receptivity in environments without either the implications of self-criticism that characterize some attitude-centered approaches, or the fragmented and sometimes trivializing generalizations of the fact-centered approach. In settings that promote an inquiry-centered approach, the concept that each individual is a cultural being can take root.

The degree of unfamiliarity a practitioner has with a client's background or the degree of difference between the client's background and that of the practitioner are not new factors to consider for some "diverse" individuals. They are instead aspects of what we must consider for each individual. In fact, the more a client seems "just like me," the more likely it is that important differences will be overlooked, with potentially negative consequences. The same holds true for relationships among professionals. Interacting with a colleague of the same profession does not ensure common values and beliefs, even though some aspects of professional enculturation will be similar. A social worker from a nursing home interacting with a social worker from an acute care facility may have very different views regarding effective transition strategies to ease a move for a client.

CULTURE BROKERS

In any situation in which cultural groups encounter each other, a few individuals step forward to assume the role of *culture broker*, or interpreter of the groups to one another. In many cases, such individuals are somewhat outside the norm for their native group, perhaps because they speak another language or have traveled more widely or received more education. Health care workers and social service providers are inevitably culture brokers because, in addition to their personal cultures of origin, they have specialized training related to both clients and the norms of practice. They must interpret for the client the organization within which they interact and, often, the bureaucracy of care. Social workers, for example, must help clients negotiate a wide array of available services and must explain potentially confusing systems of legal obligations and social supports, some of which may be at odds with clients' cultural values and beliefs (as some may also contradict the practitioner's beliefs and values).

If the culture emergent perspective is adopted, professionals in long term care organizations can view themselves as culture brokers with interpretive responsibilities in aligning practice to need. Acknowledging mutual cultural accommodation allows culture brokers to create new organizational models. Effective strategies for gathering and interpreting culturally relevant information, and using that information to facilitate change, are the tools of professional competence, part of the definition of "what professionals do" to understand organizational and client needs to best help both meet their goals. Similarly, in efforts to effect organizational change, individual practitioners may serve as brokers within the system. A social worker who has a long history of working closely with nurses and therapists may be able to frame social work expectations and needs to those disciplines and also bring information back to the social work staff from nurses and therapists.

When clients are extremely unfamiliar with these larger contexts, as in the case of recent immigrants or the newly homeless or the institutionalized elderly, the social worker must not only explain the system itself but may also need to serve as the client's advocate within it. Individuals with very different cultural backgrounds may find the larger context hostile, contrary to their own expectations and values, or directly inimical to their own well-being. Here, the practitioner may serve as the interpreter for all sorts of social institutions, assumptions, and values. It is worth noting, however, that one does not need to speak another language or come from another nationality to experience feelings of isolation, fear, powerlessness, and ignorance when confronting unfamiliar institutional communities. Even if the client and most staff appear to share many traits of race, ethnicity, language, or religion, the client may still have other aspects of his or her identity that may function as cultural factors in the process of providing care.

A good example is offered by aging gays and lesbians who may have come to adulthood in environments of hostility. Although the wider culture is now more tolerant, they may fear that such hostility is still possible from staff in residential facilities or community centers. Such individuals may not be identifiable at all on the basis of external characteristics and may be reluctant to reveal an orientation that may be stigmatized. And provider assumptions about sexual orientation or even sexuality itself among the elderly may obscure from his or her vantage any awareness of the person's identity. If the provider cannot find ways to transcend the assumptions and help the resident transcend the fear, opportunities for improved care and quality of life are lost. Expecting that people will have many different aspects to their identities and approaching this diversity from the perspective of culture emergent, using the tools of ethnographic inquiry to elicit information, and perceiving oneself as an actor with the capacity to affect the organizational culture within which the resident lives, are all, in our opinion, crucial to creating a climate of cultural competence in workplaces.

It is also well worth noting that effective culture brokers carry information in two directions. The social worker not only interprets the institutional culture for the client, but also conveys to the institution the needs, wishes, and beliefs of the client. These factors hold true for professional cultures, as well. The nursing home administration may seem unfamiliar or foreign to direct care staff. The social worker may need to observe administrative functioning dispassionately, exploring the values and patterns of that culture during the process of trying to change organizational practices.

As teams become increasingly important in the effective delivery of health care services, social workers are particularly well positioned to serve as culture brokers. Because of their specific functions, they often have more information about the clients' families and home environments than other members of the team, and can assist the other professionals to understand client needs. At the same time, because they are involved in discussion with multiple professionals involved in care of the individual, they can convey information back to the care recipients, as well.

Fadiman (1997) provides an excellent example of the way in which social workers can serve as culture brokers. In describing the case of Lia Lee, a young Hmong immigrant to central California, Fadiman gives a graphic and moving description of the dilemmas of providing care across multiple cultural boundaries. The physicians providing medical care for Lia, who has a severe seizure disorder, have difficulty communicating with the parents, who do not speak English and who do not have the same conceptualization of Lia's disorder. While the physicians perceive the Lees as difficult and inept, the social worker, who has an opportunity to observe the Lees caring for Lia at home, perceives them as caring and concerned parents. Her differing perception leads her to attempt to intervene in various health care and social service systems to better meet their needs. This differing perception as a result of observation in a more natural setting is one that is often available to social workers but not to other health care professionals.

Social workers and other practitioners are thus constantly in the role of culture brokers, and culture brokers are constantly in the forefront of culture change. Often it is the practitioner who, not just as interpreter but as change agent, can identify modifications in practice or find integrative explanations that ease the contact points between elements of the organization or between the organization and the client. In this way, over time, organizations can change and, over time, sensitive practice becomes more and more a part of organizational structure.

MUTUAL CULTURAL ACCOMMODATION

Cultures undergo constant change. There are various processes of culture change that directly affect individuals. Some may be welcome, as when a new treatment becomes available, but others may be forced, as in the case of a resident who enters a nursing home unhappily. Many aspects of culture change are outside the immediate consciousness of individuals, resulting as they do from the accumulated impact of small behavioral changes constantly made across a number of interactions, each involving different individuals. Practitioners may not realize how much interaction clients from a community have with each other concerning their individual experiences of the practitioner and his or her institution.

For example, when the first Mayan refugees and immigrants began to arrive in Indiantown, Florida in the mid-1980s, most residents there knew them primarily as "Guatemalans," rather than as members of culturally and linguistically unique groups within the oppressed Maya community that constitutes the majority population in Guatemala (Burns, 1993). As they interacted with social workers, nurses, and other social services and health providers, the Maya-speakers were addressed in their second language, Spanish, often by persons of Puerto Rican or Cuban backgrounds, whose Spanish and interactional styles were quite different from those of the refugees. Each Maya individual encountering the health care or social welfare systems learned more about the providers. Some shared that information with other members of the immigrant community, who then modified their own behaviors slightly–perhaps by adopting a form of personal address that is common to Caribbean Spanish but rare in Guatemala, or perhaps by trying to answer personal questions more directly in spite of how offensive such questions would be at home.

Meanwhile, the providers also interacted with each other, and with the sponsors of the refugee sanctuary project (mostly associated with a local church), exchanging information and trying to learn more about their new client population. With the insights of this information, they learned to phrase intrusive questions more sensitively–especially where a child was translating into the native language for a mother being treated for an intimate condition whose Spanish was poor or non-existent. They also learned more facts about the cultural and immediate political circumstances of the new arrivals, and some again modified their behaviors in the clinics and offices, especially with regard to recording personal information the refugees were anxious to keep private. Everyone in the situation was attempting to accommodate cultural differences for the greater good of their mutual goals: to deliver and receive improved care. Over time, the pattern of cultural practices across the group of refugees and practitioners changed as a result of individual shifts in behavior in specific settings, as they all worked toward mutual accommodation of their differences. We believe this process can be managed and become part of the conscious skill set of practitioners. We also believe that it can be a helpful concept for dealing with the differences among professional cultures as well.

Consider, for example, the possibility that a physician, taking seriously her Hippocratic Oath to "first, do no harm," will want to employ heroic measures to sustain the life of her terminally ill client. A social worker in the same system may be trying to institute a more palliative approach to end-of-life for residents. Careful exploration of values will be required to reach an accommodation that enables the physician to uphold her values while the social worker engages in intervention that upholds his. The social worker may be able to help the physician see that harm comes in many forms, including unnecessary suffering, while the physician may help the social worker to understand that some medical interventions can minimize suffering even while sustaining life. In the course of interaction at the boundary of the two professions, better understanding can ultimately lead to enhanced care that respects the wishes of the client and the values of both involved professions.

If successful, accommodating practitioners, like accommodating clients, will have transformed the interactional experience. They have mutually altered the culture that emerges in their encounters, perhaps successfully reaching an improved level of understanding. The changes that define this newly accommodated environment may be modest, nearly invisible to the larger structure, and are solely the work of individuals going about their individual work.

Such dynamism and responsiveness is a key dimension of culture itself and can be knowingly identified, monitored, analyzed, and mobilized to improve service. Imagine that you are the social worker in a nursing home that has begun to undergo a shift in resident demographics. The new group of residents will very likely have interests and wishes that differ in some way from those of the previous residents. To enhance quality of life for all the residents, thoughtful information-gathering regarding those interests and wishes (for all residents), and structuring of programs that address them can be much more powerful and effective than simply implementing a single "ethnic" activity, or even a series of such activities. It may develop that the key issues relate to meal schedule, forms of address, rules for visitors, or plans for community expeditions. Asking questions, with an attitude of active curiosity and an understanding of culture as dynamic and emergent, can inform effective planning.

Organizations are themselves part of the larger culture and are influenced by multiple threads from the larger context. External circumstances and the external culture impinge on the organization and its members and clients in unpredictable ways. Social workers are, for example, at the intersection of regulatory and reimbursement guidelines for long-term care facilities and the needs of care recipients. This area is one in which cultural values are often at odds, with the regulatory culture being one that values cost-containment and measurable outcomes, while care recipients are typically much more focused on harder-to-measure quality of life concerns.

CONCLUSIONS

The goal of a practitioner concerned with cultural diversity in an organization is the same as the goal of a practitioner with an individual client: a mutually satisfying environment, accommodated to the needs and purposes of its interacting participants. But achieving such an outcome is an on-going process, requiring reflection and consciousness. Skills of observation and inquiry can be taught and learned, practiced and improved. Techniques of self-interrogation, cross-checking, and program or service assessment can become part of the regular routine of work, and their implications can be experimented with and tested. But the process is never done. Goals–both those of individual clients and providers and those of organizations and communities–can be accomplished, of course. However, the nature of culture is such that satisfyingly accommodated environments are impermanent. They must be constantly reassessed, re-examined, and altered as the serving and served populations, the institutional culture, and the participating communities all change.

Cultural competence–the ability to attune to the individual while assessing the impact of community influences–is thus an integral component of professional competence. Training for skills development, opportunities for mutual support and assessment, and conscious efforts to form accommodating environments should be part of any institutional setting. They are the tools by which individual practitioners and caregivers can achieve their own highest goals. Acknowledging their continued relevance and facilitating their continued practice are fundamental to best practices.

REFERENCES

Bonder, B.R., Martin, L., & Miracle, A.W. (2001). Achieving cultural competence: The challenge for clients and healthcare workers in a multicultural society. *Generations*, XXV, 35-42.

Bonder, B.R., Martin, L., & Miracle, A.W. (2002). *Culture in Clinical Care.* Thorofare, NJ: Slack.

Brown, P.J. (1998). *Understanding and Applying Medical Anthropology.* Mountain View, CA: Mayfield Publishers.

Burns, A.F. (1993). *Maya in Exile: Guatemalans in Florida*. Philadelphia: Temple University Press.

DiversityRx. (1997). *Why language and culture are important*. http://www.DiversityRx.org/ HTML/ESLANG.htm, accessed 8/15/00.

Fadiman, A. (1997). *The Spirit Catches You and You Fall Down*. New York: Noonday Press.

Hahn, R.A. (1995). *Sickness and Healing: An Anthropological Perspective*. New Haven, CT: Yale University Press.

Hill, J.H. & MacLaurey, R.E. (1995). The terror of Montezuma: Aztec history, vantage theory, and the category of 'person.' In J.R. Taylor & R. MacLaurey (Eds.), *Language and the Cognitive Construal of the World*. Trends in Linguistics. Studies and Monographs 82. Berlin/New York: Mouton de Gruyter, p. 277-329.

Hong, Y., Morris, M.W., Chiu, C. & Benet-Martinez, V. (2000). Multicultural minds: A dynamic constructivist approach to culture and cognition. *American Psychologist, 55*, 709-720.

Law, M. (1998). *Client-Centered Occupational Therapy*. Thorofare, NJ: Slack.

Loveland, C.A. (1999). The concept of culture. In R.L. Leavitt (Ed.), *Cross-cultural Rehabilitation: An International Perspective*. London: W.B. Saunders, p. 15-24.

New Waves: Hospitals struggle to meet the challenge of multiculturalism now–and in the next generation (1993). *Hospitals, 67*, 22-31.

Pruegger, V.J. & Rogers, T.B. (1994). Cross-cultural sensitivity training: Methods and assessment. *International Journal of Intercultural Relations, 18*, 369-387.

Sleek, S. (1998). Psychology's cultural competence, once 'simplistic,' now broadening. *APA Monitor, 29* (12), December, p. 1, 27.

Spokane, A.R. (1992). Personal constructs and careers: A reaction. *Journal of Career Development, 18*, 229-236.

Urban, G.A. (1991). *Discourse-Centered Approach to Culture: Native South American Myths and Rituals*. Austin: University of Texas Press.

The Changing Consumer:
The Social Context of Culture Change in Long-Term Care

Donald L. Redfoot

SUMMARY. Sustaining "culture change" in long-term care or any other social system requires change in the underlying social structures that support a given culture. Due to the "medicalization" of contemporary long-term care, the cultural meanings of aging and disability have been increasingly defined and maintained through social structures associated with the medical professions. The "culture change" movement in long-term care is seeking to balance the power of the medical professions with more consumer empowerment. Over the next two decades, consumer empowerment will be supported by important demographic and socio-economic changes in the older population. Demographic empowerment will come from relatively small cohorts of older persons, declining disability rates, and stronger supports from informal caregivers. Socio-economic empowerment will come from higher levels of income,

Donald L. Redfoot, PhD, is Senior Policy Advisor in AARP's Public Policy Institute. His work focuses on housing, assisted living, and long-term care policy.

Address correspondence to: Donald Redfoot, PhD, AARP–Public Policy Institute, 3617 Vickery Drive, Billings, MT 59102 (E-mail: dredfoot@home.com).

The author gratefully acknowledges the assistance of Sheel Pandya in preparing this manuscript.

Much of the research included in this report comes from work found in Redfoot and Pandya (2002).

[Haworth co-indexing entry note]: "The Changing Consumer: The Social Context of Culture Change in Long-Term Care." Redfoot, Donald L. Co-published simultaneously in *Journal of Social Work in Long-Term Care* (The Haworth Social Work Practice Press, an imprint of The Haworth Press, Inc.) Vol. 2, No. 1/2, 2003, pp. 95-110; and: *Culture Change in Long-Term Care* (ed: Audrey S. Weiner, and Judah L. Ronch) The Haworth Social Work Practice Press, an imprint of The Haworth Press, Inc., 2003, pp. 95-110. Single or multiple copies of this article are available for a fee from The Haworth Document Delivery Service [1-800-HAWORTH, 9:00 a.m. - 5:00 p.m. (EST). E-mail address: docdelivery@haworthpress.com].

wealth, and educational attainment. Together these trends should provide powerful support to a more consumer-driven culture of long-term care. *[Article copies available for a fee from The Haworth Document Delivery Service: 1-800-HAWORTH. E-mail address: <docdelivery@haworthpress.com> Website: <http://www.HaworthPress.com> © 2003 by The Haworth Press, Inc. All rights reserved.]*

KEYWORDS. Long-term care, culture change, disability, socio-economic status, cohorts, informal caregiving, nursing home utilization

INTRODUCTION

Understanding the "culture change" movement in long-term care requires understanding both the "culture" of long-term care and the social structures that maintain that culture. Jennie Keith (1982), one of the pioneering anthropologists of aging, has described culture as "design for living," "a filter of patterns and meanings which defines the environment–physical, social, and cognitive–in which we live" (p. 111). These patterns and meanings that shape our lives are "transmitted socially" (p. 111) through the complex web of social structures that constitute a society.

The much-discussed "medicalization" of long-term care in contemporary society is another way of saying that the cultural meanings of aging and disability have been increasingly defined and maintained through social structures associated with the medical professions. The nursing home epitomizes the most obvious example of the extent of control exerted by medical professionals over the lives of those who enter our nation's long-term care systems. Not only are medical decisions largely ceded to professionals, but all aspects of daily living are similarly brought under professional control. Schedules for rising or going to bed, timing and content of meals, and other activities in the everyday life of long-term care institutions are controlled by medical professionals even when they do not correspond to the rhythms of an individual's life (Foldes, 1990).

Kaufman (1994) nicely summarizes the process by which the experience of disability in old age is often translated into a medically enforced definition of "frailty":

The transformation from lived problem to diagnosis, then to treatment plan, then to rules about what ought to be done, and finally to negotiated compliance is the form the social construction of frailty takes in the context of health care.

So engrained are these aspects of institutional caregiving that they are simply taken for granted as facts, "the way things are" (Kane, 1990). Indeed, from the perspective of efficiently managing an institution, they are "reasonable" ways of operating. Of course, different actors–consumers, family, caregivers, administrators, policy makers–within the social structure of long-term care have different perspectives on what is "reasonable," as Gubrium illustrated in his classic study of "living and dying at Murray Manor" (1975). Gubrium describes each of these actors as operating in a different "world," whose members share a set of understandings about how the world operates and what is "reasonable."

For example, it may be "reasonable" from a policy decision-maker's world of budgets and competing priorities to reimburse only semi-private rooms. Shared rooms may also be "reasonable" from the perspective of the nursing home owner or administrator who provides services within the limits of that reimbursement policy. On the other hand, sharing a room with a stranger is often not at all "reasonable" from the perspective of the resident–or, for that matter, from the perspective of the floor staff who must mediate endless roommate conflicts (Miles and Sachs, 1990; Kane et al., 1998).

In maintaining the cultural "facts of life" in a nursing home, the actors involved are sustaining a power relationship between providers and consumers. In particular, the medicalization of long-term care represents the power of medical institutions and professionals to define the cultural "facts of life" regarding long-term care and to enforce those definitions through the institutions of caregiving. The power relations so well described at the micro-level within caregiving institutions by ethnographers (Henderson and Vesperi, 1995) is maintained at the macro-level through the complex machinery of public subsidy programs and regulations that enforce a medical and institutional bias to caregiving.

The culture change movement in long-term care has emerged to change the cultural "facts of life" in the systems and institutions that provide support to older persons who need it. The goals of this movement have been variously described: to give "some measure of independence and responsibility" (Culture Change Now, 2001); "all elders are entitled to self-determination wherever they live" (Pioneer Network, 2002); and "medical treatment should be the servant of genuine human caring, never its master" (Eden Alternative, 2001). Each of these descriptions focus on shifting the balance of power from caregivers to consumers to give more choice in the lives they want to live. Lasting change in the cultural "facts of life" will only occur when the social structures and power relations within which they are embedded are changed. The very language emerging from the "culture change" movement reflects changes in the social structures of long-term care and the resulting power relations among the actors within those social structures.

From patient to consumer–The change in terminology reflects the goal of empowering consumers to be the active agents in choosing service options rather than the passive recipients of care under medical control.

From case manager to service broker–The goal is to transform the role of social workers "managing" cases in a bureaucracy to negotiating options on behalf of consumers.

From institution-based to community-based services–Even when the services take place within nursing homes, the goal is to promote active involvement of consumers within communities of their choosing.

From a continuum of care to a repertoire of services–The goal is to move public policy from enforcing a "continuum of institutions" through which consumers must move to an array of services options from which they can choose (Kane, 1993).

Other articles in this volume will describe these cultural changes in more detail. It is the purpose of this article to describe important changes in the demographic and socio-economic situation of older consumers that will enhance their power to make further changes in the culture of long-term care. This article will argue that relatively slow growth in the older population will combine with improved health, informal supports, education, and wealth to empower consumers and, thereby, force major changes in the culture of long-term care.

DEMOGRAPHIC EMPOWERMENT

Over the next two decades, three major demographic factors will combine to strengthen the consumer's power to demand change in the culture of long-term care:

- Relatively small cohorts will produce more of a buyer's market for service options.
- Declining disability rates will further temper demand for services.
- Stronger informal supports from family will enhance consumer bargaining power.

Cohort Size

While much has been made of the aging of the Baby Boom, those large age cohorts will not reach the high risk years of needing long-term care services for twenty years or so. What is not often noted is that the intervening years will see relatively small age cohorts coming into the high risk later years. Those born between the years of 1925 and 1945 were part of a "birth dearth" that occurred during the Great Depression and World War II. Figure 1 shows the Census Bureau's analysis of the changes in cohort sizes over the decade between 1990 and 2000. As it shows, sandwiched in between the rapid growth of the oldest age cohorts and the growth of the Baby Boom is a period of relatively low growth reflecting the "birth dearth."

The number of persons aged 75 and older grew by almost 3.5 million in the past decade. In contrast, the U.S. Census Bureau projects that the number of people in those oldest age cohorts will grow by roughly half that amount in the current decade. Smaller cohorts in the high risk years may translate into slackening demand for long-term care services, especially toward the end of this decade and into the next. Soft demand should enhance the power of older consumers to demand higher quality of services and more control over choices in the marketplace for services.

Declining Disability Rates

In a recent review of five major data sets that track functional limitations and/or dependency in activities of daily living, Cutler (2001) concludes, "Existing evidence generally suggests that disability among the elderly is falling over time." Though the surveys take different approaches to measuring "disability," Cutler notes that " . . . all of the surveys show a healthier el-

FIGURE 1. Percent Change in Population by Age Groups: 1990-2000

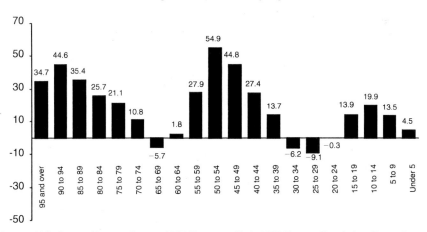

Source: U.S. Census Bureau, Census 2000 Summary file 1; 1990 Census Population, General

derly population by at least one measure." Indeed, several of the surveys show an accelerating rate of decline in disability among older persons. Figure 2 illustrates the effects of declining disability rates over the past two decades. The figure uses data over the history of the National Long-Term Care Survey to show the difference between the number of older persons with a disability that one would have expected had there been no change from the 1982 baseline and the actual number. As Figure 2 shows, the number of older persons with a disability has remained essentially unchanged over the past decade despite a substantial increase in the older population, especially among the oldest old.

While projecting future disability rates is less certain than general population aging, at least two major analyses (Manton et al., 1998; Waidmann and Liu, 2000) project flat growth in the number of older persons with a disability for the next couple of decades. For example, Waidmann and Liu (2000) report that "if they continue, declines in IADL and ADL disability prevalence . . . will be large enough to offset future increases in elderly population growth." Once again, the flat demand for services is one factor in the growing consumer power to demand culture change in the services offered.

FIGURE 2. Number of Chronically Disabled Americans Aged 65 and Over (in Millions), by Selected Years

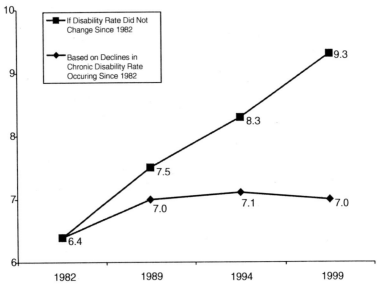

Source: Manton K., Corder L., and Stalland E. (1997); Manton K. and Gu X (2001). Prepared by AARP Public Policy Institute, 2001.

Informal Supports

Age and disability are not the only predictors of utilization patterns for long-term supportive services. The support of family and friends as advocates is also critical to the types of choices a consumer has. According to a report by the National Academy on Aging, only 7 percent of older persons with long-term care needs who have family supports are living in nursing homes compared to 50 percent of those who have no family supports (Stone, 2000).

Today's young old and near old will have more family as advocates and service providers as they make decisions about long-term care options over the coming decades. The first line of support for most older persons with disabilities is a spouse. Lakdawalla and Philipson (1999) argue that the selective growth of those most at risk of nursing home services–that is, women living alone with higher rates of disability–was the primary cause of the explosive growth in the nursing home population during the 1970s. The 1960s and 1970s saw an imbalance in longevity where the number of women over age 75 grew at twice the rate of men of that age. Indeed, the growing gender imbalance led to 900,000 more widowed older women in 1980 than would have been predicted based on 1970 rates (Lakdawalla and Philipson, 1998).

The trend toward greater nursing home utilization peaked in the late 1970s and early 1980s, then declined as disability rates declined and the gender ratio narrowed. Since the early 1980s, the mortality rate for men aged 65 and older has declined more than twice as rapidly as for women of the same ages (Sahyoun et al., 2001a). When disability rates fell and the gender ratio narrowed, fewer older women were living alone and nursing home utilization rates fell despite the rapid increase in the older population. Lakdawalla and Philipson (1998) note that increased longevity may have the paradoxical effect of decreasing nursing home utilization if it results in an increase in the supply of primary caregivers–i.e., spouses.

Figure 3 illustrates the narrowing of the gender ratio between 1990 and 2000, which is concentrated among the old and near old. The greater survival of men means that the chief supply of primary informal caregivers–namely, spouses–is likely to increase over the coming decades. Increased spousal survival may be one of the primary means of increasing consumer choice among those who encounter disabilities in late life.

Cohort differences in childbearing also have a strong impact on informal supports later in life. Those who turned age 75 in the 1970s and 1980s not only experienced high rates of disability and high levels of widowhood among older women, they also had high rates of childlessness. Having come into adulthood during the Great Depression and World War II, a period not conducive to family formation, today's oldest old cohorts were the parents of the

FIGURE 3. The Male-Female Ratio by Selected Age Groups: 1990 and 2000

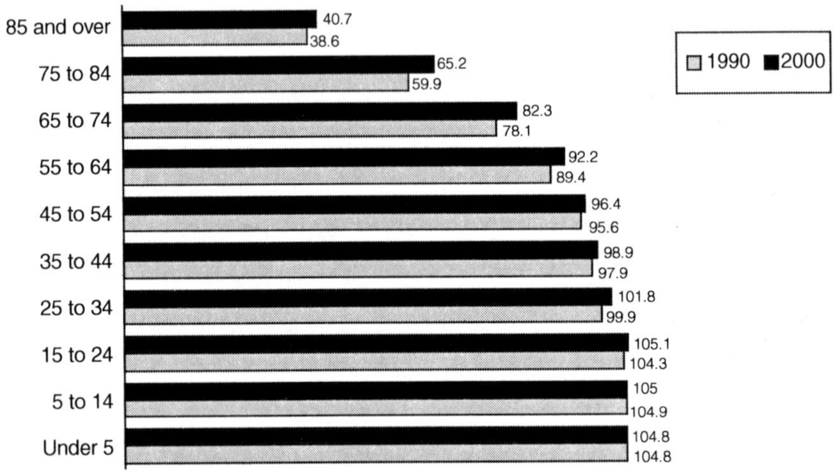

Source: U.S. Census Bureau, Census 2000 Summary File 1; 1990 Census of Population, General Population Characteristics: United States (1990 CP-1-1).

Birth Dearth Cohort. In contrast, subsequent cohorts, those who were born during the Birth Dearth years and will reach age 75 and older over the next two decades, are the parents of the Baby Boom who reached adulthood in the post-World War II era. Not only do the Birth Dearth cohorts have low rates of childlessness, they also have high average numbers of children. Indeed, roughly one-third of the women in these cohorts had 4 or more children as noted in Table 1.

The combined effects of more spouses living and more children will mean increasing potential family support for at least the next two decades. Himes (1992) projects that the percentage of persons aged 85 and older who are both unmarried and have no children will decrease by more than half between 1990 and 2020 as shown in Table 2.

In short, change in the culture of long-term care is likely to accelerate due to the demographic factors that will increase the power of successive cohorts of older persons to make choices about their care. Smaller age cohorts, declining disability rates, and improved informal supports will combine to enhance the market power and decision-making ability of older consumers. The narrowing gender ratio and the decreasing rates of childlessness will particularly benefit older women, as they are less likely to face decisions related to disability and caregiving alone.

TABLE 1. Number of Children Among Women by Birth Cohort in 2000

AGE IN 2000	PERCENT DISTRIBUTION BY # OF CHILDREN				AVERAGE # OF CHILDREN
	0	1-3	4-5	6+	
50-54	16.0	71.0	10.8	2.2	2.07
55-59	12.7	66.5	16.5	4.4	2.45
60-64	10.8	57.8	22.9	8.6	2.90
65-69	11.4	52.7	24.3	11.7	3.20
70-74	11.6	55.1	22.0	11.2	3.08
75-79	14.1	57.8	18.2	10.0	2.86
80-84	17.2	58.0	16.5	8.3	2.57
85-89	22.5	57.0	12.9	7.6	2.35
90-94	24.2	54.9	12.8	8.2	2.29
95-99	23.9	52.9	12.9	10.3	2.44
100+	21.9	50.1	15.3	12.7	2.68

Source: AARP PPI analysis of women age 40 and older in 1990 decennial public use microdata for women aged 60 and older. Otherwise the data are from Congressional Budget Office (1988).

TABLE 2. Percentage of Persons Aged 85 and Older With No Spouse and No Children by Gender and Race, 1990 and 2020

	1990	2020
White Females	22.1%	8.7%
Black Females	31.5%	14.0%
White Males	10.2%	4.8%
Black Males	17.6%	9.2%

Source: Himes (1992)

SOCIO-ECONOMIC EMPOWERMENT

Changes in the socio-economic status of older persons will also enhance their power to control decisions regarding long-term care, providing further social structural support to the culture change movement. Greater wealth and improved education levels give older consumers more means and greater sophistication in choosing service options and remaining in charge of their lives.

Some evidence for the effects of this economic empowerment come from the National Nursing Home Survey. As Table 3 indicates, there were 1.318 million older residents in nursing homes in 1985. The table compares projections of what the nursing home population would have been if 1985 utilization patterns had remained the same in 1999. Given the growth in the older population, especially among the oldest old, 1.834 million persons aged 65 and older would have been in nursing homes in 1999, 365,000 more than the actual number of 1.470 million.

In discussing declining nursing home utilization rates, Bishop (1999) rhetorically asks, "Where Are the Missing Elders?" She might have been more specific in her question to ask "Where Are the Missing 'Privately Paying' Elders?" As Table 3 indicates, the portion of the nursing home population paying privately dropped by more than half (54 percent) from the projected level. Indeed, the number of older nursing home consumers paying privately dropped in absolute terms from 570,000 in 1985 to 370,100 in 1999, a decline of more than a third (35 percent) despite the growth in the older population.

Bishop (1999) explores some of the potential explanations for this decline. She rules out limited nursing home capacity since occupancy rates have been declining during the period between 1985 and the present, indicating excess capacity in most areas of the country. Moreover, since providers generally favor the admission of private pay consumers, any limits on capacity would

TABLE 3: Nursing Home Residents Aged 65+ in 1985 and 1999, Actual and Expected, by Primary Source of Payment

	1985	1999, if 1985 rate continued	1999, Actual	Actual–Expected
Private	575,500 (43.7%)	808,300 (44.1%)	370,100 (25.2%)	−438,200 (−54.2%)
Medicaid	652,200 (49.5%)	906,600 (49.4%)	835,400 (56.8%)	−71,200 (−7.8%)
Medicare	20,300 (1.5%)	27,100 (1.5%)	227,400 (15.5%)	+200,300 (+739.1%)
Other	70,300 (5.3%)	92,200 (5.0%)	36,700 (2.5%)	−55,500 (−60.2%)
Total	1,318,300 (100.0%)	1,834,200 (100.0%)	1,469,600 (100.0%)	−364,600 (−19.9%)

Analysis by AARP Public Policy Institute based on data from the National Nursing Home Survey.

more than likely show up in fewer consumers receiving public payments. Some portion of the decline may be due to the selective impact of the demographic factors noted above–declining disability rates and stronger family supports are somewhat more common among those able to pay privately. Some portion may be due to a shift from private to public sources of payment, though the lower-than-expected numbers receiving support from Medicaid and Other do not support the notion that large numbers of older persons are spending down their assets to benefit from welfare programs. Indeed, only the number of older persons receiving Medicare benefits showed a greater than expected increase–but Medicare beneficiaries are typically receiving short-term post-acute care, not real long-term support.

Bishop concludes that most of the decline in nursing home utilization rates is likely due to older people seeking out alternatives to nursing homes–most notably home care and assisted living. Those older persons with the means to pay privately appear to be voting with their feet–and their wallets–for alternatives that they experience as meeting their needs better. Most, no doubt, prefer to remain in their homes and receive home care services. Others are opting for assisted living, an option that most view more favorably than nursing homes as the next best thing to home (Lehrer, 2001).

A substantial portion of the growth in home care was funded by Medicare and Medicaid, at least until the Balanced Budget Act of 1997 curbed that growth. But the overwhelming majority of the growth in assisted living has been among those paying privately. According to a 1998 survey of persons in assisted living facilities, only 7.9 percent received Medicaid assistance (NIC, 1998) compared to the 57 percent who received such assistance in nursing homes according to the 1999 NNHS. A 2000 survey found that 58,544 assisted living residents were receiving Medicaid assistance (Mollica, 2000) compared to 834,400 older persons receiving such assistance in nursing homes. On the other hand, more than 500,000 older persons are paying privately in assisted living compared to 370,100 older persons in nursing homes.

Future cohorts of older persons are likely to have much greater socio-economic power as measured by greater wealth and higher educational attainment. Greater socio-economic power will increase consumer choice in long-term care options. For example, in reviewing "the wealth of cohorts," Venti and Wise (1996) project "that the personal financial assets of the cohort that will attain age 76 in 28 years will be almost twice as large as the personal financial assets of the cohort that attained age 76 in 1991."

Education may be one of the strongest measures of the socio-economic empowerment of older consumers. In the first place, education levels serve as a reliable surrogate measure of economically related factors such as long-term exposure to occupation-related risks, insurance coverage, and access to health care. Education is also related to health-related behaviors such as smoking and alcohol consumption and exercise. As a result, demographers and other social scientists have found education to be a strong predictor of disability rates (Manton and Gu, 2001; Schoeni et al., 2001; Waidmann and Liu, 2000). For example, Schoeni et al. (2001) found that roughly two-thirds (65 percent) of the decline in disability rates could be explained by increasing educational levels.

In addition, education may be a good measure for choice in the marketplace of long-term care services. To the extent that more highly educated consumers are more sophisticated about options available and are more likely to have the means to pay for them, they will have greater control over long-term care services. For example, Hawes et al. (2000) found that residents in high privacy and/or high service assisted living facilities had much higher levels of education than their age peers. Only 26.8 percent of assisted living residents had less than a high school education compared to 35.4 percent of the general population aged 75 and older (see Table 4). On the other hand, 20.3 percent of the assisted living residents were college graduates compared to 13.4 percent of the general population aged 75 and older.

Further improvements in educational attainment are virtually certain given the levels attained by succeeding cohorts who will reach age 65 over the next two decades as indicated in Table 3. Waidmann and Liu (2001) project further educational improvements until at least 2020 when a quarter of the older population will have a bachelor's degree and more than 85 percent will have at least a high school education. These improvements in education are likely to result in further improvements in disability levels (Freedman and Martin, 1999) and in the sophistication of consumers in demanding control over decision-making.

CONCLUSIONS

As noted at the outset of this paper, cultural definitions of reality require the support of social structures that reinforce those definitions. The "medicalization" of long-term care reached its pinnacle in the 1970s and 1980s when the power

TABLE 4. Educational Attainment by Age, 2000

	45-49	50-54	55-59	60-64	65-69	70-74	75+
High School Grad or Higher	89.5%	88.3%	84.0%	78.8%	75.4%	71.6%	64.6%
Bachelor's Degree or Higher	30.3%	30.2%	25.0%	21.6%	18.5%	16.4%	13.4%

Source: U.S. Census Bureau, Current Population Survey, March 2000

of the medical professions was ascendant and consumers were relatively disempowered. Growth in demand came primarily from women living with higher rates of disability, weak informal supports, and few economic resources. The transformation of the demographic and socio-economic status of older consumers will be the most important driver in the creating of a more consumer-driven market that will demand change in the culture of long-term care (Kane, 2001).

Stone (2000) has declared that, "The 1990s may someday be referred to as the period when the health care and long-term care consumer came of age." The data presented in this article suggest that the age of consumer choice and control has only begun. Decisions regarding long-term care options are always difficult, but older consumers facing such decisions over the next two decades will be empowered demographically by relatively small cohort sizes, declining disability rates and stronger family supports. Increasingly sophisticated consumers will also be empowered socio-economically by greater wealth and higher education levels.

While this article focused on changes in the older population, other factors are also likely to support culture change in long-term care services. Some changes–such as legal rights (e.g., the *Olmstead* decision), improved training for professional caregivers, and market changes in the development of services (e.g., the growth of assisted living)–may be direct results of consumer demand for improved services. Other changes–such as improved medical and assistive technology and improved pharmacology–are driven by technological developments that will nonetheless contribute to consumer choice and empowerment.

Obviously, not all older consumers will be empowered by the demographic and socio-economic trends described in this article. To extend the benefits of greater choice to those with few economic resources and weak family supports will require changes in public benefit programs, especially changes in the institutional bias of Medicaid. These changes have been slow to come because of the fear of the budget implications. But the relatively slow growth in the older population during the next two decades provides the best window of opportunity to make needed changes.

The culture change movement in long-term care is both responding to the pressures of a changing marketplace and leading the market in providing innovative new care options. The movement is based on the simple but powerful idea that older people–even those with disabilities–should be treated as people who should be enabled to live life as fully as possible. But powerful ideas need powerful social support to survive and grow. Changes in the older population clearly indicate that the culture change movement in long-term care is an idea whose time has come.

REFERENCES

Bishop, Christine E. (1999). "Where Are the Missing Elders? The Decline in Nursing Home Use, 1985 and 1995." *Health Affairs*, July/August, pp. 146-155.

Congressional Budget Office. (1988). *Changes in the Living Arrangements of the Elderly: 1960-2030*. Washington, DC: Congressional Budget Office.

Culture Change Now. (2001). "Culture Change" web page at *www.culturechangenow.com*.

Cutler, David M. (2001). "Declining Disability Among the Elderly." *Health Affairs*, Vol. 20, No. 6, pp. 11-27.

Eden Alternative. (2001). "Our 10 Principles" web page at *www.edenalt.com*.

Foldes, Steven S. (1990). "Life in an Institution: A Sociological and Anthropological View." In Kane and Caplan (Eds.), *Everyday Ethics: Resolving Dilemmas in Nursing Home Life*. New York: Springer.

Freedman, Vicki A. and Linda G. Martin. (1999). "The Role of Education in Explaining and Forecasting Trends in Functional Limitations Among Older Americans," *Demography*, Vol. 36, No. 4, pp. 461-473.

Gubrium, Jaber F. (1975). *Living and Dying at Murray Manor*. Charlottesville, VA: University of Virginia Press.

Hawes, Catherine, Charles D. Phillips, and Miriam Rose. (2000). *High Service or High Privacy Assisted Living Facilities, Their Residents and Staff: Results from a National Survey*. Washington, DC: Department of Health and Human Services, Assistant Secretary for Planning and Evaluation.

Henderson, J. Neil & Maria D. Vesperi. (1995). *The Culture of Long-Term Care: Nursing Home Ethnography*. Westport, CT: Bergin & Garvey.

Himes, C. L. (1992). "Future Caregivers: Projected Family Structures of Older Persons." *Journal of Gerontology*, Vol. 47, No. 1, pp. S17-S26.

Hornum, Barbara. (1995). "Assessing Types of Residential Accommodations for the Elderly: Liminality and Communitas. In Hernderson and Vesperi (Eds.), *The Culture of Long-Term Care: Nursing Home Ethnography*. Westport, CT: Bergin & Garvey.

Kane, Rosalie A. (1990). "Everyday Life in Nursing Homes: 'The Way Things Are'," in Kane and Caplan (Eds.), *Everyday Ethics: Resolving Dilemmas in Nursing Home Life*. New York: Springer.

Kane, Rosalie A. (1993). "Dangers Lurking in the 'Continuum of Care'." *Journal of Aging and Social Policy*, Vol. 5, No. 4, pp. 1-7.

Kane, Rosalie A. (2001). "Long-Term Care and a Good Quality of Life: Bringing Them Closer Together." *The Gerontologist*, Vol. 44, No. 3, pp. 293-304.

Kane, Rosalie A. and Arthur L. Caplan (Eds.). (1990). *Everyday Ethics: Resolving Dilemmas in Nursing Home Life*. New York: Springer.

Kane, Rosalie A., Robert L. Kane, and Richard C. Ladd. (1998). *The Heart of Long-Term Care*. New York: Oxford University Press.

Kaufman, Sharon R. (1994). "The Social Construction of Frailty: An Anthropological Perspective." *Journal of Aging Studies*, Vol. 8, No. 1, pp. 45-58.

Keith, Jennie. (1982). *Old People As People: Social and Cultural Influences on Aging and Old Age*. Boston: Little, Brown and Co.

Kertzer, David I. and Jennie Keith (Eds.). (1984). *Age and Anthropological Theory.* Ithaca: Cornell University Press.

Lakdawalla, Darius and Tomas Philipson. (1999). *Aging and the Growth of Long-Term Care.* National Bureau for Economic Research, Working Paper No. 6980.

Lakdawalla, Darius and Tomas Philipson. (1998). *The Rise in Old Age Longevity and the Market for Long-Term Care.* National Bureau for Economic Research, Working Paper No. 6547.

Lehrer, Jim. (2001). "National Survey on Nursing Homes." *The News Hour with Jim Lehrer/Kaiser Family Foundation/Harvard School of Public Health.*

Manton, Kenneth G. and XiLang Gu. (2001). "Changes in the Prevalence of Chronic Disability in the United States Black and Nonblack Population Above Age 65 from 1982 to 1999." *Proceedings of the National Academy of Sciences,* Vol. 98, pp. 6354-6359.

Manton, Kenneth G., Eric Stollard, and L. S. Corder. (1998). "The Dynamics of Dimensions of Age-Related Disability 1982 to 1994 in the U.S. Elderly Population." *Journal of Gerontology,* Vol. 53, Issue 1, pp. B59-B70.

Manton, Kenneth G., Larry Corder, and Eric Stallard. (1997). "Chronic Disability Trends in Elderly United States Populations: 1982-1994." *Proceedings of the National Academy of Sciences,* Vol. 94, pp. 2593-2598.

Meyer, Julie. (2001). "Age: 2000." *Census 2000 Brief.* Washington, DC: U.S. Census Bureau.

Miles, Stephen H. and Greg A. Sachs. (1990). "Intimate Strangers: Roommates in Nursing Homes." In Kane and Caplan (Eds.), *Everyday Ethics: Resolving Dilemmas in Nursing Home Life.* New York: Springer.

Mollica, Robert. (2000). *State Assisted Living Policy: 2000.* Portland, ME: National Academy for State Health Policy.

National Center for Health Statistics. (2001). *National Nursing Home Survey.* Data analyses by Esther Hing. Hyattsville, MD: National Center for Health Statistics.

National Investment Center for the Seniors Housing and Care Industries (NIC). (1998). *National Survey of Assisted Living Residents: Who Is the Customer?* Annapolis, MD: National Investment Center.

The Pioneer Network. (2002). "Values, Vision, Mission" web page at *www.pioneernetwork.org.*

Redfoot, Donald L. and Sheel M. Pandya. (2002). *Before the Boom: Trends in Long-Term Supportive Services for Frail Older Americans.* Forthcoming from the AARP Public Policy Institute: Washington, DC.

Sahyoun, Nadine R., Harold Lentzer, Donna Hoyert, and Kristen N. Robinson. (2001). "Trends in Causes of Death Among the Elderly." *Aging Trends,* No. 1, National Center for Health Statistics.

Schoeni, Robert F., Vicki A. Freedman, and Robert B. Wallace. (2001). "Persistent, Consistent, Widespread, and Robust?: Another Look at Recent Trends in Old-Age Disability." *Journal of Gerontology,* Vol. 56B, No. 4, pp. S206-S218.

Smith, Denise I. and Renee E. Spraggins. (2001). "Gender: 2000." *Census 2000 Brief.* Washington, DC: U.S. Census Bureau.

Stone, Robyn I. (2000). *Long-Term Care for the Elderly with Disabilities: Current Policy, Emerging Trends, and Implications for the Twenty-First Century.* New York: Milbank Memorial Fund.

Venti, Stephen F. and David A. Wise. (1996). *The Wealth of Cohorts: Retirement Saving and the Changing Assets of Older Americans.* National Bureau of Economic Research Working Paper No. 5609.

Waidmann, Timothy A. and Korbin Liu. (2000). "Disability Trends among Elderly Persons and Implications for the Future." *Journal of Gerontology*, Vol. 55B, No. 5, pp. S298-S307.

Family Caregivers, Health Care Professionals, and Policy Makers: The Diverse Cultures of Long-Term Care

Carol Levine

SUMMARY. Although families and health care professionals have similar goals for the health and well-being of a patient or client, they approach care, especially long-term care, with different assumptions, values, attitudes, and behaviors. Using the popular understanding of the term, they have different "cultures." Professionals are also subject to societal and cultural influences beyond their own disciplines. In the evolving health care economy professional values have been forced to adapt to the demands of the marketplace in health care, which is governed by a corporate or bureaucratic culture. Social work's tradition of concern for

Carol Levine is the Director at the Families and Health Care Project, United Hospital Fund, 350 Fifth Avenue, 23rd Floor, New York, NY 10118.

Address correspondence to Carol Levine at the above address (E-mail: clevine@uhfnyc.org).

The author gratefully acknowledges the insights and collaborative spirit of the multidisciplinary members of The Hastings Center-United Hospital Fund Working Group on Cultures and Caregiving convened in 2000. Thomas Murray, PhD, and the author were co-directors. As noted, some of the reflections on the policy culture derive from discussions with Judith Feder, PhD, of Georgetown University, and the paper she and the author subsequently co-authored for inclusion in a volume from the project. The author alone is responsible, however, for the views expressed in this paper.

[Haworth co-indexing entry note]: "Family Caregivers, Health Care Professionals, and Policy Makers: The Diverse Cultures of Long-Term Care." Levine, Carol. Co-published simultaneously in *Journal of Social Work in Long-Term Care* (The Haworth Social Work Practice Press, an imprint of The Haworth Press, Inc.) Vol. 2, No. 1/2, 2003, pp. 111-123; and: *Culture Change in Long-Term Care* (ed: Audrey S. Weiner, and Judah L. Ronch) The Haworth Social Work Practice Press, an imprint of The Haworth Press, Inc., 2003, pp. 111-123. Single or multiple copies of this article are available for a fee from The Haworth Document Delivery Service [1-800-HAWORTH, 9:00 a.m. - 5:00 p.m. (EST). E-mail address: docdelivery@haworthpress.com].

the whole family and for justice in society make this discipline well suited to advocate for policies and practices that bridge these gaps. *[Article copies available for a fee from The Haworth Document Delivery Service: 1-800-HAWORTH. E-mail address: <docdelivery@haworthpress.com> Website: <http://www.HaworthPress.com> © 2003 by The Haworth Press, Inc. All rights reserved.]*

KEYWORDS. Family, family culture, family caregiving, home care

INTRODUCTION

Four families are seated in a nursing home (or hospital or agency) waiting room. They are speaking quietly but there is an air of anxiety in the room. If you could listen in, you would hear four different languages, including varieties of English. They are from different ethnic groups: white, Asian-American, African-American, and Latino.

One large group is multigenerational; the teenagers hold their own conversations, all the while attentive to the needs of the elderly woman who seems to be their grandmother, or perhaps their great-grandmother. Another group is made up of just two people, an elderly couple who seem to be married but they might be brother and sister. The third group includes an elderly man and his adult daughters and their husbands. The fourth group is solely female. The members of these groups have different styles of dress. Some are obviously more prosperous than others. Some wear religious symbols as pendants or pins.

What is the most distinctive characteristic of these families? Someone coming into the room might say that it is their language, their ethnicity, their social and economic class, or their religion. All these factors are important, of course, but what is often missed is that the characteristic that distinguishes these individuals from the professionals they encounter in the formal health care and social service system is that they are *families*. As people tied to each other through blood, marriage, or shared commitment, their priorities and values differ in some significant ways from those of the professionals with whom they will now begin to interact.

A DIFFERENT PERSPECTIVE ON CULTURAL DIVERSITY AND CULTURAL COMPETENCE

Nearly all the multiple versions of "caregiver burden scales" focus on the caregiver's stress that results from either the caregiver's lack of social support or the relationship with the care recipient. The "Caregiver Hassle Scale," despite its name, deals only with hassles that occur between caregiver and care recipient (Kinney and Stephens, 1989). There is hardly a mention of one of the major stressors: unsatisfactory relationships with agents of the health care system, whether they are doctors, nurses, social workers, hospital or nursing home administrators, or insurance personnel.

Although health care professionals and family caregivers have the same broad goals for a patient/relative, the relationship between them is often strained and sometimes hostile (Levine and Zuckerman, 1999). Why is this so? Usually the answer from professionals is that a particular family is "dysfunctional" or that they "don't understand" the prognosis, the treatment, or whatever has become the issue of the moment. Families are criticized when they are too involved and when they are not involved enough. For their part, families may describe a particular doctor or nurse as "cold," or "uncaring," "uncommunicative," and a social worker as "only interested in getting my father out of the hospital." But placing all the blame on individuals or personality conflicts misses a larger point.

Families and professionals have different assumptions, values, attitudes, and behaviors. In other words, using the popular understanding of the term, they have different "cultures." "Cultural diversity" has come to be equated with immigrant or minority families, yet all families have special characteristics. Every family has its own culture, a blend of group and personal characteristics developed over time and generations through both inherited factors and their shared history. And within each family's culture, different individuals have unique sets of beliefs, aspirations, strengths, and limitations.

Just as we now recognize that simplistic perceptions of what a person from a particular culture believes or would choose are outmoded and unhelpful, it is important to bring that same depth of understanding to family cultures. The early and innovative enthusiasm for bringing awareness of cultural diversity into professional training and practice at times risked stereotyping individuals according to dominant and sometimes outmoded attitudes and behaviors. While "family" is an important part of every culture, the variants are many and rich. Think, for example, of blended families, gay and lesbian partnerships, multigenerational families, newly immigrant families, non-English-speaking families, adoptive families, single-parent-headed households, and more. "Cultural competence"–the ideal to which all health care professionals should aspire–should include the ability to explore and respond appropriately to these diverse relationships without preconceived ideas about them. This is especially critical in long-term care, which strains many families' cohesion and resources.

Despite their many differences, families, as fundamental units of society, are characterized by certain values, which are manifested in family caregiving, whether it takes place in the home or in a facility. Some of the primary values inherent in family caregiving are the importance of relationships established by blood, marriage, or commitment; a shared history, often involving several generations; except in extreme cases, the absence of public oversight or involvement; emotional rather than professional or financial rewards; moral rather than legal obligations; mutual expectations of support; flexible support structures; privacy of decision making; and family rather than individual autonomy. Except in a few cases, family members are not paid for their labor. Unlike professionals who have a broad knowledge base, but know a particular patient or client in the context of his presenting problem, families know a great deal about all aspects of the person's life and history but not very much about the specific problem or issue. They are both experts but in different ways.

Some patterns do transcend different ethnicity, religion, and other cultural factors. The obligation of families to care for their ill and elderly members appears to be deep in every tradition, but the implementation may be difficult and unsupported because of contemporary circumstances. One example is the changing role of women, even in traditional families. Another is intergenerational or acculturation differences. In these cases family caregivers not only experience dissonance with the formal structure but also with their own tradition. Professionals, and caregivers themselves, may assume that support will come from the family and community, but the reality may be quite different.

In contrast to family culture, the American health care system today is dominated by the culture of Western medicine: The primary values are scientific, evidence-based data; legal or regulatory oversight; efficiency; objectivity; consistency; confidentiality of medical information; technological solutions; hierarchical organizations; and individual patient autonomy. Professionals have special knowledge of a range of pertinent issues. They are trained to understand how a specific person fits into the context of other people with similar problems, and to devise solutions based on that knowledge.

Professional care providers (such as doctors, nurses, and social workers) get financial rewards and recognition, have professional associations and community standing. Of course, not all professionals obtain these rewards in equal measure. There is an obvious gap between the status of social workers and other professionals in the health care system. While social workers are typically the intermediaries among the actors at all levels of the system and have unique expertise of value to clients and families, their special skills are not those highest on society's reward scale. Sometimes these perceived and real inequities can negatively affect relationships with those even lower on the scale.

Paraprofessionals–the indispensable home health aides and Certified Nursing Assistants–are in between families and professionals. Home health aides work in the private domain of family life, but their jobs are directed and controlled by a hierarchy of professional interests. CNAs have the most direct and prolonged contact with nursing home residents, but they too are supervised and regulated by professional and governmental agents.

Within both the broad cultures of health care and family there are of course many distinctions. In medicine, cultures vary by specialty, institutional mission and leadership; training and socialization; type of population served; and the personal background of professionals. Nurses and social workers have different cultures, but both value personal communication and building relationships. In family caregiving, families differ by structure, ethnic background, socioeconomic class, religion, degree of collaboration or conflict, and stage of life course, among other factors.

PROFESSIONALS AS FAMILY MEMBERS

Professionals also come from families, many of them like the families they serve in their agencies or institutions. Having a common background or shared experience can certainly strengthen a professional's ability to understand a family's values and to communicate with them sensitively. Many families are more trusting of a professional who "speaks their language," whether that is literal or metaphorical.

However, a professional's family background and experience can also be a barrier. Unexamined assumptions–even prejudices–about what family members "should" do may hinder an objective assessment of the situation. Gender roles are particularly sensitive in this regard. Based on their own family history or community standards, professionals can subtly or not so subtly express their opinion that a wife should quit her job to take care of her ill husband, or that a daughter should bring her mother to live with her. It is not uncommon to hear professionals describing their culture as "valuing elders" when discussing a patient's family member who, in their view, is failing to take responsibility for an elder. The family member may be a person from their own culture, who is seen as not living up to (often idealized) community standards, or a person from another culture, which is seen as inferior to one's own in this regard. While pride in one's culture is admirable, it is important for professionals to refrain from imposing their own family values and experiences on their clients and patients.

The most significant factor that comes between professionals and families, however, is most likely the professional role itself. Acting as a professional social worker, physician, or nurse, one knows and fulfills the routines, rules, and behaviors that reflect one's training and mark one's status. When a professional is put into the role of family caregiver, however, he or she often finds the situation as stressful, as unpredictable, and as frustrating as a lay family member. A recent study (Chen, Rhodes and Green, 2001) of physicians whose fathers had been ill found that "the physicians expressed concern about the care their fathers received, believing that the system does not operate the way it should" (p. 763). One physician said, "The system really didn't give me someone who I could talk to, who would understand me, understand our family, and understand the issues" (p. 763). All of a sudden professional training and know-how vanish, and all the inadequacies and uncertainties of the fragmented, discontinuous health care system loom large. Sometimes these personal experiences alter for the better the professional's outlook and behavior in dealing with patients and families. However, training and habit are powerful influences resisting change.

Professionals are also subject to societal and cultural influences beyond their own discipline. If there is a gap between professionals and families, there is another gap that is arguably even deeper–between professionals (and to the degree their views are congruent, families) and policy makers. In the evolving health care economy professional values have been forced to adapt to the demands of the marketplace in health care, which is governed by a corporate or bureaucratic culture. While some of these strictures have been valuable in reducing waste and promoting consistency, there is an inevitable tension between the primary professional value of serving individuals and families, and the economic and institutional requirements to serve larger entities, including other beneficiaries, taxpayers, and stockholders.

The culture of social work is unique in that its very name affirms the individual's place within a social network, primarily the family and community. However, social work's special role has too often been subject to the culture of these other, more powerful professions and public agencies. Given appropriate recognition and resources, social work could lead the way in closing the gap between professional and family cultures, and in bringing the policy culture more in line with humanistic values.

THE CULTURE OF PUBLIC POLICY

The category of "health policy makers" may sound abstract, but it describes real people who shape the ways medical care and social services are delivered, paid for, and regulated. Health policy makers include elected officials, like members of Congress, state legislators, governors and the President; appointed officials, like the Administrator of the Center for Medicare and Medicaid Services (CMS, formerly the Health Care Financing Administration), state Medicaid directors; the political appointees and civil servants who work for all these categories; and managers in private organizations that contract with government agencies to administer public programs. Like other health care professionals, health policy makers also have a particular culture that governs their attitudes, assumptions, and values.[1]

The gap between professional and family cultures is perhaps best illustrated by the fundamentally different perspectives of policy makers and family caregivers. Policy makers create many of the rules, regulations, and practices that govern the relationships between professionals and family caregivers. It is not that policy makers do not care about families, or that they deliberately set out to create obstacles for them. It is simply that policy makers operate at a different level of principle, responsibility, and accountability.

A fundamental principle underlying health care policy, whether public or private, is that the legal beneficiary is an individual, not a family. Even a family member covered by the same program as an individual or a dependent is still considered a separate beneficiary. Family caregivers as family caregivers are not entitled to anything beyond what they might receive as individual beneficiaries. Furthermore, while many policy makers are concerned about promoting access to quality care, their focus is on the benefits the law provides to program beneficiaries as a class of individuals, not on the varied circumstances facing individual beneficiaries and their families. Their actions reflect their responsibility to balance the legal and fiscal integrity of programs with beneficiaries' access to care. In short, their perspective is very different from the perspective of family caregivers, which looks at the specific circumstances they find themselves in. The very actions which, viewed from the policymakers' perspective, are essential to responsible program administration may be experienced by caregivers as illogical or even perverse barriers to achieving the best and most comprehensive care for their ill relatives.

Given these incongruent basic assumptions and values, it is not surprising that specific rules and regulations emerging from the policy makers' primary perspectives often baffle beneficiaries and their family caregivers. Because most family caregiving takes place in the home, along with some short-term nursing home stays, this paper will focus on Medicare–the federal program for the elderly and some people with disabilities, and in particular on its home health policies. (Most private insurance policies follow Medicare relatively closely, and in many cases are not as generous as Medicare. When Medicare is the primary insurer, a secondary or Medigap private insurer will pick up co-pays and deductibles but will not pay for a service denied by Medicare.)

In trying to obtain Medicare home health benefits, beneficiaries and caregivers are often frustrated by rules that, from the family-centered culture, seem aimed at preventing them from getting the very benefits the programs, they believe, are supposed to provide. Here another fundamental distinction determining benefits sets the parameters. This is the difference between "skilled" and "unskilled" services. In order for a beneficiary to receive "unskilled" services, such as those provided by an aide, he or she must be determined to need "skilled" services, for example, those provided by a nurse. While these distinctions are clear to policy makers, they may make no sense at all to family caregivers, who view the care recipient's needs in their totality. Some of the tasks that are classified as "skilled," such as giving an injection, may seem much less taxing than the "unskilled" job of bathing a demented or paralyzed patient. Although the full set of supports is essential to a person with impairments, insurance is far more likely to cover the services that require professionally provided or medically related care than it is to cover "unskilled" support.

The reasons for this differential treatment are neither ignorance nor meanness. In fact, Medicare's statute, enacted in 1965, explicitly prohibits coverage of what is termed "custodial care." Although Medicare pays for some limited nursing home and home health care, the program's coverage policies reflect its focus on care needs directly associated with episodes of acute illness. As a result, even when Medicare home health coverage policies were at their most expansive, in the early 1990s, only about 10 percent of elderly beneficiaries with impairments in activities of daily living who were living at home were actually receiving Medicare home health benefits. Medicare's statutory and operational limitations reflect a general aversion to insuring custodial or personal care that is almost as strong in the policy culture today as it was in 1965. Policy makers are concerned that if insurance eliminates or substantially reduces the costs of service, people will use much more of it. Moreover, they believe more people will use it who did not do so before. People will, to use policy makers' common but demeaning complaint, "come out of the woodwork" to demand these services.

Making appropriate services available by reducing financial barriers is, of course, part of the purpose of insurance. But if the potential increase in use is perceived as poorly tied to any measurable concept of need and administratively difficult to manage, then policymakers fear that costs will become uncontrollable. If that happens, the program will be unaffordable and unacceptable to the taxpayers who must support it.

Concern about the health care system's ability to control the costs of existing public programs for health care and reluctance to take on new responsibilities may lead policymakers to overstate the degree of financial risk that insurance coverage for long-term care would actually pose. And patients' and families' reluctance to have a "stranger in the house" and many family care-givers' determination to "do it myself" may limit the extent to which family caregivers rely on formal services, even when they are made available.

Nevertheless, program management has operational and political costs. Operating a program means denying service to some who would like to receive it; limiting service to those who would like more service than the program is willing to provide; and committing to expenditures that, while perhaps not uncontrollable, are certainly not easy to control. Overall, then, the insurance protection that the caregiver culture views as an investment in financial relief and service support essential to quality of life is viewed in the policy and political culture as a fiscally and politically risky course of action that they might be foolish to undertake.

MEDICARE AND LONG-TERM CARE:
NURSES, AIDES, AND FAMILY CAREGIVERS

Policy makers' ideal beneficiary is a person with a clearly defined and time-limited need, an accepted and specific set of services to accommodate that need, and an easy way to make sure that the services have been delivered appropriately. This model does not fit well with long-term care, either at home or in a facility.

Many people who are eligible for Medicare–as well as their family care-givers–are surprised and dismayed to discover the limits to its protections when they need long-term care. Among the many frustrations caregivers face, perhaps the least comprehensible are the limits and barriers posed by Medicare coverage. People in need of long-term care have a range of service requirements. Some, like housekeeping or grocery shopping, require little specialized skills or training; others, like medication management or physical therapy, require professional-level expertise.

Policy makers, and society in general, exhibit a greater reluctance to bear the risks associated with long-term care than for medical care. That is partly because of a belief that long-term care is a family responsibility (Harrington, 2000), but it is also because of some fundamental differences between medical and long-term care. In medical care, policymakers can look to professional medical standards that, at least in theory, determine who gets what service. By contrast, in long-term care, much of the care is supportive and social in nature, and the links to overall health status and functioning are not always clear or well understood. The benefit may have more to do with improving quality of life than health status, and may not be easily measured or politically acceptable because of the American emphasis on individual and family, rather than communal, responsibility.

Under Medicare, home care typically does not even begin until a nurse has made an in-home evaluation visit and completed a comprehensive OASIS questionnaire. The nurse then recommends a plan of care and requests approval. When approval is received, another nurse will call to set up services. This process means that a patient discharged from a hospital goes home without any formal home care in place (unless it was there before). During the first overwhelming day or days, until home care begins, the family is left to manage as best they can. Some approvals can be expedited, but it is not uncommon for several days or a week to pass before services are started. If there is no family member, the patient may stay longer in the hospital, be sent to a nursing home for a short-term stay, or–possibly–get a home care plan approved while in the hospital. The presence of a presumably willing (and no one knows how able) family member in this way delay the initiation of services, since it is assumed that no emergency exists.

After approval is obtained, nurses are assigned to provide the skilled care and supervise home health aides. The aide may not even be present when they visit, or there may be different aides every week. Medicare and Medicaid pay for time to perform tasks, not build caring relationships. It is left to the aide to be a constant negotiator between the supervising nurse's instructions, regulatory and economic constraints, and the family's and patient's expectations. It is no wonder that it is becoming increasingly difficult to recruit and retain home care workers. Yet these paid workers are essential if the unpaid workers–the family members–are to be able to continue to both provide care and manage the host of their other responsibilities.

Aides paid for by Medicare typically are allowed two to three hours a day three to five days a week. Home health aide care is allowed only when there is a need for "intermittent, part-time, skilled" care–in other words, not for long periods. Medicaid can be more generous or stingier, depending on the state and county or city. This kind of episodic assistance, while certainly valuable, turns family caregivers into de facto care managers, making sure the aide arrives, knows her job, is a caring and honest person. Home care agencies require a family member to attest that someone will be the "responsible party" in case there is a lapse in their service. This warning is not reassuring to family members, even though the lapse may never happen.

The relationship between home care nurses and nurses' aides and family members can be especially problematic because boundaries of what aides can and cannot do, and by different conceptions of privacy and decision making are often unclear. Here is one instance in which "cultural differences" in the sense of different language, religions, food preferences, customs, and so on really do make a difference. Respecting these differences in the context of home care can be difficult, because so many aides are from minority and immigrant groups and so many care recipients are elderly and demented and uninhibited about declaring their prejudices. But this is not simply a question of race or ethnicity. The United Hospital Fund-Visiting Nurse Service-Harvard School of Public Health survey of New York City caregivers found that African-American and Latino caregivers were twice as likely to report that they were "worried about abuse or neglect" from home health aides, who are largely from the same groups, as were white respondents (Levine et al., 2000).

Although family caregivers and home care aides often complain bitterly (and often justifiably) about each other, they are both relatively powerless in the system. Although aides are paid, their wages are low, their jobs insecure, and their working conditions are often very difficult. Many proprietary home health agencies started out as suppliers of temporary institutional help, and this outlook exists in assigning and training home care aides. This history has influenced the industry's development as many agencies have created a cadre of "temp" workers, presumably interchangeable and able to do designated tasks equally well. A system that may work in a facility as on-site supervisors monitor the work does not necessarily work at home, where there is no trained supervisor and the care is highly personal. As temporary and part-time workers, home care aides in general have not had the career benefits, job security, or training opportunities would be available to full-time, long-term workers doing the same job.

Both the home care aide and the family are invisible. At a meeting the author attended on home care, a physician showed a photograph of the "home care team"; it included a nurse, social worker, physical and occupational therapists, dietician, medical student, and no doubt a few more individuals. The two people who were closest to the patient and who carried out all the others' orders were literally not in the picture: the family caregiver and the home health aide.

Home health aides and CNAs experience many difficulties in their work. Complex family situations, unclear expectations of care responsibilities, administering painful or difficult care all are potential areas of conflict. Home health aides are often sent into situations for which they are not prepared, and left to cope on their own with these stresses when problems arise (Blaine, 2000). Carol Ann Young, who cared for her mother with Alzheimer's disease, calculated that her mother had 23 different home care aides in six months, most of them kind and caring but untrained for the job of dealing with an increasingly hostile and suspicious woman. "They needed a support group as much as I did," she said (Young, 2000). Formalized support systems are rare, although welcomed by the aides when they do exist.

Sometimes home health aides' personal lives spill over into their jobs, creating situations in which patients or family members are asked to make loans, tolerate visitors, not report lateness or absences because the aide herself had a family emergency. Especially where the aide is valued and liked, these requests are often honored, even when they exceed reasonable limits. Nevertheless, patients and aides–and sometimes family caregivers as well–can form strong bonds and caring relationships.

LONG-TERM CARE IN THE LARGER HEALTH CARE SYSTEM

Long-term care is increasingly becoming part of the larger health care world, not a separate entity with only loose ties to other health care institutions. Part of this change is a result of mergers and system building, in which various levels of care are brought together–often quite loosely–under one overall management. Part of this change is the increasing use of long-term care facilities for short-term rehabilitation. Each of these loosely connected entities has its own culture–its way of doing work–and patients and family members going from one site to another often encounter very different attitudes, behaviors, and expectations. Sometimes there are value clashes in these new arrangements, but in one regard, there is consistency. Treatment of family caregiving as free labor is a prominent value in both acute and long-term care. Changes in the health care system that have shortened stays in hospitals, for example, have relied on family members to provide care at home that used to be provided by hospital staff. Even during hospital stays, families are expected (or are forced by the shortage of staff) to provide many kinds of basic care. The result is reduced hospital expenses but increased family burdens. From society's perspective, this is a tradeoff we might choose to make. However, the existence of a tradeoff–the family costs that offset savings from shorter hospital stays–is poorly understood and rarely addressed.

In long-term care, the benefits of reducing family burdens are given short shrift. Indeed, the policy culture seems to view caregiving for impaired family members as a responsibility that families not only have to but also *ought* to cope with, with minimal if any public support. As long as the policy culture's basic presumption is that family responsibility is open-ended and unlimited, policy is likely to regard support for caregivers as unwise rather than a prudent investment. The fundamental questions that must be raised to bring the policy and caregiver cultures together is: Are we willing to spread the risks of caregiving? Is it the job of family members to bear full responsibility for the care of their own? Or is the job of society to "insure" family members as well as people with impairments against the burdens associated with long-term care? And, if we are willing to share those burdens–to spread the risk–how will we balance families' need for support against taxpayers' concern with expenditures?

CLOSING THE CULTURE GAP

What does the future hold? Gradually the family caregiver is coming out of the shadows. How the still-developing movement to respond to the needs of family caregivers will grow, and what it will select as its key agenda items, remains to be seen. However, unless the cultures of the various key actors can overcome their differences and stress their shared commitment to loving, competent care, the gaps will remain.

In this shift, social work can be a leading partner by fulfilling its original mission of helping individuals and families through a difficult time in their lives and by exposing and redressing social inequities. Social workers historically have had the skills and broad outlook that is necessary to close this gap. While this effort will not be easy, it is essential for the profession and for the people whom it serves.

NOTE

1. I gratefully acknowledge the assistance of Judy Feder of Georgetown University in developing this section. It will appear in a different form in a forthcoming volume, tentatively titled "The Cultures of Caregiving: Families, Health Care Professionals, and Public Policy."

REFERENCES

Blaine, M. (2000). Relieving stress: A short-term support group for home attendants. *Care Management Journals*, 2 (3):190-195.

Chen, F., Rhodes, L.A. & Green, L.A. (2001). Family physicians' personal experiences of their fathers' health care. *Journal of Family Practice* 50:9; 762-766.

Harrington, M. (2000). *Care and Equality.* New York: Routledge.

Kinney, J.M., & Stephens, M.P. (1989). Caregiving Hassles Scale: Assessing the daily hassles of caring for a family member with dementia. *The Gerontologist* 29(3):328-332.

Levine, C., Kuerbis, A., Gould, D.A., Navaie-Waliser, M., Feldman, P.H., & Donelan, K. (2000). A Survey of Family Caregivers in New York City: Findings and Implications for the Health Care System. New York: United Hospital Fund.

Levine, C., & Zuckerman, C. (1999). The trouble with families: Toward an ethic of accommodation. *Ann Intern Med*; 130:148-152.

Young, C. (2000). First my mother, then my aunt. In C. Levine, ed. *Always On Call: When Illness Turns Families into Caregivers*. New York: United Hospital Fund, p. 28.

Pioneer Network:
Changing the Culture of Aging
in America

Rose Marie Fagan

SUMMARY. The Pioneer Network is a national grass roots network of individuals in the field of aging, working for deep systemic change through both evolutionary and revolutionary means, using Pioneer values and principles as the foundations for change. Pioneers are individuals who work in residential long-term care settings and community based settings, in government, research, advocacy and education whose goal is to seed and cultivate a new culture of aging. In-depth change in systems requires transformation of individual and societal attitudes toward aging and elders, transformation of elders' attitudes toward themselves and their aging, changes in the attitudes and behavior of caregivers toward those for whom they care and changes in

Rose Marie Fagan is the Executive Director of the Pioneer Network. In addition, she is the Director of the Nursing Home Culture Change Project at LIFESPAN of Greater Rochester, New York.

Address correspondence to: Rose Marie Fagan, Executive Director, Pioneer Network, P.O. Box 18648, Rochester, NY 14618 <Website: PioneerNetwork.net> (E-mail: RoseMarie.Fagan@PioneerNetwork.net).

The author wishes to acknowledge the editorial assistance of many Pioneer Network board members.

[Haworth co-indexing entry note]: "Pioneer Network: Changing the Culture of Aging in America." Fagan, Rose Marie. Co-published simultaneously in *Journal of Social Work in Long-Term Care* (The Haworth Social Work Practice Press, an imprint of The Haworth Press, Inc.) Vol. 2, No. 1/2, 2003, pp. 125-140; and: *Culture Change in Long-Term Care* (ed: Audrey S. Weiner, and Judah L. Ronch) The Haworth Social Work Practice Press, an imprint of The Haworth Press, Inc., 2003, pp. 125-140. Single or multiple copies of this article are available for a fee from The Haworth Document Delivery Service [1-800-HAWORTH, 9:00 a.m. - 5:00 p.m. (EST). E-mail address: docdelivery@haworthpress.com].

governmental policy and regulation. Pioneers refer to this work as *culture change*.

While maintaining its work to recreate nursing homes, the Pioneer Network has expanded its vision, mission and focus to encourage and facilitate culture change values, principles and person-centered approaches across the whole continuum of aging services and elder living, from independent living at home to more traditional long-term care options.

In its first six years, without a formal infrastructure and largely fueled by the Pioneers' volunteer activities, the Network has been a catalyst for positive change and outcomes in the aging field across the country. *[Article copies available for a fee from The Haworth Document Delivery Service: 1-800-HAWORTH. E-mail address: <docdelivery@haworthpress.com> Website: <http://www.HaworthPress.com> © 2003 by The Haworth Press, Inc. All rights reserved.]*

KEYWORDS. Pioneer Network, culture change, values and principles, pioneering approaches, meaningful life and work, positive outcomes, champions of change

INTRODUCTION

Several significant facts create the urgency for culture change in aging and led to the formation of the Pioneer Network. First, more Americans are living longer. The growth in older American populations creates an urgent need for transformation of the experience of aging in America. Aging adults, including the millions of aging baby boomers, are looking for a different paradigm of aging in which life continues to have meaning whether they live independently, in a group setting or in a nursing home. To live meaningful lives, elders must have dignity, choice and self-determination. The issues surrounding late life–nursing home care and other living situations for elders, service delivery, societal attitudes, even death and dying–are complex and reflect our very culture.

In American history and culture there is a deep ambivalence regarding old age. On the one hand, there is the desire for respect and honor. On the other hand, there is disparagement as elders are seen as non-productive burdens, non-contributors to society or the economy, and merely consumers of costly health care. There is plenty of good evidence that this is not true, but Americans fear aging as a time of dependency and loss. Aging is often seen as a downward life change. Many elders themselves, as they become frail and more dependent, are apt to believe they are past their prime and no longer useful.

Wellness and illness are on a continuum. People who are very ill can be enormously contributory to society provided we remove the barriers of prejudice that prevent this from occurring more regularly. The overwhelming response to *Tuesdays with Morrie* is a recent example of the need we all have to learn from those who precede us, both of their take on life as well as their preparing us for our own challenging future experiences. (Unsino, 2000a)

In nursing homes, assisted living facilities and adult day programs, we supply our elders with the necessities of survival, but they are too often deprived of the necessities of living. Elders become objects of care services–disenfranchised by the regimes of service. Their caregivers are underpaid and also under valued.

The quest for meaning, relationship and participation doesn't diminish in latter years. It becomes more urgent. (Unsino, 2000b)

The Pioneer Network promotes the national movement to turn late life into a resource for elders themselves and for other generations. It is dedicated to the regeneration of the worth of elders to society as a whole. The work of transformation is not just for the sake of our elders; it is for the sake of society itself (Stein, 2001).

The Pioneer Network is a national grass roots network of individuals in the field of aging, dedicated to addressing needs and issues of aging. Pioneers are individuals who work in residential long-term care settings and community based settings, in government, research, advocacy and education whose goal is to seed and cultivate a new culture of aging. The Network's vision is to create in America "a culture of aging that is life-affirming, satisfying, humane and meaningful" (Pioneer Network, 2001).

This Pioneer vision addresses the whole continuum of living for elders, from independent living to skilled, long-term care, and all levels in between. The Pioneer Network recognizes the need to create ways of living and working together in open, diverse, caring communities that are radically different from traditional approaches.

Pioneers are working for deep systemic change through both evolutionary and revolutionary means, using pioneer values and principles as the foundations for change. In-depth change in systems requires transformation of individual and societal attitudes toward aging and elders, transformation of elders' attitudes toward themselves and their aging, changes in the attitudes and behavior of caregivers toward those for whom they care, and changes in governmental policy and regulation. Pioneers refer to this work as *culture change.*

The Pioneer Network has become a catalyst for creative change and transformation in the current American culture as it responds to aging by:

- facilitating communication, networking and learning opportunities;
- building and supporting relationships and community;
- identifying, promoting and facilitating transformations in practice, services, public policy and research and
- developing and providing access to resources and leadership.

The overall objective is to create a critical mass of individuals and organizations that are implementing such change.

> Without the Network, I would quit my work in health care as I would feel there is no avenue or group working together to change the culture of aging, that is challenging the status quo that is serving our elders so poorly. Without some group–the Network–holding out a vision and values, we are lost. (Rader, 2000)

HISTORY OF THE PIONEER NETWORK

Institutional long-term care was the entry point for the Pioneer Network. It is an especially potent point of entry because the nursing home is essentially a microcosm of our country's culture of aging and of our social and economic problems. In it, we see demonstrated the devaluation of aged people and of those who care for them. In both groups, most are women and most are poor. We see the loss of control, loss of choice and the loss of relationships that too often characterize late life in America as well as the separation of the generations from each other. And we see the dynamics of death and dying in America, characterized by avoidance and isolation.

Pioneers have been changing the way in which residents and staff live and work together in nursing homes because of concerns about the quality of life in even our most highly regarded traditional nursing homes. All over the country, pioneers have begun to create places for living and growing rather than for declining and dying.

Frustrated by having to work within the current nursing home culture, characterized by high staff turnover and resident loneliness, isolation and serious depression, and believing that there is another, better way to support elders in their last "home," Pioneers in the long-term care field began to systemically change the values, practices and culture of their facilities. In pockets across the country, four Pioneering approaches were born. While several Pioneers began their individual work in the 1970s, the networking began in the 1990s.

FOUR PIONEER APPROACHES

Each of these individuals who have become known as the early Pioneers began with the experience of the resident. Barry and Debby Barkan, of El Sorbrante, California developed *The Regenerative Community* as an antidote to institutionalization in 1977. For them, the experience of the resident was isolation, disconnectedness and a life without meaning. They demonstrated in a variety of settings throughout the continuum of elder life that a consciously conceived community can bring meaning and connection by providing to all who are involved a structure for belonging, a collective voice, an opportunity to grow and develop, and to be of service to peers (Barkan, 1995).

Charlene Boyd, administrator, and Bob Ogden, former administrator, of Providence Mount St. Vincent, in Seattle, Washington, surveyed their residents in 1990 and learned that what they missed most were their kitchens, which they regarded as the heart of the home, and control over their own decisions. *Resident-Directed Care* restores control and decision making to the resident. The organization flattened its hierarchy and traditional units were transformed into neighborhoods with country kitchens and a home environment. By decentralizing systems such as food service and laundry delivery, The Mount brought familiar, daily activities back into residents' lives (Boyd, 1994).

Joanne Rader, MSN, from Silverton, Oregon, noted that residents give up routines that are comfortable and familiar when they enter a nursing home. Her approach, *Individualized Care*, promotes the resident as a unique individual and advocates maintaining a person's familiar routines. She is especially recognized for her advocacy of restraint free care and the bathing of residents in a manner that is comfortable and familiar to them (Rader, 1996).

Bill and Judy Thomas, of Sherburne, New York identified that the three plagues of a nursing home are loneliness, helplessness and boredom. Their approach, *The Eden Alternative*, creates a healthy human habitat that is both socially and biologically diverse. Plants, animals and children restore spontaneity to daily life and encourage relationships. Residents contribute to life and are not just the recipient of services (Thomas, 1996).

Each of these Pioneers discusses their model in Section 2 of this volume.

FIRST GATHERING

Carter Catlett Williams played a key role in developments leading to the first gathering of Pioneers. As a social work consultant, she had worked closely with the National Citizen's Coalition for Nursing Home Reform (NCCNHR) and was one of the national leaders in the movement toward restraint-free care. She had first studied this approach in a Swedish nursing home that provided her initial encounter with culture change. Through her writing and speaking around the nation on care without physical or chemical restraint, she began to meet a few people who were thinking and practicing in radically different ways (Williams, 1989, 1990, 1994). What they were doing was closely related to the approach she had seen in Sweden, and she began to tell them about each other, expressing the hope that they could meet and talk together.

Sarah Greene Burger, Director of Program and Policy for NCCNHR, invited Barkan, Boyd, Rader and Thomas to speak at the annual meeting of the organization in the fall of 1995 in Washington, DC. The interest of these four trailblazers in coming together for a time of further analysis and discussion was finally realized in 1997.

In March 1997, through the efforts of Rose Marie Fagan and Carter Williams, leaders of the four pioneering approaches met in Rochester, New York. The other 28 invited participants, drawn from across the nation as well as the local area, represented regulators, nursing home administrators and directors of nursing, social workers, advocates, researchers and people in the legal field seeking change in long-term care. LIFESPAN, a not-for-profit agency in Rochester, New York whose sole mission is to provide advocacy, education and direct service to older adults, facilitated the meeting.

The goals of the meeting as set out by the funder, The Daisy Marquis Jones Foundation, were to find the common elements and values of these approaches, identify obstacles, define indicators of change and provide guidance for research and evaluation of outcomes (Fagan, Williams and Burger, 1997). During more than three days of intensive and rigorous discussion, participants harvested the essential qualities of the four Pioneering approaches to nursing home culture change and the common values and principles that formed the framework for culture change work.

Participants recognized that meaningful and lasting change can only occur when all players are involved, and the change is deep and systemic. On the gathering's final day the decision was made to continue to meet semi-annually in different regions of the country to find kindred spirits, grow the network and promote the movement. As one attendee exclaimed: "I feel like I have found my lost tribe" (see Table 1).

TABLE 1. Pioneer Vision, Mission, Values and Principles

Vision:

The Pioneer Network envisions a culture of aging that is life affirming, satisfying, humane and meaningful.

Mission:

The Network advocates and facilitates deep system change in our culture of aging.

Values and Principles:

We commit to the following values and principles as the heart of all culture change work within the diversity of elder living and aging:

- Know each person
- Each person can and does make a difference
- Relationship is the fundamental building block of a transformed culture
- Respond to spirit, as well as mind and body
- Risk taking is a normal part of life
- Put person before task
- All elders are entitled to self-determination wherever they live
- Community is the antidote to institutionalization
- Do unto others as you would have them do unto you
- Promote the growth and development of all
- Shape and use the potential of the environment in all its aspects: physical, organizational, psycho/social/spiritual
- Practice self-examination, searching for new creativity and opportunities for doing better
- Recognize that culture change and transformation are not destinations but a journey, always a work in progress

---

GROWTH OF THE PIONEER NETWORK

At the next gathering, the original group was joined by forty others from around the nation who believed in this vision of culture change and the Network was born. LIFESPAN became the incubator, providing leadership and coordination to the movement. Subsequent gatherings offered the opportunity for the participants to explore how to work together on the goal of putting values and principles they held in common, into practical, day-to-day changes in how care is regulated, delivered and received.

In 2000, recognizing that some clients feel institutionalized by the system in their own homes and how they don't want to be viewed as a "case that is managed," the Pioneers broadened the organization's focus and changed the organization's name from Nursing Home Pioneers to the Pioneer Network. The broader implications of aging in America required that although the Network would continue its work to re-create long-term care, Pioneers needed to take on the mission of making a positive change in the entire culture of aging.

In 2001, The Pioneer Network incorporated and received tax exempt status as a 501 (C) (3) and elected its first board of directors. In 2002, the organization began to seek foundation funding to hire staff and develop a plan to sustain itself. Its primary activities are education, consultation and research.

The Pioneer Network hosted two major national conferences in Rochester, New York: *From "Frustration to Pride"* and *"Everything Challenged Everything Gained."* Each was attended by over 300 participants from 28 states and Australia. The third, *"Becoming A Champion of Change: Transforming Eldercare and Our Own Aging"* was scheduled for summer 2002 in Chicago, Illinois with major funding support from The Hulda B. and Maurice L. Rothschild Foundation, Retirement Research Foundation, The Commonwealth Fund and Mather LifeWays. The purpose of this conference was to identify leaders in the field of aging, to mobilize them and to create networks to expedite culture change. In addition, the Network has established a web site, PioneerNetwork.net, a speakers' bureau, and has begun developing a central clearinghouse. Network publications are also widely disseminated (Fagan, Williams, and Burger, 1997; Lustbader, 2000; Williams, 2001).

THE PIONEER MOVEMENT AND NETWORK AS A CATALYST FOR CHANGE

In its first six years, without a formal infrastructure and largely fueled by the Pioneers' volunteer activities, the impact of the Pioneer movement has been experienced throughout the country. A sampling of the rippling effect of the Pioneer movement and Network, based on anecdotal reports, includes:

- Eight states are in varying stages of forming networks for culture change;
- Increase in long-term care facilities starting on the path to culture change;
- Several multi-facility organizations have committed their homes to culture change, among them are Apple Health Care, Avon, CT and The Evangelical Lutheran Good Samaritan Society;
- Research, looking at new ways of gathering and feeding back information about culture change outcomes, is being conducted (Dannefer & Stein, 1999, 2002);
- Regulators are starting to take notice of and developing interest in long-term care transformation. The Center for Medicare and Medicaid Services is producing a video about the Pioneer Network values, principles and practices for surveyors in the country;
- Improved quality and retention of front-line workers.

PRACTICES THAT EXPRESS PIONEER VALUES AND PRINCIPLES

Table 2 contrasts the practices of the cultures of the medical model and the community model.

> I just feel like a nobody . . . they are very nice to me . . . it's always clean . . . Life for me, as far as being comfortable, couldn't be better, you know, if I just wanted to sit around and do nothing. I'm told what to do and when to do it. I'm very well fed and I'm comfortable, but that's not living. (Dannefer and Stein, 1999)

These are the words of a nursing home resident. But they reflect the lives and the feelings of many elders in our communities, wherever they live. Contrast them with the words of a social worker who puts Pioneer values and principles into practice.

> There's a general tendency to see elders primarily as having problems and as being frail. I believe that despite those losses, there is something else–that essence is there. We just have to uncover it–go through the layers to find it, and hope to develop this relationship with each person–a partnership–to rediscover meaning in life. (Meyers, 2001)

Culture change seeks to transform life in all its aspects. Behavioral symptoms are viewed as the interaction of a person's feelings with the external, physical, psycho-social and organizational environment in which he or she lives.

TABLE 2. Practices That Express Pioneer Values and Principles

Medical Model Culture	Community Model Culture
Staff provide traditional care and "treatments"	Individualized care that nurtures the human spirit
Residents follow facility and staff routine	Staff follow resident's routine
Staff rotate	Consistent assignments
Staff make decisions for residents	Residents make their own decisions
Facility belongs to staff	Facility belongs to residents
Structured activities	Spontaneous activities around the clock
Departmental focus	TEAM focus
Staff know resident by diagnosis	Staff have personal relationships with the resident

Reprinted with permission of Susan Misiorski, Long Term Care Operations Specialist for Paraprofessional Healthcare Institute.

For example:

- The organization and daily operations are restructured to support relationships between elders and workers who care for them.
- Residents are making their own decisions about diet, when to get up or go to bed, activities and bathing.
- The experience of bathing through individualization and exploration of a variety of ways to maintain cleanliness is becoming one of comfort and pleasure for residents. The practice of bathing people against their will and having them scream, fight and beg their way through baths is no longer considered a "normal" and "necessary" practice in facilities involved in culture change.
- Transforming facilities are implementing individualized care practices, including care plans written from the resident perspective, the "I" format, where the resident speaks directly to the caregiver about her/his care.
- Meal times are changing to family style dining and other alternative methods that maintain the way and the times that residents dined in their own homes.
- Front-line caregivers, who know the residents best, are participating in care planning.
- Certified Nursing Assistants, with residents, participate in interviewing candidates for positions.
- Certified Nursing Assistants are serving as presenters in conferences and forums and as teachers in CNA training classes.
- Career ladders are providing front-line workers with opportunities to advance within their chosen profession.
- Community meetings create new opportunities for relationships, exploring common interests and goals. The meetings are utilized to provide residents, including those with dementia, with a regular forum to help connect with the world around them, their pasts and their futures, and wrestle with common problems.
- Pets and plants contribute to spontaneity in daily life.
- New and/or renovated buildings are developing alternative design models creating neighborhoods and households versus institutional units and long double-hung hallways.
- Facilities are changing the rituals around death and dying. In culture change, the community celebrates the life of the resident who has died and has the opportunity to say good bye in a bedside memorial service. In the medical model, death is a clinical experience without acknowledgment of meaning and relationship. In effect, the one who died essentially just "disappeared."

The values and principles at Fairport Baptist Homes in Fairport, New York, include believing in the sanctity of life and sacredness of death. My personal experience illustrates how the staff at Fairport put that value into practice with a Bedside Memorial Service for deceased residents.

> My mother lived at Fairport only for a brief few months before her death on February 21, 2000, my birthday. Our family was with her when she died. Staff encouraged us to stay with her as long as we wanted and gave us privacy. When we were ready, a bell was chimed three times over the intercom system to inform other staff and residents throughout the house that a resident had died. After the third chime, my mother's name was given, *Yolanda Capanna*.

> Within 10 minutes, staff and residents gathered in my mother's room with us for a brief prayer service that was led by a member of her household staff. After prayers, staff and residents shared their memories of my mother. Our family was amazed at how well they had come to know her during her brief time there. This occasion gave our family an opportunity to express our thanks for the care and friendship she experienced while living there. We thanked them for making us feel part of her life there. We were especially grateful to staff for making it possible for us to enjoy our final Thanksgiving and Christmas with her at our home. This was a gift to us, and we owed it to the staff for the care she received.

> As staff and residents left the room, they approached my mother's bedside to say their good-byes to her. This was like calling hours in a funeral home and was an important and meaningful experience for all who participated.

> Next, my mother's body was draped in a beautiful embroidered shroud. Staff and family accompanied her to the side door where the hearse was parked.

> My family and I found this ritual respectful and dignified. It gave family, staff and residents the opportunity to bring some closure to her life at Fairport Baptist Homes. But most of all, the Bedside Memorial Service honored the humanity in all of us. (Fagan, 2000)

POSITIVE OUTCOMES

"Despite the lack of research on culture or its relationship to outcomes in long term care, culture change initiatives have been implemented in the hopes of improving both work and care quality" (Bowers, 2001). Long-term care facilities that are transforming themselves through Pioneer culture change approaches report that they are experiencing positive changes in resident quality of life. Most of the data are anecdotal and have been collected from Apple Health Care, Avon, CT; Crestview Nursing Home, Bethany, MO; Evergreen Retirement Community, Oshkosh, WI; Fairport Baptist Homes, Fairport, NY; Lakewood Rehab and Nursing Center, Milwaukee, WI; Live Oak Living Center, El Sorbante, CA; Providence Benedictine Nursing Center, Marian Estates, Sublimity, OR; Providence Mount St. Vincent, Seattle, WA; Teresian House Nursing Home, Albany, NY.

For example, there is reduced use of resident medications, including antipsychotic medications for behavioral symptoms related to dementia. That disengaged "nursing home look" disappears from resident faces–you can see that they are more involved in life. People who haven't talked in years begin to talk. Families are involved in meaningful ways.

Costs are lowered because homes are reducing or eliminating the use of agency staff. Staff turnover is reduced, and there is less absenteeism. Homes report a higher occupancy rate; most have waiting lists. Other outcomes which have been reported, many of which are detailed in the case study (Section 3) of this volume, include:

- A more positive reputation in the community
- Increased levels of resident activity, most notable in specialized care units, including units for people with dementia
- Greater continuity in personal relationships, resulting in improved quality of resident life
- Reduction in the number of special diets
- Reductions in all categories of incidents (falls, fractures, skin wounds) and in weight loss and dehydration
- Less depression
- Stability in health and Activities of Daily Living indicators
- Increased resident mobility; residents demonstrating a willingness to "do for themselves"
- Lower resident mortality
- Front-line caregivers with increased positive feelings about their work
- Increased recognition on the part of staff that for residents visits with family and friends and choices in their schedules are a *first priority*
- Greater resident involvement in decision making
- Increased resident, staff and family satisfaction
- Increased intergenerational contact and understanding in facilities that have incorporated children in day care and school children as intentional visitors
- Reduced state survey deficiencies
- Increased private pay census

RESEARCH AND EVALUATION

A three-year study, from 1998-2001 (Dannefer and Stein, 1999, 2002) of two nursing homes in Rochester, New York, was funded by the New York State Department of Health and the van Ameringen Foundation. The evaluation of the culture change effort was focused on two fundamental questions: (1) *Does the intention to bring about culture change actually lead to a changed culture,* and (2) *To the extent that culture change does occur, what are the consequences for staff and residents?*

Culture was evaluated by several dimensions, including: (a) level of activity and social interaction; (b) shared knowledge; and (c) shared sense of residential belonging. Staff change was evaluated by means of a survey concerning job commitment and work stress, through informal interviews, and by measuring staff turnover. Resident change was evaluated by means of health, mortality and identity coherence on the individual level, and by data from incident reports on the collective level.

Substantial culture change was documented by researchers at one or both facilities by the following indicators:

- Relationship-building among and between staff and residents, facilitated by (1) use of continuous assignment policy and (2) aging in place (eliminating the requirement that residents move to a different floor when their needs change)
- Increased amounts of social activity; decreased amount of residents asleep, completely inactive or agitated
- Evidence of "ownership of space" and sharing of life experiences across individuals, both staff and residents

Several indices of resident health and well-being and of staff attitudes and behavior support the hypothesis that positive culture change has beneficial consequences for residents and staff. With regard to residents, these include

- Identity coherence–enhanced ability to integrate present life with a resident's sense of life history
- Incidents (fractures, falls, etc.) decreased over the time of the project
- Mortality also decreased over the time of the project
- Greater levels of interaction with family members

With regard to staff, these include:

- Enhanced staff concern with residents' self-expressed needs and concerns
- Substantially reduced staff turnover

GETTING STARTED

Culture change begins within ourselves. "We must become the change we want to see in the world" (Ghandi, 1869-1948). The process in long-term care, for example, begins with education about culture change values, the change process and journeys of others on the path. The work is about learning to align an organization's practices with the Pioneer values and principles. Organization leaders must own the vision and be totally committed. This cannot be only a top-down approach. Everyone must be involved in the process of writing the vision, mission and values statements for the organization. Residents, staff, family members and leadership together must assess daily practices to be certain that practice expresses values. This requires looking at practice in every aspect of the organization including: admission, hiring, staff orientation, food service, bathing, aging in place, staff assignments, resident schedules, and death and dying (see Table 2). Culture is an organic, on-going process that has the potential for change, growth and development. There is no "cookie cutter" way to turn an organization around. Each facility must develop its own non-prescriptive approach that recognizes the existing culture and its implications for administrators, staff, residents and families.

> Aging baby boomers find the 19th century culture of aging service organizations to be obsolete. And a 21st century work force cannot thrive under the yoke of 19th century supervision and management practices. (Unsino, 2000c)

Therefore, each home sets out on its own journey, entering the path at varying points. While most in the Pioneer Network believe it is prudent to begin with small changes so staff can see and celebrate successes and feel comfortable taking risks, there is a growing opinion that the deep systemic change needed can best be achieved through more radical approaches. Whether one advocates an incremental or more radical initial approach, there is one point of agreement: It is necessary to rigorously re-orient the organization's compass over and over again to the new vision, values and principles. This is most successfully achieved when management encourages the voices of residents and staff and organic positive change. Once a home begins to make changes in the way staff and residents live and work together, the challenge is to change all systems to support this new way. The journey continues by always asking "how can we do it better," while continuing to enjoy the journey and celebrate successes along the way.

BECOMING CHAMPIONS OF CHANGE

Anyone who ascribes to the principles and values of the Pioneer Network is encouraged to become involved in the movement. Pioneers are individuals not seeking membership, but *opportunities* to grow their skills, and enhance the effectiveness of the work of culture change.

Culture change is going to happen. It is the right thing to do. Baby boomers are coming along and will drive change as consumers and as residents. Most of us, if we are really honest, do not want the current system for ourselves, let alone our loved ones. If we work to create something new, we can create something that will meet everyone's needs. The outcomes are so positive that we believe the Pioneer Network–cultural transformation–gives hope to people in an industry that is feeling very defeated.

REFERENCES

Barkan, Barry. (1995). *The Regenerative Community: The Live Oak Living Center and the Quest for Autonomy, Self-esteem, and Connection in Elder Care.* In *Enhancing Autonomy in Long Term Care*, Gamroth, L., Semradek, J. Tornquist, E. (Eds). New York: Springer Publishing Co.

Bowers, Barbara. (November 2001). University Wisconsin-Madison, School of Nursing "Organizational Change and Workforce Development in Long Term Care," paper prepared for Technical Expert Panel Meeting, Washington, DC.

Boyd, Charlene. (1994). Residents First. *Health Progress*, 75 (7): 34-39, 50.

Dannefer, Dale, & Stein, Paul. (1999). Warner Graduate School, University of Rochester, Rochester, New York, "Systematic Change in Long Term Care." Report to the NYS Department of Health.

Dannefer, Dale, & Stein, Paul. (2002). Warner Graduate School, University of Rochester, Rochester, New York, "From The Top to the Bottom, From the Bottom to the Top: Systemically Changing the Culture of Nursing Homes" Report to the van Ameringen Foundation.

Fagan, Rose Marie. (March, 2000). American Society on Aging Conference, San Diego, California, "Pioneering Approaches in Long-Term Care."

Fagan, Rose Marie, Williams, Carter & Burger, Sarah. (March 1997). *Meeting of Pioneers in Nursing Home Culture Change.*

Ghandi, Mahatma, 1869-1948, aphorism attributed to Ghandi.

Lustbader, Wendy. (March 2000). *The Pioneer Challenge: A radical change in the culture of nursing homes.* In Noelker, L.S. & Harel, Z. (Eds.), *Qualities of caring: Impact on quality of life.* New York: Springer Publishing Company.

Meyers, Sandy. (November 2001). Jewish Home and Hospital, Bronx, New York, in taped discussion with Mrs. Beatrice Taishoff about her Ethical Will. Mrs. Taishoff is 99 years old and lives in the Jewish Home.

Pioneer Network Brochure, *Vision Statement*, 2001.

Rader, Joanne. (January 2000). Personal conversation.

Rader, Joanne. (1996). Maintaining Cleanliness: An Individualized Approach. *The Journal of Gerontological Nursing*, 22 (3): 32-38.

Stein, Paul. (August 2001). Warner Graduate School, University of Rochester, Rochester, New York, personal conversation.

Thomas, William. (1996). *Life Worth Living*, Acton, MA: VanderWyk & Burnham.

Unsino, Catherine. (April 2000a). Keynote: Culture Change in Aging, First New York State Conference on Alzheimer's Disease, sponsored by the NYS Department of Health and Eddy Alzheimers. Albany, New York.

Unsino, Catherine. (September 2000b). Edna Gates Annual Conference on Alzheimer's Disease, Keynote: "Meaningful Living with Alzheimer's Disease." Detroit, Michigan.

Unsino, Catherine. (April 2000c). "Elders and the 21st Century Workforce: The Culture Change Imperative," Public Policy Forum for PANPHA administrators, Harrisburg, Pennsylvania.

Williams, C.C. (1989). *The Experience of Long-term Care in the Future. The Journal of Gerontological Social Work*, 14 (1/2), 3-18.

Williams, C.C. (1990). *Long Term Care and the Human Spirit, Generations*, XIV (4): 25-28.

Williams, C.C. (1994). *Days and Years in Long-term Care: Living versus Surviving, Journal of Geriatric Psychiatry*, xxvii (1): 97-112.

Williams, Carter Catlett. (March 2001). *Relationship Is the Heart of Care.*

SECTION 2
MODELS OF CULTURE CHANGE
IN LONG-TERM CARE

Evolution of Eden

William H. Thomas

SUMMARY. The American Nursing Home is in the center of a "perfect storm" as a result of financial, workforce and liability issues. To date, conventional approaches to quality improvement have been ineffective at fundamentally changing our notions of care and treatment for our Elders.

Begun in 1992 as an effort to transform life in a single New York State nursing home, The Eden Alternative has, a decade later, more than 5000 Eden Associates and 200 organizations as members.

William H. Thomas, MD, is President of The Eden Alternative, Sherburne, NY.

Address correspondence to: William H. Thomas, MD, President, The Eden Alternative, 742 Turnpike Road, Sherburne, NY 13460 (E-mail: info@edenalt.com).

Editors' Note: Many of the articles included in the volume include a specific reference to either The Eden Alternative or to Bill Thomas as its visionary. In asking Bill to participate in this collection, it was our goal to emphasize that the history and evolution of The Eden Alternative philosophy and the Green House concept were central to creating an understanding of the urgency of change in our system of long-term care.

[Haworth co-indexing entry note]: "Evolution of Eden." Thomas, William H. Co-published simultaneously in *Journal of Social Work in Long-Term Care* (The Haworth Social Work Practice Press, an imprint of The Haworth Press, Inc.) Vol. 2, No. 1/2, 2003, pp. 141-157; and: *Culture Change in Long-Term Care* (ed: Audrey S. Weiner, and Judah L. Ronch) The Haworth Social Work Practice Press, an imprint of The Haworth Press, Inc., 2003, pp. 141-157. Single or multiple copies of this article are available for a fee from The Haworth Document Delivery Service [1-800-HAWORTH, 9:00 a.m. - 5:00 p.m. (EST). E-mail address: docdelivery@haworthpress.com].

10.1300/J181v2n01_10

Its impact has been international. Building on the principles of Eden and its direct response to loneliness, boredom and helplessness, the Green House concept has subsequently evolved.

This is more than an iteration or improvement on the Eden Alternative. Rather, its premise is that change, however well intentioned and profound, in our current system of long-term care is inadequate. *[Article copies available for a fee from The Haworth Document Delivery Service: 1-800-HAWORTH. E-mail address: <docdelivery@haworthpress.com> Website: <http://www.HaworthPress.com> © 2003 by The Haworth Press, Inc. All rights reserved.]*

KEYWORDS. Elders, Eden Alternative, nursing homes, innovation, empowerment, Green House, long-term care

TRANSCENDING LONG-TERM CARE

The Eden Alternative
The idea is simple.
Total institutions damage people.
Nursing Homes are total institutions.
Nursing homes damage people.

The modern American nursing home is being crushed between the intrinsic weaknesses of the institution and the rising expectations of a new generation of elders. We are witnesses to its destruction. Like the leper colony, the tuberculosis sanitarium and insane asylum, the nursing home is about to be heaved onto the ash heap of history. The crisis is apparent even to the casual observer.

American nursing homes and assisted living facilities are in the midst of a "perfect storm." They face a combination of financial, workforce, and liability issues that will destroy them in their current forms. Conventional approaches to quality improvement and risk management are clearly over-mathed. These extraordinary times call for extraordinary measures. A metamorphosis is essential.

In order to survive, long-term care facilities must become places where elders feel at home, family members enjoy visiting, staff are respected, listened to and appreciated, the care is good, life is worth living, and legal action is unnecessary.

Our generation confronts a challenge that is both noble and difficult; we must transcend the legacy of the nursing home as a therapeutic institution. We must resist the temptation to "fix" long-term care.

A Japanese folktale reveals the distinction between fixing and transcending.

> A sage took a young man as his student. The youth was exceptionally energetic and diligently studied his teacher's every word. This disappointed the teacher and so he resolved to teach the young man a valuable lesson.
>
> The sage cast about until he found a broken roof tile lying on the dusty earth. Taking the shard in hand, he went to find his student. When he found the young man, he began polishing the roof tile with a fold of his robe. The student found this behavior quite strange and he immediately asked the master what he was doing.
>
> The sage responded, "I am polishing this roof tile and I am going to keep right on polishing it until it becomes a jewel."
>
> "But master, it doesn't matter how long you polish that thing, it will never become a jewel." "How true," the sage responded, "and you will never find wisdom as long as you insist on changing only what you know. True wisdom is available only to those who willingly go beyond what they know and change what they are."

We must go beyond the best practices and continuous process improvement. These techniques, while valuable in polishing existing processes, cannot change what long-term care and its affiliated institutions are. An honest accounting of the damage which institutions are doing to our elders must be our starting point. This article will describe the evolution of The Eden Alternative and its philosophic metamorphosis into the Green House philosophy; others in this collection describe the actual implementation of The Eden Model in detail (see for example Mackenzie and Monkhouse).

A BRIEF HISTORY OF THE EDEN ALTERNATIVE

The Eden Alternative has grown in size, scope and complexity since it inception in 1992. What began as an effort to improve quality of life for residents in a single nursing home, has emerged as a worldwide movement to reform the structures and practices of long-term care as a whole. The importance of the Eden Alternative can be found in three of its most enduring characteristics. First, the Eden Alternative is founded on 10 principles. These ideas are the purest expression of what Eden is. They do not change. The techniques that Eden makes available to those who wish to pursue these principles, on the other hand, continue to evolve. The methods used by Edenizing organizations today are substantially different from what was in use in 1996 and will, the author hopes, be substantially different from what works best in 2006. Finally, the Eden Alternative has powerful devotion to the art of replication. Innovations in long-term care are valuable only when they can be practiced effectively by many different organizations in many different situations so that a fundamental culture change can be brought about, not merely a new system. The Eden Alternative frequently fails to take root in an organization that embraces the philosophy. These failures have offered some of the most valuable lessons of our decade of experience.

EDEN VERSION 1.0–ONE FACILITY

The Eden Alternative began as a grant project funded by the New York State Department of Health. The project was conducted in 1992 and 1993 at the Chase Memorial Nursing Home in New Berlin, New York. This 80-bed not-for-profit facility brought to the project a record of quality care and a willingness to innovate. The grant underwrote a small evaluation program that yielded some startling results. Powerful associations between the implementation of the Eden Alternative and improvements in staff turnover, resident infections, polypharmacy and resident longevity were identified. These highly statistically significant findings hinted that radical changes in the physical and social environment inhabited by the residents could have substantial positive impacts on the well-being of staff and elders alike (Thomas, 1994).

EDEN VERSION 2.0–REPLICATION IN UPSTATE NEW YORK

The next major effort was an attempt to replicate the work done at Chase Memorial. In 1994 three progressive facilities in Upstate New York were recruited–The Ideal Senior Living Center, Vestal Nursing Center and Tioga Nursing Center. Work followed to help them adopt the principles and practices of the Eden Alternative. This experience is where the crucial difference between innovation confined to a single facility and the task of replicating innovative methods in different organizations became quite clear. One size cannot fit all.

This project demonstrated the importance of meeting organizations "where they are." The dominant inspection/penalty culture of survey and regulation has bred the fallacy that all organizations can and should resemble all other facilities. In response to this myth, we have embraced the idea that the Eden Alternative should offer a unique expression wherever it is practiced. Because of the prevalent fear in long-term care, many facilities possess a hair trigger sensitivity to the issue of "being told what to do." Defensiveness of this kind is one of the chief barriers encountered by any serious attempt to "change the culture of long-term care." This defensiveness can lead them to reject information and indeed guidance that could be very helpful. The result can be wasted effort and resources. This replication project ran from 1994 through 1995.

EDEN VERSION 3.0–
CREATION OF THE EDEN ALTERNATIVE ASSOCIATE TRAINING PROGRAM

In 1996, Jude Thomas developed a three-day course on the Eden Alternative philosophy and its practices. Building on sustained efforts to improve the replication process, the Eden Alternative Associate Training marked a new phase of development. Our efforts were concentrated on teaching others how to lead the Eden Alternative process in their own organizations. We now had a viable mechanism with which we could bring the Eden philosophy and implementation to organizations outside of Upstate New York.

The course is built around the principles of the Eden Alternative. Each principle is reviewed and a variety of techniques for understanding it, teaching it and practicing it are presented. There is a great emphasis on participation. Art, music and theater are part of the experience in every course we offer.

EDEN 4.0–
THE REGIONAL COORDINATOR AND TRAINING PROGRAM

By late 1998, the demand for Eden Associate training was far outstripping capacity. In order to respond to the growing number of people who wanted to begin with Eden, we developed the Eden Regional Coordinator model. The United States and Canada were divided into a dozen regions and a highly skilled Eden educator was placed in each region. The result was a great improvement in the availability of Eden education. We had been reaching only about 100-200 people a year. With the regional system we began to reach about 1,000 people a year.

A year later, with The American Association of Homes and Services for the Aged (AAHSA), the Eden Across America Tour was launched. The Tour lasted 31 days in the summer of 1999 reaching 27 cities and spanning 10,000 miles. In order to advance the cause of Eden in the cities we visited, we arranged public lectures, meetings with government officials and rallies for people practicing Eden in long-term care organizations. We also developed partnerships with local elder-centered charities. In the evening we presented a two act play that described the creation of the Eden Alternative philosophy (in dramatic form). The proceeds were donated to the partner charity.

By 2002, there were over 7,000 Eden Associates and more than 200 organizations which had joined the Eden Alternative organization and display its official seal.

EDEN 5.0

The next version of the Eden Alternative will maintain the emphasis on education and research while broadening the approach to the problem of fostering healthy change in the field of long-term care. New training materials and new strategies for helping organizations find the path to Eden are in development.

The most exciting thing about being part of an emergent social phenomenon (in this case the fundamental reform of an antiquated approach to the care of our elders) is that the organization that undertakes this work must itself change, grow and evolve. For as long as we are able, we will be in the garden, helping it grow.

The reader is encouraged to read additional work describing the evolution of the philosophy of The Eden Alternative model including *Learning from Hannah* (Thomas, 1999), and *Life Worth Living* (Thomas, 1996).

EDEN 6.0–THE EMERGENCY OF THE GREEN HOUSE MODEL

As pleased as we are with the successes of the Eden Alternative, there is a need for an even more daring approach to the problem of reinventing the long-term care environment for the 21st century. We must change the way we think about, regulate and deliver services to people who are coping with difficult changes that often accompany old age. The facility-based approach, which has dominated American long-term care for the past three decades, is not keeping pace with society's rising demands for quality of care and quality of life.

The Green House Project, conceptualized in the last years of the 20th century, is an attempt to design, build and test a radically new approach to residential long-term care for older people. It is founded on the idea that the physical and social environments in which we deliver long-term care can and should be warm, smart, and green. The Green Houses themselves will be small (6 to 8 person) community homes where people requiring skilled nursing services can live and receive the care they need. We will link them with a sophisticated health care delivery network that can ensure quality, provide expertise, organize back up staffing, and deliver back office (e.g., account/billing) support. The first Green Houses began construction in Tupelo, Mississippi in the summer of 2002. Occupancy was planned for early 2003.

The houses will fit the character of the neighborhoods in which they are built. We will know we have it right when we can drive down a street and not know which house is the Green House. Inside, we will create warmth through the floor plan, furnishings, décor and, most importantly, the people. A small number of caregivers will share ongoing responsibilities for the elders and the house. Developing close personal relationships will be made easier by the fact that each Green House will provide a minimum of 36 hours of staffing a day (6 hours per elder per day), a standard well above that provided in conventional, facility-based long-term care. The house will be filled with useful but unobtrusive technology that ensures safety, promotes quality of care, rigor in record keeping, and community and family involvement. It will be the Einstein of smart houses. Finally, we recognize that people find great pleasure in the company of animals, the laughter of children and the growth of green plants. Our work with the Eden Alternative has shown, time and again, that contact with the living world is a major factor in both quality of life and improved clinical outcomes. The Green Houses must indeed be green.

We believe that the Green House can become a high-quality, safe, cost-effective alternative to institutionalization for frail and disabled people who require skilled care. The difficulty lies in designing them to operate within the parameters of existing funding and regulation and ensuring that they adhere to the general regulatory schema laid out for skilled nursing facilities by CMS and seeking the minimum possible number of waivers that are consistent with our goals in this project. They will accept and operate within the funding constraints imposed by Medicare and Medicaid reimbursement.

CONCEPTUAL MODEL

The foundation of the Green House model is drawn from the lessons we have learned through our extensive work with existing long-term care institutions. The Eden Alternative has given us the opportunity to educate and advise some of the most gifted leaders and forward thinking organizations in the nation. We have seen many of them make dramatic progress. In fact a comprehensive study of the Eden Alternative conducted by Southwest Texas State University examined staff stability and clinical outcomes in seven "Edenizing" homes in Central Texas. The results reveal substantial, highly significant improvements in these areas (Ransom, 2000).

- A 60% reduction in behavioral incidents: This is defined as altercations between two or more residents
- A 57% decrease in decubitus ulcer formation
- A 25% decrease in numbers of bedfast residents
- An 18% decrease in use of restraints
- An 11% increase in census sustained over two year period
- A 48% decrease in staff absenteeism: This means that we have the same staff members there day to day taking care of our beloved elders
- A 59% increase in self scheduling.

Even with this data, we know there can be more. While the teaching of the Eden Alternative has, as noted above, been significant, only 2 percent of nursing homes in the United States have adopted The Eden approach. If America was truly satisfied with its system of long-term care, this would be acceptable, but that is clearly not the case. Residents, regulators, family members and professionals routinely rail at the failings of the status quo. The reason that the Eden Alternative (like all other efforts to "reform" long-term care) has such limited penetration lies with the structure of the nursing home itself.

Therapeutic institutions are notoriously difficult to reform. Efforts to effect deep-seated and lasting change generally require tenacious visionary leadership and the sustained investment of energy, enthusiasm and educational resources. To make matters worse, even with skilled leadership the institution is in constant danger of relapse. It is a hard truth that the default state of a nursing home is that of a cold, sterile, technically focussed service delivery entity. Good leaders using ideas like the Eden Alternative can blunt that fact and do much good for all involved, but the truth remains. There has to be a different way.

By critically examining the reality of skilled nursing facilities and both the strengths and weaknesses of the Eden Alternative, we have been able to define a new conceptual model for the care of frail elders and the chronically ill. The Green House model is founded on three key ideas. It is worth summarizing the major components of each concept in this model.

WARM

Human beings thrive in warm, loving environments; they wither in cold, sterile and institutional settings. This is more than common sense.

The work of designing, creating and maintaining warm environments is a subtle and difficult art. Warmth demands persistence, patience, forgiveness, tolerance and respect. These virtues never come naturally to human organizations, indeed that may be more broadly true about our society, but that is not a universal truth. They flourish only when cultivated. The task of sustaining these values inside facility-based long-term care organizations is made especially difficult by the bedrock of institutional thinking and bureaucratic procedure that underlie conventional practice.

Decades of reform and advocacy have resulted in substantial improvements in safety and quality of care in nursing homes. Unfortunately, there is little evidence that the current system can be modified, reformed or improved so that it consistently yields the warmth we all want for the people we love or for ourselves. Large, hierarchical, policy driven organizations foster intimacy the way an elephant dances, poorly if at all. When it comes to warmth–small, flat and informal is best.

THE NEW LOGIC OF SMALLNESS

What I wish to emphasize is the duality of the human requirement when it comes to the question of size: there is no single answer. For his different purposes man needs many different structures, both small ones and large ones, some exclusive and some comprehensive . . . For constructive work, the principal task is always the restoration of some kind of balance. Today, we suffer from an almost universal idolatry of gigantism. It is therefore necessary to insist on the virtues of smallness–where this applies . . . (Schumacher, 1999)

The larger a human group, the harder it is to maintain warmth among the people attached to the organization. Human beings are incapable of maintaining and nurturing large numbers of simultaneous, intimate relationships. It would seem a matter of common sense that the places we create for our elders would be constructed on a small scale. In fact, in the pre-Medicaid era, many of them were. Before we succumb to a haze of 1950s nostalgia, however, we should remember that those years also gave rise to horrendous examples of abuse and neglect. Small size does not guarantee warmth.

Since 1964, the trend toward large facilities has been driven, in part, by a desire to standardize service and improve safety, but the most important factor has been financial performance. The skilled nursing facility's concentration of expertise, labor, equipment and elders has made sense for the same reason that a gigantic steel plant makes sense. These arrangements help the staff carry out necessary tasks in the quickest most efficient manner possible. Greater operational efficiency opens the door to improved financial performance. Economic imperatives and the needs of professionals, not the desires of elders, have fostered largeness in long-term care. The idea of being cared for alongside one to two or even three hundred other similarly situated people for the rest of one's life will never rank with Mom and apple pie as an American ideal.

RETHINKING HIERARCHY

The impulse toward hierarchy and the power of bureaucratic authority grow stronger as human organizations grow larger. Outside of national armies, few people inhabit organizations that are as rigidly compartmentalized and uniformly hierarchical as the American nursing home. The work of caring for our elders has been transformed into an exercise in which "established policies guide an assembled staff in the efficient execution of the sequence of task and procedures delineated by the interdisciplinary care plan document." This is care filtered through the sieve of bureaucracy. Worse, the slope of the skilled nursing facility's organizational pyramid is steep and the people at the bottom tend very much to stay at the bottom. Careful observers have noted how these institutions socialize staff and residents in ways that encourage them to accept the "chain of command" as an unavoidable fact of life.

Far from being an imperative of long-term care, bureaucratic hierarchy obstructs the work of caring. The small size of the Green House allows us to reconsider the role of hierarchy in our work. A council of elders, caregivers and family members will oversee the social environment of the Green House. The council will be led by a community elder who possesses the life experiences and skills needed to help this group of people identify and resolve interpersonal conflicts as well of the dilemmas of daily life in a communal setting. (See Barkan and Norton, this volume, for related strategies.)

For those seeking to sustain human warmth, flat is better.

THE POWER OF ROOTEDNESS

All social organizations have rules. These rules exist though they may be both unspoken and unwritten. Our culture often struggles as it seeks a satisfying balance between written rules and regulations and unspoken but clearly understood norms of behavior. An imbalance in either direction carries with it many harmful effects.

The novel "The Lord of the Flies" offers a telling literary illustration of this dilemma. It is the tale of a group of schoolboys, reared within the rigid confines of industrial society, and their plunge into chaos after a plane crash strands them on a deserted island without adult supervision. In the novel's despotic vision, the absence of formal rules and authoritarian figures to enforce those rules quickly leads to mayhem and death. This is a fear that lives in all of us, and there is truth to it.

Codifying and enforcing rules of conduct that protect the weak, the infirm and the frail is a cardinal virtue of a just society. In the world of long-term care, government officials and advocates have long shared the sense that these written protections need strengthening. I support the protections that have been put into place and see them as necessary bulwarks against the specters of abuse and neglect. They do, however, carry with them a pernicious and unintended consequence. As we slide ever deeper into the arena of regulating speech and behavior among those who provide care for the frail elders, we foster the idea that compliance with those regulations is the equivalent of quality. Over time the steady application of such rules erodes internal, unspoken, unwritten, heartfelt ideals. While they are clearly meant as minimum standards, official approval is offered in equal measure to those who merely comply with published standards and those who soar above them. We are living in an age when officially prescribed standards are slowly, silently replacing unspoken and deeply personal commitments to elders and the work of meeting their needs.

This trend is understandable in part because managing people is devilishly difficult work. Officially sanctioned codes of behavior offer an appealing refuge from the prickly aspect of creating and maintaining human relationships. This is why even the most spiritually driven organizations experience a gradual descent into formalized policies and procedures. The road to organizational formality is well worn. Much less traveled is the path that teaches us to defend a deeply rooted commitment to frail elders and their well being against the might of imposed policies and procedures. When it comes to sustaining human warmth, we must master the art of balancing formal and informal codes of conduct.

SMART

The technology revolution that is remaking life, work and leisure in the 21st century has left long-term care behind. This is both unfortunate and correctable. The potential for off the shelf technology to improve our ability to care for frail elders and the chronically ill is tremendous.

1. We have to seek out the best in assistive technology. Too little attention has been paid to the ways we can use new technologies to help elders do more for themselves. Such tools carry a double-edged benefit. First, they can help us reduce the burden on caregivers by adding an important element of self-care experience of daily life. Second, and perhaps more

importantly, they can help maintain and even grow the self-efficacy of the elders.

2. Conversations with long-term care professionals often come around to the concern that "paperwork" consumes valuable time that might better be spent actually caring for those about whom we are documenting. If the large parcel delivery services were forced to return to the level of technical sophistication found in most long-term care settings today, they would collapse overnight. "Paperwork" is a poor use of increasingly scarce staff expertise and energy. The Green House will employ advanced technology that can free the staff from pencil pushing and ensure that the clinical record is complete, accurate and up-to-date.

3. The technology we use must help the people who live and work in the Green House stay in close contact with the rest of the world. Relationships, educational opportunities and personal growth can all be fostered through the appropriate use of e-mail and the World Wide Web.

In all of this, we must make every effort to make the tools we use as unobtrusive as possible. Technology works best when it is woven seamlessly into the fabric of daily life.

GREEN

The Eden Alternative has demonstrated that it is better to live in a garden. Human beings need close and continuing contact with the living world, and it is wrong to deny it to them. The main problem we have encountered with our work with the Eden Alternative is that the vessel with which we are working (the conventional long-term care institution) is so large and inflexible that the process of "Edenizing" becomes a titanic struggle. The greenness to which I am referring is something we all seek in our own lives. We manage it in our own homes without policy committees, executive approvals and regulatory waivers. The small size, flattened structure and shared ethos of the Green House should make it possible to give the gift of life, laughter and companionship in ways that are less strenuous and more enduring.

FUNDAMENTAL CONCERNS

Any new idea in the field of long-term care that is less safe, produces lower quality, or costs more than conventional institutional care is doomed from the start. The Green House will meet and exceed existing standards in each of these areas.

Safety

The question of whether previously institutionalized people can be returned to the community to take up residence in small group homes has been examined intensively over the past two decades. The primary concerns have revolved around fire safety, need for prompt and effective medical attention, the risk of elopement and the risk of abuse and neglect. Experience has shown that people who care for the chronically mentally ill and developmentally disabled have been able to meet and overcome these concerns. We believe that the Green House will allow us to do the same for frail and demented elders.

Fire Safety

Fire safety concerns remain with us and are a legacy of the unregulated era of boarding home care where older people were often placed in upper floors of homes that had no fire warning or suppression systems. In response to these concerns, the project in Tupelo, Mississippi will adhere to the building standards and fire safety procedures embraced by the New York MR/DD de-institutionalization movement.

Medical Attention

While it is conventional wisdom that prompt access to effective medical attention is a vital component of quality long-term care, time studies have shown that nursing home residents spend only a small portion of their day receiving such care. The challenge lies in ensuring the following for our Green House residents.

1. Rapid response to emergent medical conditions. The emergency medical response system depends on attentiveness, skillful assessment, rapid communication and, rapid transportation when necessary. We propose to staff each Green House with a licensed practical nurse around the clock. We will make a specially trained RN available by phone and video with no more than a ten-minute response time when paged. Interestingly, in the state of Texas it is common practice to have an RN available onsite for only one shift a day, even in large facilities. This practice led the Texas Nurses Association to develop a comprehensive curricu-

lum that includes a training manual, a skills checklist and an algorithm for when to call for help and what to do while it is forthcoming. It has been used widely in Texas and many other states, and we will follow its example.

2. Consistent, well-trained medical staff will be available.

3. Physical therapy, speech therapy and occupational therapy will be provided to the elders just as they are now. There will be no dimunition in assessment or delivery of services. A vast body of experience in this country has already demonstrated that these services can be delivered to people in contexts outside of the conventional skilled nursing facility.

Elopement

Much of the elopement related literature concentrates on the person's drive to elope. We believe that the combination of small size, a truly homelike interior, close relationships between staff and elder, true integration into the community and high technology exit monitoring can reduce the risk of elopement relative to the classic skilled nursing facility. The comparatively high staffing ratio will serve as an additional protective factor as will the community location of the Green Houses. Many skilled nursing facilities are located in areas that are zoned for commercial enterprises and are thus nearly deserted during the very hours when the danger of elopement is greatest. Interestingly, the opposite is true in most residential neighborhoods.

Abuse and Neglect

The specter of elder abuse and neglect continues to haunt our system of long-term care. Its persistence compels us to continue taking actions that are likely to reduce its prevalence. Some observers have raised the question of whether the small size and decentralized nature of the Green Houses will increase or decrease the potential for mistreatment of elders. We are confident that the potential for mistreatment will be significantly less than that experienced in conventional facilities. We think that an environment that expressly supports the creation of meaningful relationships between caregivers, elders and their family members is likely to deter many forms of abuse and neglect. Further, we are examining a web cam capacity in the houses that will operate much like those already in use of children's day care centers. This approach is distinct from the "granny cam" model of surveillance that we find intrusive and demeaning for staff and elders alike. Properly password protected video access via the web browser will enable professionals, family members and state officials to "stop by" any time of the day or night. This is the electronic equivalent of the friendly visit that should, of course, never be restricted. We believe that this system will enable even geographically distant family members to remain aware of the happenings and people that surround their family members. Use of off the shelf web based technology will keep the price low.

SUPERIOR CLINICAL OUTCOMES

We believe that the Green House approach can yield superior clinical outcomes for those who live in them. The model is being designed expressly for the most frail and chronically ill of all our citizens. We are committed to caring for any patient who is qualified to receive skilled nursing care. The Green House will not "skim" the more able, less ill patients into this setting.

Our confidence in this area finds a firm foundation in published work which links quality to high staff/elder ratios, small facility size and continuity of care (Teno et al., 1997). We will focus on each of these factors. Substantially more staffing hours will be dedicated to direct patient care than the conventional institutional facility can offer. We anticipate improvements in communication and documentation based on the intimate understanding of the individual that this setting affords. We will track all standard parameters of quality of care and compare them to the facility, state, and national standards. We have also developed a standardized system for recording and tracking complaints. These measurements and comparisons can be shared with the all stakeholders on a regular basis.

SUPERIOR QUALITY OF LIFE

The signs are everywhere from mental health to MR/DD to public housing to real estate development. Smaller, community oriented options are replacing larger institutional organizations. Our proposal simply extends this widely recognized trend to a group of people who are trapped, often for life, in large bureaucratic organizations. In order to maximize quality of life for people in this setting, we will pay particular attention to giving staff special training in the area of dementia. We will also provide advanced education in the areas of end of life and palliative care. We look forward to partnering actively with the Hospice movement in this area.

Finally, we must consider the question of social isolation. Would people living in a small community based home actually suffer from isolation and a sense of confinement? Is it truly possible to build meaningful relationships between frail elders and members of a real neighborhood? Much has been done in this area by the MR/DD movement but much more needs to be done. A Green House living environment that fails to connect with its community will never reach its full potential. We will conduct an active and ongoing outreach program for the neighborhoods where our Green Houses are situated. Volunteers are going to contribute to the success for the Green House in ways that have never been possible in the traditional nursing home. We envision the active recruitment, training, support and recognition of a cadre of volunteers spanning all age groups in every Green House.

COST CONTAINMENT

Almost all involved in or touched by long-term care would like to see an increase in funding. The truth is that any advance in practice must take place in the context of existing funding. If it won't work with the money we have, it won't work. The good news is that we propose to deliver a higher level of care and an improved quality of life for the same daily per diems we are now receiving in existing facilities. The proposed Green House model is clearly viable in a high Medicaid reimbursement state like New York and in the hands of an established and well run not-for-profit organization. We have also been able to work out a Green House structure that is feasible in Mississippi as well. Much more needs to be done to build sophisticated and flexible business models that translate to other environments. We are currently working with the Robert Wood Johnson Foundation to develop a detailed business case analysis of the Green House model.

RESEARCH INITIATIVES

In addition, rigorous research and evaluation will assess care standards, quality of life and staff satisfaction. As of summer, 2002, the Green House Project was proposed for Faxton–St. Luke's in Utica, New York. Faxton–St. Luke's hoped to test the model and to develop seven Green Houses in surrounding residential neighborhoods. Each home will house 6 residents. As a result of this pilot project forty-two elderly and disabled Uticans will have the opportunity to leave the SNF where they have been living and move into Green Houses built in 2002-2003.

REFERENCES

Ransom, S. (2000). *Eden Alternative: The Texas Project.* IQILTHC Monograph Series 2000-4. San Marcos, Texas: Texas Long-Term Care Institute, Southwest Texas State University.

Schumacher, E.F. (1999). *Small is Beautiful: Economics as if People Mattered: 25 Years Later with Commentaries.* London, England, Hartley & Marks, p. 54.

Teno, J. et al. (1997). The Early Impact of the Patient Self-Determination in Long-Term Care Facilities: Results from a 10 State Sample *Journal of the American Geriatrics Society,* Vol. 45, No. 8, pp. 939-944.

Thomas, W. (1999). *Learning from Hannah: Secrets of a Life Worth Living.* Acton, Massachusetts: VanderWyk & Burnham.

————(1994). *The Eden Alternative: Nature, Hope and Nursing Homes.* Columbia, Missouri: University of Missouri Press.

————(1996). *Life Worth Living: How Someone You Love Can Still Enjoy Life in a Nursing Home.* Acton, Massachusetts: VanderWyk & Burnham.

Culture Change in Long Term Care: The Wellspring Model

Mary Ann Kehoe
Betsy Van Heesch

SUMMARY. While embarking on a journey to learn how to survive in the permanently altered health care marketplace, a group of eleven Wisconsin not-for-profit providers learned that the true keys to sustained organizational quality include teaching line staff best clinical practices and, more importantly, in changing the typical long-term care culture of control.

Wellspring Innovative Solutions for Integrated Health Care emerged in 1994 as a pro-active response to the trend toward "managed care," decreased reimbursement, limited human resources, increased resident acuity, and increased consumer demand for quality. Despite increased challenges in these areas, today Wellspring members have continued to be totally committed to providing quality care and quality of life to those served.

At its core Wellspring believes that few individuals are working in long-term care today for the pay. Rather, individuals are attracted to the field because they want to make a difference. Wellspring focuses on showing line

Mary Ann Kehoe, RN, NHA, is the Executive Director of Wellspring headquartered at Good Shepherd Services in Seymour, Wisconsin.

Betsy Van Heesch, BS, is the Resident Services Director at Fond du Lac Lutheran Home in Fond du Lac, Wisconsin.

Address correspondence to: Mary Ann Kehoe, Executive Director, Wellspring, 607 Bronson Road, Seymour, WI 54165 (E-mail mak@goodshepherdservices.org).

[Haworth co-indexing entry note]: "Culture Change in Long Term Care: The Wellspring Model." Kehoe, Mary Ann, and Betsy Van Heesch. Co-published simultaneously in *Journal of Social Work in Long-Term Care* (The Haworth Social Work Practice Press, an imprint of The Haworth Press, Inc.) Vol. 2, No. 1/2, 2003, pp. 159-173; and: *Culture Change in Long-Term Care* (ed: Audrey S. Weiner, and Judah L. Ronch) The Haworth Social Work Practice Press, an imprint of The Haworth Press, Inc., 2003, pp. 159-173. Single or multiple copies of this article are available for a fee from The Haworth Document Delivery Service [1-800-HAWORTH, 9:00 a.m. - 5:00 p.m. (EST). E-mail address: docdelivery@haworthpress.com].

staff employees in all departments the difference they can make on a daily basis. Wellspring culture values and respects not only the individual resident, but also each employee, no matter their department nor function.

This article describes the philosophy of the Wellspring approach, its history, implementation and initial outcomes. *[Article copies available for a fee from The Haworth Document Delivery Service: 1-800-HAWORTH. E-mail address: <docdelivery@haworthpress.com> Website: <http://www.HaworthPress.com> © 2003 by The Haworth Press, Inc. All rights reserved.]*

KEYWORDS. Wellspring, culture change, nursing homes, long-term care, clinical protocols, care resource teams

WELLSPRING OVERVIEW

Wellspring Innovative Solutions for Integrated Health Care emerged in 1994 as a pro-active response to the trend toward "managed care" and the permanently altered marketplace of decreased reimbursement, limited human resources, increased resident acuity, and increased consumer demand for quality. Despite increased challenges in these areas, today Wellspring members have continued to be totally committed to providing quality care and quality of life to those served.

The Wellspring movement began as a cooperative effort between two Wisconsin organizations, Evergreen Retirement Community in Oshkosh and Good Shepherd Services in Seymour. The founding Wellspring members (known as charter members) also include Benevolent Corporation Cedar Campuses, West Bend; Christian Home & Rehabilitation Center, Waupun; Fond du Lac Lutheran Home, Fond du Lac; Iola Nursing Home, Iola; Lutheran Homes of Oconomowoc, Oconomowoc; Northland Lutheran Retirement Community, Marinette; Odd Fellow-Rebekah Home Association, Green Bay; St. Paul Elder Services, Kaukauna and Sheboygan Retirement Home & Beach Health Center, Sheboygan.

This charter Wellspring group is an alliance of eleven independent not-for-profit organizations located in Eastern Wisconsin. Wellspring Inc. itself is a 501(C)(3) not-for-profit corporation. The eleven skilled nursing facilities range in size from 63 to 415 beds with the average home having 135 beds (see Table 1).

The charter facilities are unionized (1) and non-unionized (10) and are located in urban as well as rural areas of Wisconsin. Wellspring homes have the same overall and nursing care hours as other homes in Wisconsin (see Table 2).

TABLE 1. Comparison of Wellspring and Other Wisconsin Facilities

	Wellspring	Non-Profit Non-Govt.	All Non-Wellspring
No. of Facilities	10	144	416
Avg. Bed Size	145	102	110
Median Bed Size	103	93	98
% Medicaid	59.0%	57.2%	64.2%
% Medicare	5.1%	11.6%	9.9%

Source: OSCAR data from 2/98-11/99. Data from 132 facilities are from 1998.
Table authored by staff of the Institute for the Future of Aging Services.

TABLE 2. Average Staff Hours Per Day in Wellspring and Non-Wellspring Wisconsin Facilities

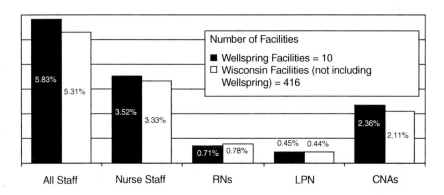

Source: OSCAR data from 2/98-11/99.
Table authored by staff of the Institute for the Future of Aging Service.

WHY CHANGE?

In the opinion of the charter Wellspring members, the current system of nursing home care in the nation is broken. Long-term care facilities are in crisis in terms of quality care and staff availability (Stone and Reinhard, 2001a). The typical organization has an autocratic management structure with high staff turnover and low staff morale. These challenges have been exacerbated by the shortage of nurses, nursing assistants and other front-line workers.

For many years there has been a reliance on a system of federal survey enforcement to address and respond to these problems. Despite voluminous regulations, poor providers are still operating. More regulation and draconian enforcement are not, in these authors' opinion, the answer. Rather, national policy must move beyond the deficiency/correction cycle to a model of true quality assurance. There needs to be increasing recognition that true quality improvement requires both efficient clinical intervention and transformation of the traditional organizational culture. Now and in the future, organizations need to provide high levels of quality at the lowest possible human and financial cost. That philosophy is the backbone of the Wellspring approach.

At its core Wellspring believes that few individuals are working in long-term care today for the pay. Rather, individuals are attracted to the field because they want to make a difference. Wellspring focuses on showing line staff employees in all departments the difference they can make on a daily basis. Wellspring culture values and respects not only the individual resident, but also each employee, no matter their department nor function.

Despite its rather concise culture and values statement, Wellspring is a complex model for nursing home reform. Wellspring homes have formed a quality enhancement alliance, integrated the federal quality indicators, nationally defined best clinical practices and a new management paradigm to dramatically improve staff efficiency and hence resident outcomes. "The dual focus on changes in clinical practice and changes in the nursing home culture distinguishes the Wellspring model of quality improvement from other nursing home programs" (Stone and Reinhard, 2001b).

ALLIANCE STRUCTURE

Wellspring believes that the keys to organizational viability in the future are:

- collaboration and cooperation among facilities
- staff empowerment
- data based decision making
- accountability between partner organizations for improved resident outcomes
- assigning permanent staff to groups of residents

In order for these concepts to succeed, the traditional management paradigm must be replaced by an environment where managers become team builders, coaches, mentors and enablers. This is in sharp contrast to the more traditional roles as controllers and disciplinarians.

In 1994, when the group of Wellspring charter organizations first came together, it was determined that a typical "business" merger was not a desirable outcome. Rather the group worked in an effort to address future challenges and to share resources to become more effective with clinical care (the core business). Wellspring defines this group as an alliance. Each charter Wellspring facility contributes a standardized monthly fee to cover the costs for an advanced practice nurse and other clinical experts in geriatrics who work with facility staff to translate research-based best practices into everyday care of residents. These clinicians work with facilities as consultants on at least a quarterly basis. The alliance also generates standards and works to ensure consistency of goals and understanding among facilities.

Since 1994, Wellspring Inc. chief executives and administrators have met monthly and the nursing directors, Wellspring coordinators (RNs who serve as facility Wellspring coaches), and the nurse practitioner have met at least quarterly.

The original Wellspring premise was that long-term care facilities generally are clinically inefficient and do not provide line staff in all departments with the appropriate education/support to do their jobs. Wellspring theorized that greater staff education and efficiency would lead to higher customer satisfaction, would allow time for quality of life interactions for residents and staff, and would not be more costly. Charter Wellspring members also theorized that such front-line worker empowerment would also translate to higher staff retention and lower staff turnover.

In establishing the alliance model, Wellspring also predicted that the support and accountability provided by groups of homes working together was key to nurturing and sustaining the process. The research findings as described later support the original premises (Stone and Reinhard, 2001b).

The role of the alliance is therefore:

- one of leadership
- identifying and sharing information and best practices
- translating best practices into action
- providing a focal point for accountability.

The alliance structure works to minimize competitive behavior and encourages facilities to work in partnership to achieve jointly held goals. Wellspring becomes the permanent way of doing business in the organization. "An intervention of this magnitude and complexity requires careful alignment of the Wellspring model philosophy and structure with the organizational structure in the facility" (Stone and Reinhard, 2001b).

WELLSPRING REPLICATION

Since 1998, in addition to the charter alliance, six other groups have formed alliances and have been working with Wellspring to replicate the model in their organizations. These alliances have begun in Texas, Wisconsin, and Illinois and involve forty-seven facilities in addition to the charter Wellspring group. At the end of 2001, over ten thousand nursing home residents were impacted annually by the Wellspring model.

Currently Wellspring Inc. charges a licensing fee to each home in an alliance. This fee covers the cost of materials, clinical experts to train the alliance staff, a data reporting system, and Wellspring support during the two-year implementation process.

Creating local (groups within two hours driving distance) alliances is the first step for a region's implementation of Wellspring. Alliances consist of from five to twelve nursing homes. Once an alliance has been formed, building trust and cooperation among group members is key. It is recommended that top facility administrators begin monthly meetings in order to

1. assess their readiness for implementation
2. determine the formal relationship between group members (such as establishing a corporation)
3. appoint a representative to interface with Wellspring corporate staff
4. begin the task of recruiting an advance practice nurse
5. begin the task of permanently assigning staff to groups of residents.

Most often several facilities among the group will tour charter Wellspring facilities in order to gain a better understanding of the process. The facilities are encouraged to ensure that line staff members are part of each tour group.

Once fees are paid and an advance practice nurse is secured, the process of training staff begins through the management and clinical modules described below. Staff of different disciplines attend each education module. The implementation of Wellspring generally requires a major organizational change; therefore, the process occurs in facilities over at least a two-year period.

While Wellspring is being implemented in all charter facilities, there is variation across the charter homes. Wellspring works best in facilities where teams have become effective agents of authority and accountability at the unit level. Staff empowerment is central to Wellspring. In practice, however, empowerment is supported differently in each organization. The most successful Wellspring homes have the clearest authority/accountability structures.

In the most successful facilities (e.g., those with the most positive outcomes), empowerment means that CNAs and representatives of other traditionally lower level disciplines have high level positions in these authority/accountability structures and that these structures were integrated at the unit level. That is, a CNA might be a care resource team member, with nurses and other unit staff reporting to him/her.

MANAGEMENT MODULE

Fundamental to the Wellspring process is the concept that the definition of quality care is created by top management, but that the best decisions about how care is delivered to each resident are made by the front-line staff who know the residents best. A key determinant in the success of facility implementation is the commitment of middle managers and especially staff nurses to working with and mentoring front-line staff.

In order for the Wellspring process to be sustained over time, managers need to provide opportunities for staff to learn new skills, establish the parameters for change, and refrain from blaming line staff for mistakes that may occur during implementation. The practical approach taken by Wellspring is to provide both management and line staff education.

The first Wellspring module session is for top and middle managers in all alliance facilities. The session takes place at a retreat/conference center over a three-day period with the objective of teaching managers how to become coaches, mentors and enablers of the culture change that needs to occur in traditional organizations in order for Wellspring to succeed. The module is taught by a management consultant and follows the general format of the clinical modules. Areas of focus include staff empowerment, change, coaching, and problem solving according to Wellspring. A personality profile is also administered to managers as a means to assist with team building within their respective facilities. Upon completion of this module, managers must return to their facilities and assess the organizational readiness for Wellspring. Ongoing communication is established between each alliance and the charter Wellspring organizations.

The requirement to assign staff to permanent groups of residents serves to create a "family atmosphere" in Wellspring facilities.

CLINICAL COMPONENT

The clinical module component is based on nationally defined "best practices" in areas of care that affect the elderly. Seven clinical modules have been created that include:

- geriatric physical assessment
- elimination/continence
- skin care
- nutrition
- dementia care
- falls prevention
- restorative care.

Wellspring also strongly recommends that alliances seek out the Palliative Care Program created by the Medical College of Wisconsin (Weissman, 1996) as their eighth clinical module.

In Wellspring's view, the real key to providing sustainable quality over time is teaching line staff to collect relevant data, to critically evaluate information and to finally implement processes that improve care. The initial process of staff planning takes place at the module educational sessions.

GERIATRIC NURSE PRACTITIONER (GNP)

In order for facility staff to learn "best clinical practices," Wellspring utilizes the services of a team of advance practice clinicians headed by a geriatric nurse practitioner. The GNP and other clinical experts (e.g., dietician, speech therapist, enterostomal therapist) develop material for the modules by researching best practices and assembling information for presentation at the training modules. The advanced clinicians serve as the primary source of "best practices" knowledge for facility staff over time. These individuals visit each facility on at least a quarterly basis to review data, analyze documentation, and ensure that staff are implementing the model effectively. Each alliance must secure the services of their own advanced practice registered nurse prior to Wellspring implementation. The alliance advance practice nurse interfaces with Wellspring and functions as an on-going consultant to individual alliance facilities.

CARE RESOURCE TEAMS

Each facility establishes "care resource teams" for each clinical module. The teams have the responsibility for ensuring that each organization is utilizing "best practices" in resident care.

Care resource teams serve an essential role with Wellspring implementation in each organization. The teams are groups of professional and line staff from each facility who are educated in nationally defined best clinical practices in the care of the elderly. There is a care resource team from each facility for each clinical module. The size and composition of the individual teams depends on the module content (e.g., dietary staff for the nutrition module, activity staff for falls) and is at the discretion of each facility. Generally, each organization sends approximately five to six different line staff to each clinical module retreat session.

The teams are immersed in best clinical practices for two full days including an overnight stay. The education takes place at a comfortable location central to the alliance facilities such as a hotel or retreat center.

During the module retreat, teams not only learn best clinical practices, but they bond with one another and with the teams from the other Wellspring facilities in attendance. This inter-facility staff networking is a key component of Wellspring. Each facility pays for their own staff expenses at the module education, and they share the costs equally for the retreat center/hotel.

When teams return to their respective organizations, it is their task to educate the other facility staff in the best practices. Teams become *facilitators* (e.g., they don't "do it all" themselves) of best clinical practices and culture change in their respective organizations.

In addition to best clinical practices, each module teaches staff to utilize personality profiles in building self-directed teams. Essentials of proper clinical documentation, infection control, resident rights, and communication are also a part of each clinical module. The teams report to management, make recommendations to department heads and begin the process of education throughout the facility. Implementation follows with changes in process, policy and procedures to reflect best practices. Following the clinical module, staff have six months in which to assess and provide enhanced care to each resident affected by the clinical condition. The implementation process mirrors the facility RAI/MDS schedule. Evaluation of overall clinical practice takes place at least quarterly.

WELLSPRING FACILITY COORDINATOR

The role of the "Wellspring facility coordinator" is a critical component in each Wellspring organization. Since nursing assessment is a key portion of each clinical module, this individual is an RN (not the director of nursing). The Wellspring coordinator is essential in guiding the care resource teams through the implementation process. He/she is usually not the team leader, but attends all of the module education and becomes an overall coach and internal mentor to the teams. The coordinator assists in defining the organizational structure and often serves as a bridge between management and line staff during the implementation process. The person selected for this role is also at the discretion of each facility based on a position description that is provided by Wellspring. Most often this individual is the education coordinator or the assistant director of nursing.

PERFORMANCE IMPROVEMENT

The data collected by each Wellspring facility compliments, but is in addition to, the MDS data. Wellspring data include such elements as the number and pattern of incontinent episodes, the time of day that falls most often occur, the type of incontinence exhibited by a resident, and the category of severity of a fall. Staff are required to collect Wellspring defined data on each resident for each clinical area of care on at least a quarterly basis.

With the assistance of the coordinator and the clinical experts, line staff review their data, identify challenges and plan changes in practice to ensure improved results. Facility successes are celebrated and challenges are addressed.

The "Wellspring Program" has been enhanced over time in a joint effort between a team of clinical experts in geriatric care, a management consultant and staff from the charter Wellspring facilities. This relationship serves as the glue to ensure inter-facility accountability for positive resident outcomes. The clinical experts also visit each facility on a quarterly basis to review resident care, to evaluate clinical outcome data, and to ensure that staff is implementing best practices as taught in the modules.

COMMONWEALTH FUND RESEARCH PROJECT

In June of 2000, the American Association of Homes & Services for the Aging (AAHSA) through the Institute for the Future of Aging Services (IFAS) received a grant from the Commonwealth Fund of New York to do intensive research in the charter Wellspring homes. The researchers evaluated the charter Wellspring facilities both quantitatively and qualitatively as compared to a group of similar not-for-profit homes who are members of the Wisconsin Association of Homes and Services for the Aging (WAHSA) in order to understand the impact of this model on residents, staff, and family members.

The charter Wellspring members and other Wisconsin Association of Homes and Services for the Aging (WAHSA) homes have been participating in a Provider Initiative Program (PIP) with the Center for Health Care Policy and Research (CHSRA) at the University of Wisconsin for approximately eight years. The PIP project involves receiving and analyzing OBRA quality indicator reports. These same reports are now part of the federal survey process and are used as part of pre-survey preparation for state and federal surveyors.

From July 2000 through November 2001, the IFAS researchers assessed the charter facilities pre- and post-Wellspring. In their evaluation the group reviewed OSCAR (online survey, certification and reporting system) and MDS (minimum data set) data, facility survey history, staff turnover rates, quality indicator reports, and Medicaid cost reports.

> The Wellspring program has withstood the most intensive, detailed scrutiny of any quality improvement model that this research team has ever been involved in–and they have come though it with very strong marks–warts, flaws, and inconsistencies for sure–but very strong marks. (Stone and Reinhard, 2001b)

IFAS preliminary research data (see Table 3) indicated that charter Wellspring homes have higher immunization rates, fewer bedfast residents, lower restraint usage, more preventive skin care, fewer psychoactive medications, less resident incontinence, fewer tube feedings and more altered diets than comparison homes. The charter Wellspring homes have the SAME staffing levels as the PIP group (Table 1).

The researchers also found that in comparison with other Wisconsin facilities, charter Wellspring homes had fewer survey deficiencies both pre- and post-Wellspring. During implementation these organizations had slightly more deficiencies than the comparison group which, according to the researchers, suggests that something occurs around the initial implementation of the Wellspring model. Anecdotally, the charter homes report that during the initial implementation, state surveys became more intense than prior experience.

Following implementation of the modules, however, the charter facilities have substantially fewer deficiencies than their Wisconsin peers whose performance stayed approximately the same over the research period.

> Wellspring exhibits a slightly higher percentage of no-deficiency facilities in the pre-period, virtually the same percentage in the period during which the modules were being implemented, and a 50% higher percentage in perfect surveys during the period following module implementation. (Stone and Reinhard, 2001b)

Following Wellspring module implementation, the charter homes also had no severe deficiencies (see Table 4) compared with other Wisconsin facilities that had a severe deficiency average of seven percent.

TABLE 3

| | Wellspring | Non Wellspring | |
		NFP/Non Gov't	All Non-Wellspring
Number of facilities	10	144	416
% Flu Immun.	41.4	28.2	31.2
% Pneumonia Vaccine	27.7	12.1	12.9
% Ambulatory w/ Assist	51.3	44.2	42.7
% Bedfast	1.0	2.7	2.9
% Restrained	9.6	13.6	13.1
% Prevent. Skin Care	64.4	53.5	51.5
% Psychoactive Meds	41.4	48.4	50.9
% Pain Management	31.4	29.5	25.8

Source: OSCAR data for Wisconsin facilities from 2/98-11/99.
Table authored by staff of the Institute for the Future of Aging Services.

The IFAS researchers also found that the charter Wellspring facilities ex-celled in the area of staff retention. With Wellspring implementation, the char-ter homes were able to reverse the state trend toward increases in nursing staff turnover. In 1999, following implementation, Wellspring homes were thirteen percentage points better than the comparison group with a 43% staff turnover rate versus 56% for the PIP group.

> Wellspring facilities were also able to improve their retention of nursing staff following program implementation with greater success than their peers. The consistency of the findings across nursing categories suggests greater success of facilities implementing Wellspring in retaining nurs-ing staff and limiting the general increase in turnover rates following im-plementation. (Stone and Reinhard, 2001b)

These findings were not unexpected given that the Wellspring foundation supports staff and by extension, their retention.

FACILITY EXPERIENCES

Through Wellspring implementation, staff at Fond du Lac Lutheran Home have grown to expect to be part of the discussion and part of the decision-

TABLE 4. Exhibit 5: Percent of Facilities with Severe Deficiencies: Wellspring vs. Other Wisconsin Facilities

Table authored by David Zimmerman as part of the Institute for the Future of Aging Services Grant No. 20000483.

making process. Each employee is accountable for quality customer service. For example, implementation of Wellspring has changed the hiring process.

While hiring practices have always been "value based," since Wellspring, the organization has left positions open rather than fill them with the "wrong persons." At Fond du Lac Lutheran Home quality standards have been increased and therefore employee performance expectations have increased as well. The facility now seeks individuals who believe in quality and who want to be part of defining quality today and in the future.

When the culture changes so that information is shared with all employees, those employees become willing to risk sharing their opinions with management staff in the best interest of the residents. This approach accomplishes two things:

1. When the organization has knowledgeable staff, those staff members take pride in their daily work.
2. When members of the management team take time to help line staff understand how they impact organizational outcomes, the staff are more receptive to change.

A goal of Wellspring is to make daily facility operation more efficient. With greater staff efficiency there is time for increased staff creativity. An example of this type of innovative program is "Walking with the Beat" at Good Shepherd Services in Seymour, Wisconsin. The life enrichment coordinator created an interdisciplinary program that began as a quality assurance study.

The goal of the program was to determine if music combined with a rhythmic beat matched to the tempo of a resident's gait might positively impact walking distance, quality of gait and the resident's response to ambulation. Results have been very positive. One resident was able to increase his ambulation distance from seventy-five to over three hundred feet. This resident, who had cardiac disease, was able to increase the distance he walked and yet was less short of breath during the exercise. A second resident was able to return home following her progression to independent ambulation. A third resident progressed from walking fifty feet with the assistance of two to three staff members to three hundred feet with the assistance of only one person. These positive results have been replicated with many other residents since the program began. Today "Walking with the Beat" is featured on the State of Wisconsin Bureau of Quality Assurance web site as a part of their "Best Practices Program." This creative program has benefited residents and given the staff a sense of pride with their accomplishments.

CONCLUSION

The Institute for the Future of Aging Services (IFAS) has completed the project that evaluated the Wellspring Program as a model for promoting quality of care in nursing homes. The research determined that

> Wellspring has an explicit approach to quality improvement that focuses on both clinical care and organizational culture change, with a high degree of interaction between these two core concepts . . . Wellspring does mesh clinical and cultural change together in an intentional model of quality improvement in nursing homes. (Stone and Reinhard, 2001b)

In order for the program to work the organizational culture and the Wellspring process must be compatible. Every department and every employee in the organization has a role in ongoing quality assurance.

When Wellspring is fully implemented within a facility, managers must be totally committed to the process on an ongoing basis, front-line staff must feel empowered to make critical decisions about the work they do, and information sharing is crucial in daily activities.

Wellspring, in its seven year tenure, has successfully responded to the institutional long-term care crisis and in so doing has created a model of culture change rooted in clinical best practices, which has the potential to be replicated on a national basis.

REFERENCES

Stone, R. & Reinhard, S. (2001a). Promoting Quality in Nursing Homes: The Wellspring Model. The Commonwealth Fund. *Field Report.*

Stone, R. & Reinhard, S. (2001b). Evaluating the Wellspring Program as a Model for Promoting Quality of Care in Nursing Homes. Institute for the Future of Aging Services. *Grant No. 20000483 Final Report.*

Weissman, D., www.mcw.edu/pallmed.

Models for Individuals with Alzheimer Disease: Beyond the Special Care Framework

Douglas Holmes
Mildred Ramirez

SUMMARY. For the past two decades much attention has been given to the definition and evaluation of special care units for nursing home residents with dementia. Beyond their potential as a marketing device, the controversy rages regarding the qualities, qualifications and benefits of special care.

Inasmuch as 80-90% of nursing home residents suffer from some form of cognitive impairment, the debate would be better focussed on the quality of care and living for all residents. In that regard a fundamental restructuring of all nursing home care and life is a more appropriate direction than the continued debate on this more narrow theme. *[Article copies available for a fee from The Haworth Document Delivery Service: 1-800-HAWORTH. E-mail address: <docdelivery@haworthpress.com> Website: <http://www.HaworthPress.com> © 2003 by The Haworth Press, Inc. All rights reserved.]*

Both authors are affiliated with the Research Division of the Hebrew Home for the Aged at Riverdale (RD/HHAR): Douglas Holmes, PhD, is Administrator of Research and Development, HHAR, and Director of the National Alzheimer Center of the HHAR, and Mildred Ramirez, PhD is Research Associate RD/HHAR.

Address correspondence to: Dr. Mildred Ramirez, Research Division, HHAR, 5901 Palisade Avenue, Riverdale, NY 10471.

[Haworth co-indexing entry note]: "Models for Individuals with Alzheimer Disease: Beyond the Special Care Framework." Holmes, Douglas, and Mildred Ramirez. Co-published simultaneously in *Journal of Social Work in Long-Term Care* (The Haworth Social Work Practice Press, an imprint of The Haworth Press, Inc.) Vol. 2, No. 1/2, 2003, pp. 175-181; and: *Culture Change in Long-Term Care* (ed: Audrey S. Weiner, and Judah L. Ronch) The Haworth Social Work Practice Press, an imprint of The Haworth Press, Inc., 2003, pp. 175-181. Single or multiple copies of this article are available for a fee from The Haworth Document Delivery Service [1-800-HAWORTH, 9:00 a.m. - 5:00 p.m. (EST). E-mail address: docdelivery@haworthpress.com].

10.1300/J181v2n01_12

KEYWORDS. Long-term care, dementia, special care units, nursing homes

INTRODUCTION

Before exploring the directions in which they are *going*, one well could ask: "Where did Special Care Units for nursing home residents with dementing illness (SCUs) come *from*?" The answer is that they really grew out of the efforts, in the 1980s, to improve the lot of nursing home residents (Berg et al., 1991). For example, beset by the scandals of the early 1970s, the New York State Department of Health (NYSDOH) undertook a regulatory function, most visible in terms of regular, routine surveys of all Nursing Homes in the State; this was accompanied by a "premium" paid for the maintenance of residents with dementing illness. This step was particularly important, as the NYSDOH is responsible for all 673 nursing homes in New York State (approximately 4% of all the nursing homes in the United States). However, there was little available by way of a "tight" definition of what constituted, or did not constitute, a Special Dementia Care Unit (SCU).

A later step in the developmental chain of SCUs was provided by the National Institute on Aging (a constituent part of the governmental National Institutes of Health), which undertook a collaborative evaluation of eleven SCU intervention programs; this major effort, which extended over one decade, was spearheaded by the "best and the brightest" from within the government and from without, seeking to establish definitively the necessary constituent parts, the impacts, and the costs of SCUs.

As developed in 1993 by a national panel of experts[1] working in profit and non-profit academic and commercial organizations convened by the National Institute on Aging as part of its Collaborative Studies of Dementia Care, in order to be identified as a SCU, a unit had to include at least: (1) additional staffing; (2) special activities staff; (3) location in a unit dedicated entirely to persons with dementing illness; (4) a specially designed environment; (5) specific, written admission criteria; and (6) specific, written discharge criteria. In a survey conducted in the early 1990s, Leon found that approximately 12% of all nursing homes in the United States reported the maintenance of a special dementia care unit (SCU) (Leon, 1991); by the time of his second survey, a decade later, this proportion had almost doubled, to 22% (Leon & Teresi, 2000).

While the final meta analyses of the emergent data are still forthcoming, results to date further suggested that SCUs are really extremely heterogeneous, subject to local conditions and local interpretation of what is "good" for which residents. In other words, the controversy still rages regarding the qualities and the qualifications of Special Care which, to this day, remains a "best effort" at quality of care and quality of life for some facilities, and little short of a marketing gambit for others.

At this juncture, one may more generally ask what is "special" about services which are, ostensibly at least, to be made available to the *majority* of residents in nursing homes? That is, between 80% and 90% of nursing home residents suffer from some degree of cognitive impairment, and perhaps 65% to 80% of them exhibit cognitive impairment to a degree which is consistent with their categorization as "demented" (most frequently senile dementia of the Alzheimer's type) (Teresi & Holmes, 1997). Given this situation, in which we are speaking of services to the *majority* of nursing home residents, is it not more appropriate to speak not of "special" care, but of *quality* of the care meted out to all residents? Such a designation would remove any residual stigmas associated with the identification of a resident as being "SCU-ready," and would reinforce the provision of adequate care–even quality care–to all residents.

This having been said, the authors would be remiss if they did not first make note of the most recent trend, i.e., effecting some degree of change in the cultures of the institution so as to make it (the nursing home) less institutional and more home-like and, in so doing, to render the concept of the SCU borderline obsolete. In other words, renewed attempts are being made to make the entire nursing home culture more homelike, in which there is (a) greater engagement of *all* residents in activities; (b) greater (longer) retention of staff; (c) relaxation of "rules," e.g., those which mandate "three square meals a day," only at specified times, to be replaced by an "open kitchen" 24/7; (d) involving all staff in all activities, at all times, instead of maintaining rigid definitions of what members of one profession can, and cannot, do; and (e) creating permanent assignments of staff to specific residents. There is quantitative evidence in support of some of these notions (Teresi et al., 1993), and anecdotal, clinical evidence in support of others. The bottom line, as stated succinctly by the creator of the *Eden Alternative* (New York State Department of Health, 1994), during a recent meeting of persons involved in the provision of long-term care services to elderly persons: "We are boring our residents to death" (Thomas, 2002). While this represents an admittedly extreme view, the fact does remain, however, that the (advertized) presence of an SCU for persons with dementing disease may constitute little more than a marketing tool (Holmes, 1996; Holmes & Teresi, 1994) and, as such, may accomplish none of its stated goals. That is, some nursing homes advertize themselves as providing SCUs, when in fact, there is little "special" about the care actually being provided.

RECOMMENDATIONS

This information suggests two (possibly conflicting) points of view, namely, that there is some doubt as to the applicability of the term "Special" to the care of nursing home residents with dementing illness, although the prevalence of "Special" dementia care has doubled over the last decade, with more promised to come. Therefore, let us speak now less of SCU care for residents with dementing illness, and more of Quality Care (QC) for *all* residents, borrowing overtly and directly from that which has been learned from the SCU trials and evaluations of the last decade (Teresi et al., 1997; Teresi et al., 2000a; Holmes et al., 2000b). First, we know that care can (and probably should) come in "many flavors." That is, not only should there be differing levels of *dementia* care in any single nursing home (Teresi et al., 1993), this concept should be extended to all types of care, i.e., there should be available a menu of placement options so that each resident can be situated in the company of his/her peers. Second, staff (with the necessary professional credentials) should be sufficient and available to fulfill all resident needs; this will mandate differing staff configurations for different units, to include staff who are specially-trained and with orientations specific to such additional special activities as are deemed appropriate for each sub-group of residents. Third, the nursing home environment, itself, should be "cleaned up." That is, the traditional hospital/institutional "cookie-cutter" approach should be abandoned entirely . . . even such environments that have been changed to become (putatively) more "dementia friendly." In other words, tacking on a wandering path (straight or circular) to a pre-existing nursing home corridor-focused environment will not suffice. Instead, there is urgent need for new construction which, from the ground up, seeks to replicate in spirit and in fact, the "home environment." This is not to say that nursing home environments should seek to replicate communities (which may never have really existed); however, each should constitute a place in which the resident can feel at home.

Speaking practically, it will prove economical in the long term to plan for the several trends we now have identified as relating particularly to long-term care. In addition to the fact that the majority of facilities rely on public (largely Medicaid) support and that the great majority of residents in these facilities are demented, these "trends" suggest that, as a function of demographic imperatives, there will be a growing crescendo of demand for long-term care, including nursing home care, for elderly persons, of a magnitude with which society is not prepared to deal; among the burgeoning numbers of nursing home applicants will be growing numbers of minority elders–it is projected that the proportion of elderly Hispanics will greatly outstrip the proportion of non-Hispanics by the year 2020 (Kaye et al., 1990)–which, after all, is less than two decades away–the point here is that not only will we have to further develop and expand existing facilities and programs, but will have to further differentiate among programs so as to target a larger, more diverse, number of specific sub-groups, as well (Arbepimpe, 1994). Further, given the potential enormity of programmatic needs coupled with the inability of society to pay for emergent programs, it will become necessary to focus on the creation and/or refinement of alternative modalities of care, possibly to include reliance on technological innovation.

As an example of non-technological alternatives we have only to look at the growth of the assisted living "industry"–noting that in this, as in nursing homes, there is an purported effort to develop "special dementia care" although, in at least some instances, this is little more than an attempted marketing tool. Here the authors do not seek to comment on the current status of assisted living facilities, but only to cite them as potential alternatives to more traditional forms of institutional long-term care. Turning to technology, society is–or should be–on the brink of launching many innovations which will both improve care and reduce total cost. For example, telemedicine is being used to monitor and generally "reach" elderly diabetics who live in hard-to-serve areas (Shea et al., (PI) Ongoing). Another technological "first" will permit ongoing passive electronic monitoring of persons for possible falls and/or deviations from usual routines, e.g., leaving the bed every night for a predetermined "average" time duration. Such technological innovations may well make it possible for greater numbers of impaired dependent elderly persons, including those with mild or moderate dementia, to receive higher quality care, and for society to provide such care at reasonable cost (Shea et al., 2002). Or, "technological innovations" can be very simple . . . as simple as removing a door threshold for easier passage of a wheelchair, or of "medium simplicity," e.g., having installed a panic alarm system, or an automated locking system in order to prevent wandering.

In conclusion, a simple suggestion: We should each look at our own self in the mirror and ask a straightforward question relative to the nursing home with which we are connected: "Would *I* like to spend the last days of my life in this nursing home?" If not, there is something terribly wrong with the situation . . . because, willy-nilly, a nursing home resident must spend his/her last days in . . . not his/her home, but in the institution for which we are responsible.

Perhaps our in-depth discussions about the benefits of special care units and related heterogeneous versus homogeneous placement of residents in long-term care have distracted us from the more fundamental restructuring of the basic nursing home model of care and living–that would indeed be a more valuable goal.

NOTE

1. Panel convened in 1993 by the Coordinating Center to the NIA Studies of Special Dementia Care. Panel members included Leonard Berg, Kathleen Buckwalter, M. Powell Lawton, Joel Leon, Katie Maslow, Douglas Holmes, and Jeanne Teresi.

REFERENCES

Abepimpe, V. (1994). Race, Racism, and Epidemiological Surveys. *Hospital and Community Psychiatry,* 45(1), 27-31.

Berg, L., Buckwalter, K.C., Chafetz, P.K., Gwyther, L.P., Holmes, D., Koepke, K.M., Lawton, M.P., Lindeman, D.A., Magaziner, J., Maslow, K., Morley, J.E., Ory, M.G., Rabins, P.V., Sloane, P.D. & Teresi, J. (1991). Special Article: Special care units for persons with dementia. *Journal of the American Geriatrics Society,* 39, 1229-1236.

Holmes D., & Teresi, J. (1994). Characteristics of Special Care Units in the North East Five State Survey: Implications of Different Definitional Criteria. *Alzheimer's Disease and Associated Disorders: An International Journal* 8, Suppl. 1, S97-S105.

Holmes, D. (1996). Special care units: What makes them special? *Nursing Home Economics,* February/March, 28-31.

Holmes D., Teresi, J., & Ory, M. (2000b). Special Care Units for People with Cognitive Impairment, Including Alzheimer's Disease and Related Disorders: An Overview. *Research & Practice in Alzheimers Disease,* Vol. 4, 7-18.

Kaye, J., Lawton, P., & Kaye, D. (1990). Attitudes of Elderly People about Clinical Research on Aging. *The Gerontologist,* 30(1), 100-111.

Leon, J. (1991). The National Survey of Special Care Units in Nursing Homes, in Holmes, D., Ory, M., & Teresi, J. (Eds.). *Alzheimer's Disease and Associated Disorders: An International Journal,* 8,1, S72-S86.

Leon, J., & Teresi, J. (2000). A Demographic Profile of Nursing Home Residents Suspected of Having Dementia with Confirmed Cognitive Impairment: Findings from the National Institute on Aging Special Care Unit Initiative Studies, in Holmes, D., Teresi, J., & Ory, M. (Eds.). Special Care Units, *Research & Practice in Alzheimer's Disease (RPAD)* 4, 105-116.

New York State Department of Health (1994) grant to the Chase Memorial Nursing Home (in New Berlin, New York) for a demonstration project involving the provision of animals (cats and dogs) and birds (parakeets) in the nursing home. This project, of which the PI was William Thomas, MD., became known as the Eden Alternative.

Ory, M. (1994) in Teresi, J., Lawton, P., Ory, M. & Holmes, D. (Eds.). (1994). Measurement issues in chronic care populations: Dementia special care. *Alzheimer's Disease and Associated Disorders: An International Journal,* 8, Suppl. 1, S144-S183.

Shea, S. (PI) (Ongoing) IDEATel Demonstration, funded by the HCFA (now the Center for Medicare/Medicaid).

Shea, D., Starren J., Weinstock, R., Knudson, P., Teresi, J., Holmes, D., Palmas, W., Field, L., Goland, R., Tuck, C., Hripcsak, G., Capps, L., & Liss, D. (2002). Columbia University's Information for Diabetes Education and Telemedicine (IDEATel) Project *Journal of the American Medical Informatics Association, 9*(1), 49-62.

Teresi, J., Holmes, D., Benenson, E., Monaco, C., Barrett, V., Ramirez, M. & Koren, M. (1993). A primary care nursing model in urban and rural long-term care facilities: Attitudes, morale, and satisfaction of residents and staff. *Research on Aging, 15*, 667-674.

Teresi, J. & Holmes, D. (1997). Reporting source bias in estimating prevalence of cognitive impairment. *Journal of Clinical Epidemiology, 50*(2), 175-184.

Teresi, J., Lawton, P., Holmes, D., & Ory, M. (1997). Guest Editorial: Measurement in Older Chronic Care Populations. *Journal of Mental Health and Aging, 3*(1), 3.

Teresi, J., Holmes, D., & Ory, M. (2000a). The Therapeutic Design of Environments for People with Dementia: Further Reflections and Recent Findings from the National Institute on Aging Collaborative Studies of Dementia Care. Invited Commentary: *The Gerontologist, 40*(4), 417-421.

Thomas, W., Presentation sponsored by the Jewish Home and Hospital for the Aged, at the New York Academy of medicine, as part of a day-long conference on November 1, 2001, dealing with culture change in nursing homes.

Peer Mentoring of Nursing Home CNAs: A Way to Create a Culture of Caring

Carol R. Hegeman

SUMMARY. A carefully-crafted peer mentoring program for CNAs may be an appropriate component of any culture change movement in the long-term care setting. This paper contains a detailed description of the peer mentoring program developed by the Foundation for Long Term Care (FLTC) and how peer mentoring may affect culture, with or without a formal cultural change movement within the facility. In it, we suggest that peer mentoring is likely to (a) improve CNA retention rates; (b) improve orientation processes so that they reflect the values of the facility; (c) reinforce critical skills and behaviors; (d) teach the value of caring; (e) use exemplary aides to role-model exemplary care; (f) support new staff as they make the transition to being part of the facility team; and (g) provide recognition and a career ladder for experienced nurse aides. The nurse aide subculture is critical to a supportive nursing home

Carol R. Hegeman, MS, is the Director of Research at the Foundation for Long Term Care, Albany, NY.

Address correspondence to: Carol R. Hegeman, MS, Director of Research, Foundation for Long Term Care, 150 State Street, Suite 301, Albany, NY 12207 (E-mail: chegeman@nyahsa.org).

The author acknowledges the work of Carolyn Ryan, who refined the tri-part peer mentoring curriculum described here, and the project trainer, Francis Battisti, CSW-R. Also acknowledged are the contributions of other authors of peer mentoring manuals (listed at the end of the article).

[Haworth co-indexing entry note]: "Peer Mentoring of Nursing Home CNAs: A Way to Create a Culture of Caring." Hegeman, Carol R. Co-published simultaneously in *Journal of Social Work in Long-Term Care* (The Haworth Social Work Practice Press, an imprint of The Haworth Press, Inc.) Vol. 2, No. 1/2, 2003, pp. 183-196; and: *Culture Change in Long-Term Care* (ed: Audrey S. Weiner, and Judah L. Ronch) The Haworth Social Work Practice Press, an imprint of The Haworth Press, Inc., 2003, pp. 183-196. Single or multiple copies of this article are available for a fee from The Haworth Document Delivery Service [1-800-HAWORTH, 9:00 a.m. - 5:00 p.m. (EST). E-mail address: docdelivery@haworthpress.com].

10.1300/J181v2n01_13

environment and a culture of caring, and hence, must be considered in any culture change movement. *[Article copies available for a fee from The Haworth Document Delivery Service: 1-800-HAWORTH. E-mail address: <docdelivery@haworthpress.com> Website: <http://www.HaworthPress.com> © 2003 by The Haworth Press, Inc. All rights reserved.]*

KEYWORDS. Peer mentoring, CNAs, culture change, long-term care, staff retention, staff orientation, role model

INTRODUCTION

This article contains a discussion of why a carefully-crafted peer mentoring program for CNAs may be an appropriate component of any culture change movement in the long-term care setting. It also contains a detailed description of the peer mentoring program developed by the Foundation for Long Term Care (FLTC) and how peer mentoring may affect culture and cultural change, with or without a formal cultural change movement within the facility.

This FLTC peer mentoring program, entitled "Growing Strong Roots" in recognition of a powerful poem written by CNA Connie Trendel (see Box 1) is designed to (a) improve CNA retention rates; (b) improve orientation processes so that they reflect the values of the facility; (c) reinforce critical skills and behaviors; (d) teach the value of caring; (e) use exemplary aides to role-model exemplary care; (f) support new staff as they make the transition to being part of the facility team; and (g) provide recognition and a career ladder for experienced nurse aides. It is a program in which experienced and excellent CNAs share values and their practice wisdom with new aides to help the new aides succeed in, and stay with, the facility. By being identified as an excellent worker and by being compensated for their peer mentoring, the experienced aides also benefit.

For the purposes of this project, we define mentoring as a process by which an expert (in this case an exemplary and experienced CNA) acquaints a novice (in this case the newly-hired CNA) with the customs, resources, and values of the organization (Madison, 1994, parentheses added).

The FLTC is a not-for-profit research entity affiliated with the New York Association of Homes and Services for the Aging (NYAHSA), an association of not-for-profit and governmental providers of elder-care services in New York state. The author hopes that the FLTC's enthusiasm for this concept will resonate throughout this paper.

BOX 1

The Caring Tree

Nursing facilities are like trees . . .
The residents are the leaves . . .
growing, changing and falling away from the tree.
The branches are the homes,
giving the leaves a safe, nurturing environment to do their growing,
the other staff are the limbs,
they keep the branches sturdy,
the administration is the trunk of the tree,
supporting the limbs and branches.
I'm sure you are
wondering where nursing assistants fit into this analogy . . .
they are the roots.
Leaves fall, branches and limbs may break in a strong wind,
you can even cut into the trunk of a tree but if the roots are strong,
growth will continue.
Have you ever seen a tree that has a root disease?
The leaves will die without the nourishment the roots provide.
The limbs, branches and trunk will remain for a while but they too eventually die.
They are the roots of every facility.
In the past, they've been called the 'lowman.'
I guess they are, after all, roots are the lowest part of the tree . . .
also one of the most
vital.

By Connie Trendel, CNA
Printed with permission.

Connie Trendal lives in Michigan where she has been a Certified Nursing Assistant in long-term care for over 20 years. She is a Certified Eden Associate and serves as her facility's NAGNA (National Association of Geriatric Nursing Assistants) Chapter Chairperson. Connie has taken advantage of many opportunities to write about, and teach others, her powerful message–that a CNA is not "just an CNA," but a professional caregiver.

THEORETICAL AND RESEARCH BACKGROUND

A FLTC survey of 345 nursing homes from three states (New York, Pennsylvania, and Illinois) in 1999 revealed that 69 percent of respondents have some form of self-defined mentoring or peer support program for their CNAs, but only 13 percent of respondents reported mentoring programs which focus not only on expediting initial training, but also on *supporting* new aides so that they remain with the facility (Hegeman, 2001). This expanded concept of peer mentoring is the one used in this article.

Based on information and concepts from these respondents, other extant models, a literature search and suggestions from our consultants and advisory board, the FLTC developed "Growing Strong Roots." At the time this article is being written, the FLTC is rigorously testing its impact in 15 New York state not-for-profit nursing homes.

There are three key ways by which a peer mentoring program relates to culture change: (1) it has the potential to improve retention of staff; (2) it is a cultural change movement of its own, focused on the CNA subculture; and (3) it supports other principles of culture change. Each of these responses is discussed below.

Improving retention: With turnover rates of nursing home CNAs cited as high as 105 percent (Wilner and Wyatt, 1998), it can be difficult to begin and support culture change. Historically, aides do not remain at a facility long enough for meaningful education, not only to the cultural change environment, but to the very basics of care. The revolving door of CNAs is a self-perpetuating problem. Aides leave in frustration because staffing is short, and staffing is short because aides are leaving.

Peer mentoring promises to be part of the solution to this disheartening downward spiral. Straker and Atchley (1999) report that in a survey they conducted "both nursing home and home health care agencies with low turnover rates were more likely to mention programs to *improve co-worker relationships* than their high turnover counterparts." Developing good co-worker relationships is, of course, at the core of peer mentoring. A study of one peer mentoring program found turnover was reduced from 53.7 percent to 17 percent once the program started (Shemansky, 1998).

Reducing costs: There is also a potential for considerable cost-saving. One study estimates the cost of turnover in a nursing home at $4,000 per position per year in 1992 dollars (Straker and Atchley, 1999). When translated to a facility level, just one facility with a high turnover rate could spend more than $240,000 on recruiting and replacing staff. This project may therefore result not only in improved care, but also in savings that can be used for direct care of residents.

PEER MENTORING AS CULTURAL CHANGE FOR CNAs

Peer mentoring is also–in itself–a way to create a culture of caring among aides within a long-term care facility. When carefully-selected, experienced CNAs who embody the caring values of their facility become successful peer mentors, there are clear potential organizational changes:

- aides who demonstrate and embody a culture of caring are acknowledged and recognized. It is a program expectation that this acknowledge-

ment will increase their own satisfaction and retain them within the facility. Therefore, we are rewarding the skills we most value;
- the behaviors and attitudes of staff that support a culture of caring are the behaviors and attitudes the new CNA is exposed to, making it more likely they will be the traits which are learned and emulated; and,
- the facility establishes a formal process to develop a positive CNA subculture.

The nurse aide subculture is critical to a supportive nursing home environment. It interacts separately from and often in reaction to the corporate culture of the entire nursing home. Deal and Kennedy [in Ramirez (1990)] define the culture of a nursing service organization as just "the way we do things around here." If the "way we do things around here" is perceived as supportive, work redesign is more productive (McDaniel and Stumpf, 1993). If CNAs perceive "the way we do things around here" as supportive of both them and the residents they care for, there is likely to be a positive CNA culture.

By contrast, a negative perception of "the way we do things" can aid and abet a negative subculture of the nursing aide within the nursing home. A Website devoted to CNAs (*http://www.nursingassistant.org/HorizV1.html*) used the term "horizontal sabotage" for negative CNA-to-CNA behaviors which are in reaction to a facility culture that is seen as punitive. Examples included setting the next shift up for failure or blaming a previous shift for mistakes or omissions made by the current shift.

A negative CNA subculture can also occur by omission. In an observational study, Bowers and Becker (1992) noted that experienced CNAs were, while not hostile to the new CNAs, quite passive about making any effort to help them, commenting frequently on whether they believed a new employee would make it or not, but rarely offering any assistance to help the new hires be successful. This kind of studied indifference to the real challenges of starting work in a long-term care unit (which in some cases can also be seen in management staff) is what some advisory board members of "Growing Strong Roots" describe as a system in which nursing homes "eat their young." A peer mentoring program in which aides are empowered when they support each other may well reduce the deleterious "horizontal sabotage" and "eating their young" effects on CNAs.

Another approach to the nursing home CNA subculture was developed by Tellis-Nayak and Tellis-Nayak (1989). It focuses on how the culture CNAs bring *to* the facility affects the culture *within* the facility, classifying inner-city aides into two types: (a) the determined "strivers" and (b) the disaffected "endurers." Needless to say, the "strivers" are hired more frequently, but tend not to stay.

The typical facility, Tellis-Nayak and Tellis-Nayak (1989) assert, with its middle-class management, often does not respond to the needs of this larger second group and reinforces their disaffection. The authors suggest that poor administrators ignore the affective needs of these aides, but excellent administrators foster a family spirit that compensates for the challenges of their personal world. Peer mentoring may be a way to create this family spirit.

SUPPORTING ELEMENTS OF CULTURAL CHANGE

A third way peer mentoring can relate to cultural values and cultural change in the nursing home setting is by supporting other principles of culture change. Certainly, one cornerstone of cultural change in nursing homes is greater autonomy of both residents and staff. Bowers and Becker (1992) found that strategies developed by individual nurse aides to plan and implement the way they deliver care affected the quality of care they give. If, as would be logical, nursing home management selects mentors who embody *both* caring behaviors and excellent care planning/time management skills, new CNAs will learn a critical, but often untaught "trick of the trade"–effective management of their work load so that they work and respond to the collective needs of residents rather than work around a rigid task list.

The speed of the acquisition of knowledge will also be impaired. Instead of learning time and resident management by trial and error (or even worse, not learning it at all and quitting in frustration), new aides will learn important "tricks of the trade" faster. Peer mentoring is an ideal way to teach positive "practice wisdom" management not formally taught in the clinical skills component of the CNA certification program.

DESCRIPTION OF THE FLTC'S PEER MENTORING PROGRAM

"Growing Strong Roots" is a project supported by funding from the Fan Fox and Leslie R. Samuels Foundation. The overall goal of the project, funded in March 2001, is to create an effective, replicable, and sustainable peer mentoring program for new nursing assistants which encourages their retention and commitment to explicit caring values of long-term care.

Measurable objectives are:

1. to develop a training intervention based on the "best of the best" of peer mentoring programs that have shown promise in nursing homes across the country;
2. to test this intervention in 15 nursing homes in New York state in terms of costs, feasibility and outcomes; and,
3. to disseminate findings through the World Wide Web, national conferences, specific trainings and through a Web and print-based "how-to" manual.

Consistent with the objective to build upon "the best of the best" of extent models, those models (see Appendix A) were reviewed, analyzed, synthesized and broadened with input from the project's advisory board (see Appendix B) and refined following experience at the pilot site.

The model that was ultimately developed has five core organizational components:

- training for facility coordinators;
- an orientation for the mentor and mentee's supervisor to assure their support;
- mentor training;
- follow-up booster training of mentors; and,
- a formal evaluation.

It is important to note that two of these components (facility coordinator and supervisor training and orientation) provide an essential facility-wide context for the peer mentoring training. It is, in the view of the advisory board and project staff, naïve and counterproductive to try to fix a system-wide problem by targeting resources solely on training of CNAs, who are often the victims of larger management problems (short staffing, scheduling, case mix) rather than its cause. A peer mentoring program is designed for aides, but it is also a statement that the entire facility has core values it wishes to impart to the new aides and is willing to reward experienced aides who embody these core values through a special program. Therefore, it is a project that should be "owned" by the entire facility. This facility-wide ownership, of course, is a prerequisite of any culture change endeavor.

The training for facility coordinators, called "facility liaisons" in this project, focuses on assuring facility "buy-in," an overview of project training content and a checklist of the myriad of logistical issues inherent in a project of this size. These logistical issues include: a process for recruiting and selecting mentors; union involvement; project oversight; training logistics; and evaluation.

The training program for the mentors requires a full six-hour day; it is recommended that the selected aides receive this training off-site, in the same way nurse supervisors and administrations attend workshops. This "away from work" training accomplishes two things:

1. it sets this training apart from the familiar in-services; and
2. avoids the CNA being called back onto the unit.

The educational goals of the peer mentoring training are to:

1. identify the four main roles of a mentor (role model, social support, tutor, peer resource);
2. describe how a positive attitude sets the tone for the social and professional integration of mentees into the facility;
3. demonstrate the use of effective communication skills;
4. describe ways to use leadership skills to recognize and manage potential conflicts and solve problems;
5. recognize situations when information or guidance is needed from other sources and be able to access the appropriate resources and references (a critical component here is that the mentor *does not* teach clinical skills);
6. describe how to use reinforcement strategies to assist the in-service coordinator and mentee to identify, plan, and reinforce learning experiences; and
7. apply mentoring skills to real-life situations.

The supervisor training is a one-hour overview which is intended to build support for the project. Without such an orientation, supervisors may resent or block mentors and mentees from spending extra time together because it is perceived as a disruption of work or as a diminution of their authority. The training content includes a review of the rationale and goals of the project and allows time for supervisors to make suggestions on the project implementation, therefore assuring increased support.

The booster session is an additional one-half day of training for the mentors scheduled after they have been working with their mentees for approximately four weeks. With a trained facilitator, the challenges, joys and frustrations of working in the program are shared. Several typical challenges are shared and joint solutions found. In addition, there is a review of important skills introduced in the training program.

The evaluation is described in a subsequent section of this paper.

TIME-FRAME AND PROCESS

"Growing Strong Roots" is organized so that:

- The person assigned to coordinate the project within the nursing home receives five hours of focused orientation, using the facility liaison manual designed for this purpose.
- Each nursing home selects from 5-15 mentors to provide mentoring to at least 10 but no more than 30 "mentees" (The number range is large to reflect the different sizes of facilities and different sizes of new CNA cohorts).
- Mentoring takes place *after* the CNA certification is complete. This mentoring is intended to supplement, not replace or duplicate, the usual training of new CNAs.
- Each mentee-mentor has an active relationship for eight weeks (more if needed). The intensity of the relationship will be highest in the beginning, then reduces incrementally.

The mentor is working on four areas with the mentee: role model; social support; tutor; peer resource. In the first week, the mentee and mentor work together on the same shift, with the mentee initially observing care and gradually taking on a more significant role in care. In weeks two to four, both mentor and mentee have a full complement of residents, but about two hours a week is devoted to mentee support by the mentor. In weeks four to eight, only one week of direct contact is involved.

- Mentor training makes clear that the mentor does not teach or re-teach clinical skills. Formal education remains the responsibility of the in-service educator, and the mentor is encouraged to notify training staff when re-training seems indicated.

At each stage, all four roles (detailed in training) are covered. The mentor is modeling correct clinical skills and attitudes, time management, reinforcing formal policies and procedures, explaining the far more subtle and informal policies of breaks, lunches, telephone usage, encouraging the new CNA to use the facility resources to make the job easier and more understandable, and being a good friend and advocate.

- The FLTC suggests that the mentor and the mentee(s) be on the same shift and on the same unit, as all other options will complicate logistics. If this option is not possible, however, each facility will have to decide who moves: the mentee or mentor.

- Each facility provides a 10-20 percent salary increase for the extra work the mentors will have. For some models, the extra work of the mentors simply cannot be accomplished in the usual shift. In that case, the facility must decide whether to change the honorarium to an overtime payment or to reduce the workload of the liaison.

This specific structure will not work for every nursing home. Therefore, one of the many responsibilities for the facility liaison is to determine which operational changes, if any, need to be made in this model so that it will work well. Even in a demonstration project, nursing home structures and needs may differ and nursing homes may operationalize the project differently.

We envision that this eight-week cycle will be repeated each time a new class of CNAs enters the facility. This time frame excludes the initial planning time as well as the preliminary work the facility will have to do to develop its own protocol for recruitment and selection of mentors. Timing for these activities will be at minimum a few months, and probably more for most facilities, especially those which involve a union.

COSTS

Grant funding is being used to develop and refine the training materials, orient and train the participating sites across New York, and conduct the evaluation. It does not support costs at each site, and in fact, each site is required to contribute matching funds toward the cost of the project. Each site is also monitoring costs as one of the evaluation activities.

Because, at the time this article is being written, we are in the early stages of the project, formal cost information for participating nursing homes is not yet available. However, some costs are predictable: management staff time in planning and implementation; training (an outside trainer is recommended); extra payment for mentors (either in the form of a temporary salary increase or honorarium); extra staffing costs when the mentors are being trained to cover their units; and depending on how the mentor-mentee relationship is designed, extra staff costs during the eight-week mentoring program.

OUTCOMES

Outcome data are not yet available. However, a comprehensive project evaluation has been implemented. The 15 New York state nursing homes in this project are divided into one pilot site (which received the training first and provided feedback so that the training material could be refined); seven intervention sites at which the program will first be implemented; and seven "wait-comparison" sites which will implement the program after the first intervention sites are completed. For evaluation purposes, however, data at the wait-comparison sites will be collected at the same time the intervention groups are completing the peer mentoring program.

The evaluation design consists of:

- Comparison of retention rates of new CNAs being mentored with CNAs in wait-comparison group at (1) baseline, (2) post-test, and (3) post-post-test intervals; and,
- Comparison of attitudinal scores of mentees at (1) baseline, (2) post-test, and (3) post-post-test intervals.

At the end of the three-year intervention, we intend to answer such important process questions such as:

1. What barriers (organizational, administrative, fiscal, etc.) assist or impede effective implementation of the intervention?
2. What staffing and deployment strategies assist or impede effective implementation of the intervention? and,
3. What are the cost benefits of this intervention as compared to the hidden costs of doing nothing about high turnover?

The heart of this project evaluation, however, is to determine its impact on the new CNAs, since their longevity and nature of the care they give is critical to quality. This part of the evaluation will answer the following questions:

1. When implemented in a sample of New York state nursing homes, does the FLTC's model of peer mentoring have a positive impact on the retention of participating nurse aides?
2. When implemented in a sample of New York state nursing homes, do the "peer-mentored" aides demonstrate more knowledge of the importance of their role, their resident-staff relationship, and more effective caring behavior than comparable aides who were not mentored?

RELEVANCE TO SOCIAL WORK PRACTICE AND VALUES

There is a natural potential affinity between social work and a peer mentoring program in nursing homes. In terms of conceptual affinities, both look for and build upon the strengths of a target population. Mentors' strengths are ac-knowledged and used to develop new aides. Both value empowerment. Peer mentoring of aides empowers the mentors to supplement their caring nature to extend from residents to peers. It empowers the new aide by providing a locus of support.

On a more practical level, participating in the design and training of a CNA peer mentoring program may present an expanded role for the long-term care social worker. Social workers are always relied upon to enhance the residents' integration into the facility. It seems a logical extension for the long-term care social worker to be called up to enhance the integration of new staff into the fa-cility as well. The interpersonal skills of the professional social worker can be well used in this manner, and foster interdepartmental cooperation in pursuit of a common goal.

REFERENCES

Bowers, B. and Becker, M. (1992). Nurses Aides in Nursing Homes: The relationship between organization and quality. *The Gerontologist*, 32, 360-366.

Hegeman, C. (2001). Peer Mentoring by and for Certified Nurse Aides in Nursing Homes: A Synthesis from a Tri-State Study and the Literature. *The Gerontologist*, 41, 93.

Madison, J., RN, MPH. (1994). The Value of Mentoring in Nursing Leadership: A De-scriptive Study. *Nursing Forum*, 29, 17-23.

McDaniel, C. and Stumpf, L. (1993). The Organizational Culture: Implications for nursing service. *Journal of Nursing Administration*, 23, 54-60.

Ramirez, C. (1990). Culture in a Nursing Service Organization. *Nursing Management*, 21, 14-5.

Shemansky, C.A., Med, RNC. (1998). Preceptors in Long-Term Care: 1997 NGNA In-novations in Practice Award Winner. *Geriatric Nursing*, 19, 232-234.

Straker, J. and Atchley, R. (1999). *Recruiting and Retaining Frontline Workers in Long-term Care*. Oxford: Scripps Gerontology Center, Miami University.

Tellis-Nayak, V. and Tellis-Nayak, M. (1989). Quality of Care and the Burden of Two Cultures: When the world of the nurse's aide enters the world of the nursing home. *The Gerontologist*, 29, 579-80.

Wilner, M.A. and Wyatt, A. (1998). *Paraprofessionals on the Front Line: Improving Their Jobs–Improving the Quality of Long-term Care*. Washington DC: AARP.

APPENDIX A

Other Resources for Peer Mentoring of Nursing Home CNAs
Used in the Development of "Growing Strong Roots"

Krause-Barrett, H., Biklin, P., and Findley, D. (n.d.) *For Those Who Mentor*. Des Moines: Iowa Caregivers Association.

Maruschock, Roberta G. (1999). *Certified Nursing Assistant Mentor Program*. Rochester: Kirkhaven Nursing Home.

Pillemer, K., Hegeman, C., Dean, C., Albright, B. and Meador, R. (1997). *Partners in Caregiving*. Ithaca: Cornell Applied Gerontology Research Institute.

Pillemer, K., Hoffman, R., Meador, R., and Schumacher, M. (n.d.) *CNA Mentoring Made Easy*. Somerville: Frontline Publishing.

Shemansky, C. (1999). *Nursing Preceptor Handbook*. Burlington: Masonic Home of New Jersey.

Nursing Assistant Mentor Program Handbook. (1998). Quincy: Quincy United Methodist Home.

APPENDIX B

Advisory Board
Fan Fox and Leslie R. Samuels Foundation

Diane Findley
Executive Director
Iowa Caregivers Association
1117 Pleasant Street, Suite 221
Des Moines, IA 50309
Phone: 515-2418-697
Fax: 515-248-587
E-mail: iowacga@aol.com

Edward (Ned) Hirt
Director of Human Resources
United Helpers Management Company
732 Ford Street
Ogdensburg, NY 13669
Telephone: 315-393-3074 ext. 220
Fax: 315-393-3083
E-mail neduh@northnet.org

Ann Gignac
Director of Education
Baptist Health Nursing and
Rehabilitation Center
297 North Ballston Avenue
Scotia, NY 12302
Telephone: 518-370-4700 ext.161
Fax: 518-370-5048
E-mail: gignaca@nycap.rr.com

Sara Joffe
Paraprofessional HI
100 Yale Ave
Swarthmore, PA 19081
Phone: 610-544-3768
Email: HCASara@aol.com

Kathy Knee
Owner
Specialty Seminars
587 Sturbridge Drive
Highland Heights, OH 44143
Telephone: 440-461-7370
Fax: 440-461-7370
E-mail: kne@prodigy.net

Ann Rotz
Director of Staff Development
Quincy United Methodist
Homes and Village
6596 Orphanage Road
Quincy, PA 17247
Phone: 717-749-3151
Fax: 717-749-2013
E-mail: qhome@innernet.net

Peola Small
Director of Patient Care Services
Dr. Susan Smith McKinney Nursing
and Rehabilitation Center
594 Albany Avenue
Brooklyn, NY 11203
Phone: 718-245-7231
Fax: 718-245-7060
E-mail: peesmall@aol.com

Nancy Tucker
Director of Nursing Facility Policy
NYAHSA
150 State Street
Albany, NY 12207
Phone: 518-449-2707
Fax: 518-449-8210
E-mail: ntucker@nyahsa.org

Linda G. Morrison
Outreach Program Manager
Wisconsin Alzheimer's Institute
7818 Big Sky Drive, Suite 215
Madison, WI 53719
Ph: 608-829-3306
Fax: 608-829-3315
E-mail: lgmorrison@facstaff.wisc.edu

Cindy Shemansky
Director of Education
Masonic Home of New Jersey
902 Jacksonville Road
Burlington, NJ 08016
Phone: 609-239-3924
Fax: 609-386-1199
E-mail: cas@njmasonic.org

Robyn Stone
Executive Director
Institute for the Future of Aging Services
AAHSA
901 E Street NW, Suite 500
Washington, DC 20001
Phone: 202-783-2242
Fax: 202-783-2255
E-mail: rstone@aahsa.org

Mary Ann Wilner
Paraprofessional HI
349 E 149 Street, Suite 401
Bronx, NY 10451
Phone: 718-402-7226
Fax: 718-585-6852
E-mail: maryann@paraprofessional.org

The Live Oak Regenerative Community: Championing a Culture of Hope and Meaning

Barry Barkan

SUMMARY. The Live Oak Regenerative Community has been applying a new culture of aging throughout the continuum of life for elders since 1977. Among a number of models for culture change, the Live Oak Regenerative Community is distinguished by its focus on building a healthy culture for aging rather than on mitigating the negative effects of aging. This paper tells the story of the development of the Live Oak Regenerative Community. It describes the values, the processes and the roles that enable the model to impact the lives of elders and to transform institutions. It describes the theoretical framework for the Regenerative Community and presents stories that illustrate how the approach has

Barry Barkan has been developing the Live Oak Regenerative Community since 1977. Director of Live Oak Institute and Co-CEO of Regenerative Health Systems, Inc., he is a founding member of the Pioneer Network Board of Directors and a co-founder of the Spiritual Eldering Project.

Address correspondence to: Barry Barkan, Live Oak Institute, 2150 Pyramid Drive, El Sobrante, CA 94803 (E-mail: barbarkan@aol.com).

Dedication: My wife Debora Cushman Barkan is my soul partner and my best friend in the work of Live Oak Regenerative Community Development. She has kept the light burning when I might have given up and continues to create much of the best of what we do. This paper is dedicated to her.

[Haworth co-indexing entry note]: "The Live Oak Regenerative Community: Championing a Culture of Hope and Meaning." Barkan, Barry. Co-published simultaneously in *Journal of Social Work in Long-Term Care* (The Haworth Social Work Practice Press, an imprint of The Haworth Press, Inc.) Vol. 2, No. 1/2, 2003, pp. 197-221; and: *Culture Change in Long-Term Care* (ed: Audrey S. Weiner, and Judah L. Ronch) The Haworth Social Work Practice Press, an imprint of The Haworth Press, Inc., 2003, pp. 197-221. Single or multiple copies of this article are available for a fee from The Haworth Document Delivery Service [1-800-HAWORTH, 9:00 a.m. - 5:00 p.m. (EST). E-mail address: docdelivery@haworthpress.com].

worked. A vision is offered for the Live Oak Elders Guild, an approach to creating a new role for elders of the new millennium. *[Article copies available for a fee from The Haworth Document Delivery Service: 1-800-HAWORTH. E-mail address: <docdelivery@haworthpress.com> Website: <http://www.HaworthPress.com> © 2003 by The Haworth Press, Inc. All rights reserved.]*

KEYWORDS. Culture, transformation, regenerative community, community developer, Live Oak Institute, Live Oak Living Center, mastery path

PURPOSE OF PAPER

The purpose of this paper is to inform the reader of the values, history, methodologies, expanded roles and evolving body of work that are intrinsic to the Live Oak Regenerative Community. On a deeper level it is the intention to transmit an experience of the Live Oak Regenerative Community that recruits the reader to seed regenerative community development in all settings where elders are served.

The form and language of an approach to cultural transformation, such as the Live Oak Regenerative Community, is as much metaphoric and poetic as prosaic, and this is reflected in the form and style of this paper. More than anything this paper is the story of an evolving body of work. It is interpreted through the heart of one person who has been privileged to be inspired by a vision of a new culture of aging in which the old and abandoned are transformed into the elders of society, connecting past and future and leaving the world as a better place. Like any good story, each person who lives in the midst of its unfolding will tell it from a unique point of view. The aggregate of the points of view defines the culture, conveying the episodic events, heroic actions and living truths that support the life of the community.

DEFINITION OF MODEL

The Live Oak Regenerative Community is not so much a model based on a structured, replicable design as it is a consciously cultivated culture, a living system, formulated with the intention of creating a healthy culture of aging within the long-term care environment and ultimately within the wider society. For purposes of defining the Live Oak Regenerative Community, a living culture provides an environment in which the people who are an integral part can achieve their greatest possible potential, by bringing past, present and future into harmony. The people are constantly interacting with and influencing one another and the larger systems with which they are connected, thus expanding their collective potential and assuring that those who come after them will thrive.

The Live Oak Regenerative Community is one of a number of approaches within the emerging "culture change movement" that focuses on building a new and healthy culture within long-term care organizations. Among these approaches are the Eden Alternative, resident directed care, resident centered care and Wellspring (see other models within this volume). William Thomas, MD, founder of the Eden Alternative, explains the difference between the Live Oak approach and these other models:

> The basis of the Eden Alternative and all these other models is that they sought to mitigate problems connected to aging and institutional life. For example, the Eden Alternative, was developed in response to the three plagues of hopelessness, loneliness and boredom. Although these approaches share many common values and approaches, the Live Oak Regenerative Community approach is differentiated by its concentration on regenerating a culture in which elders evolve and transform, not as a mitigant to problems, but as a healthy context for aging. (Thomas, 2002)

Structurally, the core components of the Regenerative Community are (1) values, which keep the organism on course and promote a dynamic homeostasis within the community; (2) methodologies for community development which provide the context for people to grow and fulfill themselves; and (3) creation of a role for people who consciously take responsibility for promoting the culture's values and championing change and renewal.

The heart of the "model" is the conscious and consistent cultivation of a community developed with the intention of connecting people to who they are, to one another and to a positive vision of what it means to be an elder in this culture. Beginning with residents at the center of culture, community development also involves the full range of stakeholders within the long-term care setting, including family members; staff on all levels and in all departments; volunteers; governing body; advocates; ombudsmen; and state surveyors. The community provides the people with a cultural context through which they can form relationships and do the naturally occurring "things" that people have done in healthy cultures and healthy communities since the beginning of time. They care for one another. They celebrate life and its seasons. They mourn together. They informally teach one another how to belong. They solve problems. They promote a healthy future so that those who come later will benefit from the experience of their life together.

The resident community meeting which is described later in this paper is the keystone of the Regenerative Community. Once the community meeting is established, the culture takes on a life of its own as the stakeholders begin to feel its impact and identify with it. A significant variable is the extent to which management embraces the values promoted by the Regenerative Community and seeks to make decisions and relate to people based upon these values.

The Regenerative Community culture is based on the working assumption that all the stakeholders share such basic human needs as friendship; recognition; self esteem; connection to one another; integrity in relationship; the experience of being heard; respect for one's origins and traditions; joy; meaning; preparation for the future; and pride in what one does and in one's affiliation. The more these needs are met, the more the quality of life, the quality of care and the quality of belonging within the long-term care organization flourish.

The building blocks of the culture are its lore and stories; songs and jokes; collective memory; hopes and aspirations; initiations and roles; vision and dreams; values and principles; ethos and traditions; practices and rituals that enable the heart and soul of a community to drive an organization towards its highest purposes.

The Regenerative Community is a living system, connected to a universe of other interconnected living systems, in which the whole is greater than sum of its parts and the parts are constantly informed by the larger context. Thus, for example, the Live Oak culture which has been cultivated for a quarter of a century and the culture of the emerging Pioneer movement share a common source and common future with one another. And these share a common source and common future with the many movements with which they have been and will be connected.

DESCRIPTION OF VALUES

When we talk about "values" in the Regenerative Community, we refer to the core beliefs that, through their acceptance and practice, define the culture and support its evolution in a way that promotes the well being of its members. The values and mission of the Live Oak Regenerative Community are intrinsically connected. From the moment we began conceptualizing the Live Oak work in the mid-seventies, the renewal of the culture of aging and of elder care was at the heart of our mission.

From the outset we understood that the culture of elder care is awry because both the role of institutions and the role of elders in society were off kilter. The core values of the Regenerative Community were distilled to bring healing and renewal to the culture of aging and of long-term care by creating a new vision of the role of elder and empowering a shift in the way stakeholders in long-term care environments relate to themselves, to one another and to the long-term care environment.

Formally, the values of the Regenerative Community are transmitted to stakeholders through: community meetings with its songs and rituals of initiation; in-service education; orientation; intake interviews; the educational process of progressive discipline, etc. Informally, the values are communicated on a person-to-person basis. Because they speak to what is real and meaningful in the lives of the people, they are readily owned and shared through the informal networks of communication that exist in every community.

The core values of the Live Oak Regenerative Community follow.

- The people who live in long-term care environments are the elders of the people. The Live Oak "Definition of an Elder" has been printed on a poster and distributed to more than 2,000 individuals and organizations. It is promoted as the central creed of the *Spiritual Eldering Institute*. Spiritual Eldering Institute is an organization that was begun by Rabbi Zalman Schachter Shalomi in 1993 to promote conscious aging. Live Oak Institute community developers were actively involved in the development of the spiritual eldering and conscious aging concepts and program design and were among the founders of the Spiritual Eldering Project which was ultimately incorporated as the Spiritual Eldering Institute.

The Live Oak Definition of an Elder

An elder is a person who is still growing, still a learner, still with potential and whose life continues to have within it promise for, and connection to the future. An elder is still in pursuit of happiness, joy and pleasure, and her or his birthright to these remains intact. Moreover, an elder is a person who deserves respect and honor and whose work it is to synthesize wisdom from long life experience and formulate this into a legacy for future generations. (Barkan, 1977)

The Definition of an Elder battles the negative self image and negative stereotypes promoted by institutionalization and that have been consistently reinforced by a society that has yet to discover the importance of its elders to our collective well being. The avowed mission of Live Oak has been to begin on the ground on which we stand in the nursing home to work to restore the role of elder to society.

- Basic and universal values such as love, joy, meaning, friendship, hope and sharing of blessings are the binding force that holds the community together.
- Regeneration is a life long process which can occur even as we are in physical, emotional or mental decline. It is constantly occurring within all living organisms as long as life flows within them. Among the very frail, one's regenerative potential can be diminished by undermining one's will, spirit and autonomy through unkindness and lack of respect. It can be enhanced through listening to what a person needs and responding accordingly.
- Learning, growing and developing is a naturally occurring process, even among people with cognitive loss and disability. Among staff members, in most cases, education is the most effective vehicle for replacing activities that run counter to the culture with those that are consistent with the values of the community.
- In the Regenerative Community, we are all equal participants. The common denominator among residents and staff is that we are all people with the same needs, aspirations and emotions.
- Participation in community is intrinsically healing. Belonging to something greater than ourselves connects us to one another and to the future and provides meaning in our lives.
- Life is good, even when we are challenged. This is a fundamental article of faith within the culture. We acknowledge pain, suffering and loss and pay it its due. But we constantly advocate for a positive view of life.
- Concentrate on what is healthy, positive and potentiated. Traditionally, the medical model has seen people in terms of what is wrong with them, and this has defined our institutional vision of the people who are receiving care. While it is important to anticipate and respond to problems, healing comes from the place where well being exists. In a wound, the healing grows from the healthy tissue in, rather than from the damaged tissue out. While we address needs and problems, if a person has three percent that is healthy, that is where we concentrate as we strive to move that to four percent or five percent.
- Diversity is a blessing. Diverse origins, traditions and wisdom of residents and staff are the wealth of community. By honoring and celebrating each person and each group and from where they come, communal unity emerges and the diverse elements feel a sense of belonging and ownership.
- Treat one another as we would want to be treated. If we expect staff members to be kind to residents, honoring their individual needs, then we need to treat staff members the same way.

- In the Regenerative Community we are part of a movement for human dignity and empowerment. Each of us, particularly when we join together, has the capability to significantly change and improve the world around ourselves, to build something new together, something that will alter our lives and the lives of those we touch. When enough people in enough places identify with this movement, we will have significantly improved the very nature of society.

Our core values are the basic assumptions upon which the Regenerative Community has developed. Our belief is that the more we act as if they are true, the more they are manifested in the community and the more reality shifts to conform to our vision.

BRIEF HISTORY OF IMPLEMENTATION

The Live Oak Regenerative Community approach to community development has been the vehicle through which we have seeded a culture that has brought hope, meaning and renewal to a number of environments in which dread has defined our shared perception of reality. This Live Oak community building has gone on throughout the continuum of living for elders, from nursing homes and rehabilitation units to nutrition sites and senior centers. The Regenerative Community approach was first cultivated by Live Oak Institute in 1977 and has been thriving at the Live Oak Living Center in El Sobrante, California, since 1986.

There are two organizations primarily involved in the implementation of the Regenerative Community approach: Live Oak Institute, a 501 (c) (3) non-profit organization, seeded with the Live Oak Project in 1977 and incorporated in 1981 for the purpose of developing models to impact the way society ages; and Regenerative Health Systems, Inc. (RHSI). RHSI is a proprietary company that has operated the Live Oak Living Center since 1986, when 21 supporters of the Live Oak concept invested $180,000 as a down payment for the purchase of a long-term lease on the facility. Renamed the Live Oak Living Center, the facility includes a skilled nursing facility licensed for 60 people and an assisted living facility that is licensed for 37 people. When it was acquired, the facility was in the midst of a Medicare and Medi-Cal decertification process and faced an imminent strike, all of which were averted as the management team worked quickly and effectively to establish the Regenerative Community and win the confidence of all the stakeholders.

Housed in a plain, old building built in the late 1960s in a residential neighborhood in El Sobrante, about 20 miles northeast of San Francisco, the Live

Oak Living Center has demonstrated that one need not have a new or reno-vated building to establish a dynamic culture that empowers stakeholders and creates a joyful and lively environment. From 30 to 50 people each day partici-pate in the daily community meeting. Friendship Circle, a community devel-opment program aimed at people with Alzheimer's related diseases, is held each day in late afternoon to reduce agitation and wandering. To meet the needs of people who can't or won't participate in group activities, the *Pleasure of Your Company*™ (POYC) was developed at the facility as an approach to providing meaningful and individualized one-on-one programming. Hundreds of facilities in the United States and Canada have purchased the POYC.

One of the strongest aspects of the Live Oak Living Center is the commu-nity that exists among staff members who come from many nations around the world and work together harmoniously. They routinely solve problems on their own and bring constant joy and celebration of the facility.

Perhaps nowhere is the power of the Regenerative Community culture more apparent than in the fact that the Live Oak Living Center is still thriving today despite a series of financial crises in recent years that have threatened its exis-tence. Family members, staff members and residents have stood by the facility during these difficult times with virtually no interruption in the quality of ser-vices and quality of life.

Despite a seemingly unrelenting succession of daunting circumstances, the facility has had remarkable success. The retention rate among line staff in 2001 is 80 percent. The occupancy rate in the skilled nursing facility ranges from 98 to 100 percent. The number of people paying privately in skilled nursing is the highest in the area, having increased from 13 percent to 33 percent two years later. According to the facility's December, 1999 Quality Indicators, with the exception of the prevalence of anti-psychotic drugs for a population that pre-sented a high number of psychiatric problems upon entry, all the indicators are better than average. Even though the licensed staff was challenged during a nine month period in which four licensed nurses regularly worked double shifts because they didn't want to trust their residents to registry nurses, the most recent survey showed no deficiencies more serious than Level E, related to occasional short staffing and insufficient documentation of TB testing.

The Regenerative Community was launched in 1977 with the independent Live Oak Project at the Home for Jewish Parents in Oakland, California, where the routine of daily community meetings was begun. Although considerable time was spent in conceptualizing the model, nothing prepared us for how daunting the task of creating that first Regenerative Community would be when we began our first community development effort at the Jewish Home. The first community meeting was chaotic, disjointed and disorienting. Most of the people were suffering from the cumulative effects of isolation, disconnection and lack of meaning in their lives. Most had cognitive loss. Many were survivors of the Holocaust and the pogroms that preceded it. Those people who weren't encapsulated in their own world were often angry and aggressive.

Nonetheless, we stood with the residents and struggled to create a center of calm in the midst of the chaos and to express our utmost belief in the deep social transformation we anticipated would come out of this experience of Regenerative Community building. At our first community meeting we arranged seating in a circle and spoke to the residents from the center and said:

> We are the Live Oak Project and we intend to join you every day, right here at the same time to build a community that will bring joy and meaning to our lives . . . Many of you may feel abandoned and put away into a warehouse . . . But to us, you are the elders of the people . . . and right here, today, we will begin a movement that will transform the culture of aging in America . . .

One man, Kenneth Fox, a lifelong activist who was the last Jewish member of the Berlin legislature as the Nazis came to power, was perhaps the one person who really understood the full ramifications of our assertion. Unable to speak because of a stroke that ravaged his body, he placed himself in front of this author after the meeting and with his forefinger, he made a circle in the air around his temple. And then he drew his arm in an arcing circle pointing to everyone in the group, and once again repeated the gesture of a circle around his temple. And then his whole body shook with laughter as he limped away enjoying his own private joke.

The next morning he was there early waiting to see if we would be back. He presented me with a barely legible typewritten note on a quarter sheet of paper. "If you think you can do that with those people, you're crazier than they are," he had typed. But every day he came back with a daily note to the community. Mute and paralyzed and hungering to still be a part of that great movement for social justice, he emerged as the first indigenous leader of our Live Oak Regenerative Community.

Over a period of less than a year, the daily community meeting grew from a chaotic enterprise that barely lasted 20 minutes with a handful of participants to an hour and a half event in which 50 or more elders participated voluntarily each morning in a home that housed 115 elders.

In 1979, in an evaluation commissioned by the Evelyn and Walter A. Haas, Jr. Fund, a team from the Andrus Gerontology Center, University of Southern California, reported on the first Live Oak Project:

> . . . the model as demonstrated, has definite potential, shifting the emphasis of long term care from viewing its role as a custodian of ill people to one of rehabilitating and regenerating people for new roles within an institutional setting . . .

> . . . although no concrete evidence exists, the Live Oak Project appears to have had some economic benefit in terms of reduction of medications, better use of staff time, lower staff turnover and overall heightened morale which lessens staff absenteeism . . .

> . . . It is our feeling that Live Oak could alter conceptions about what is possible in old age . . . and thereby ultimately alter the reality of aging itself. The oft expressed slogan of the Live Oak founders that they are out to "revolutionize" old age in America may not be so far-fetched. (McConnell, Cohn and Kobata, 1979)

In the early 1980s, with funding from a number of local foundations, Live Oak Institute developed applications of the model in three long-term care settings in Northern California. This cohort of facilities was selected after a rigorous process that identified a high level of facility commitment to participate in Regenerative Community participation. Outcomes were positive.

> The model has been successfully transferred to three nonsectarian facilities. "In-kind" resources of using a facility's own staff to implement the regenerative community has been developed. The project has gained entry into the professional community of gerontology . . . Live Oak is to be commended not only for its success, but specifically for the upbeat positive influence it brings much neglected nursing home facilities. (Cohn and Bolduc, 1982)

In 1983, Live Oak Institute received a major grant from the Gulf+Western corporate foundation as a result of a national competition to identify models that had the potential to change the way America ages. The Live Oak Regenerative Community was one of three organizations funded from a field of some 950 applicants. The idea was to entrepreneurialize Live Oak and market the Regenerative Community to private sector nursing home companies. That effort was far less successful. In those days before OBRA, the concept of building a resident centered, non-medical-model culture in long-term care held little or no appeal to nursing home operators. This attitude had also filtered down to management and staff in the few facilities in which the Regenerative Community was introduced.

This last year, the project attempted economic self-sufficiency. It has grown, changed staff and repeatedly refined its model, while maintaining its original values and enthusiastic stance in what was, at times, an admittedly difficult working environment.

The outcomes of this year were mixed. The pluses were the further development of the model and the opportunity to actually conduct work in a facility for renumeration. These achievements, however, were countered by the eventual recognition of the poor suitability of these facilities for Live Oak. Given the difficulties of the year, the staff should be applauded for their unending efforts, innovative thinking, and visibility in an arena in which few other projects have been willing to venture. (Cohn and Bolduc, 1985)

In 1985, the Live Oak approach to developing a values driven corporate culture for a proprietary nursing home company did find a receptive environment in American Medical Services (AMS). AMS, a Wisconsin and Southern California based company that was identified by Forbes magazine as one of the best run small companies in America, sought out Live Oak Institute to play a major role in its effort to create a culture based in the values similar to those expressed within the Regenerative Community. Live Oak personnel worked with staff members on all levels and in all departments to articulate resident-centered values and design a system of performance management. Because there was a major and consistently visible commitment by top management, the problems encountered under the Gulf+Western grant were virtually non-existent and the Live Oak community development efforts were embraced corporate wide.

Other efforts at Regenerative Community development in the late 1970s and early '80s occurred at the following Northern California settings: Posada de Colores, a HUD sponsored senior housing project operated by the Spanish Speaking Unity Council in Oakland; a Title Seven Nutrition Site at the Jewish Community Center in Oakland; the senior program at the Berkeley Jewish Community Center; the acute rehabilitation unit at Mills Peninsula Hospital in Redwood City; and a small adult day care center for people with Alzheimer's disease in San Carlos. Regular community meetings were established in each of these settings. In the Oakland nutrition site where the people were independent and healthy, the community meeting spun off programs in holistic health, self defense for elders and a Yiddish folk chorus that became part of the Jewish Community Center's core programming. Live Oak Regenerative Community programming continued in these facilities for varying lengths of time depending on commitment of management and staff. Today, some of the facilities no longer exist and there has been so much management and staff turnover, that at best, only vestiges of this 20 year old community development remain.

In recent years, the National Citizen's Coalition for Nursing Home Reform identified the Live Oak Regenerative Community as one of four core approaches that were pioneering a new culture of nursing homes in America; others included resident directed care, the Eden Alternative and resident centered care. The coming together of principles from these approaches provided a direct antecedent for the launching of the Pioneer movement which has touched thousands of people across the country and has opened up a number of opportunities for the Live Oak Regenerative Community to have impact in a number of organizations around the country. Among these in which Live Oak programming continues today:

- Live Oak Regenerative Community developers were for years the only outside consultants to work with Connecticut based Apple Health Care (see Hagy, this volume). Working with senior management they helped the company to prioritize "culture change" as the driving force of its bottom line and to bring managers on all levels aboard. With key personnel from all facilities, the community meeting was seeded throughout the company.
- Regenerative Community development was a core component of the foundation and NY State sponsored culture change research project at the Jewish Home of Rochester and Fairport Baptist Homes.
- At Lakewood Health and Rehab in Milwaukee, WI, community meetings occur daily.

CLOSE ENCOUNTERS OF A VERY PAINFUL KIND

My first encounter with the culture of nursing homes was in the late '60s when I visited my old friend and grandmother, Lottie Barkan. I covered a civil rights beat first for the United Press International and later for the Richmond, Virginia, AFRO AMERICAN newspaper and had visited such culturally bankrupt environments as segregated rural southern schools and women's and men's prisons. Nothing in my experience prepared me for what I encountered in that nursing home. As I wrote:

> I remember clearly going to visit her for the first time . . . Exiting the elevator at the third floor, my sensation was akin to experiencing some grim science fiction story in which I entered the elevator in one reality dimension and emerged in another. There was absolutely no correlation be-

tween the name and the facade of the home and what I experienced when the elevator door opened.

The smell of disinfectant was overwhelming. The ambiance of the place was that of a hospital. Not quite so clean and spic and span, but a hospital nonetheless.

. . . (The nurses) were formal, aloof and not very friendly. Clearly it was their turf. Not ours. Not grandma's. But theirs. Without speaking to one another, my mother, father, brother and I assumed the posture of less than welcome guests, anxious and careful, lest we offend.

Grandma, who for the whole of her adult life was an impeccable home-maker, who in recent years had moved King Lear-like from the home of one child to the home of another, but always with a space of her own, now shared a room with a stranger. Neither woman was actively interested in knowing the other. Each kept her distance.

. . . It was two in the afternoon, and grandma lay in a hospital bed wearing a nightgown. Her teeth were not in her mouth. She had aged considerably since I had last seen her a month or so before. She was visibly smaller.

As a boy, I used to spend hours on end sitting in grandma's rocker, talking with her about the family, about world affairs, especially as they related to the Jews, about the old days–just chatting.

Now there wasn't much to say. I couldn't find the way to transcend the sorrow which now became a barrier between my grandmother and the rest of us.

She didn't want to live anymore. She said it again and again. Not as a person letting go of the sweet gift life and preparing for a mysterious connection to the G*D to whom I remember her frequently praying, but as a person betrayed.

Her life was culminating in a stiff and cold, formal environment that had no knowledge and respect of who she had been and, moreover, had not time to care. She was disconnected from her past. Her future had been presumed to be nonexistent, and her present was relegated to a limbo state–not by the True Judge to whom she prayed–but by a culture which at best had lost its way and at worst was corrupt, profiting usuriously from the infirmity of elders.

> As a family we never really recovered from our inability to find an appropriate response to the cumulative series of late life crises that culminated in her institutionalization. The once tight knit extended family had disintegrated. (Barkan, 1979)

First, I was simply haunted by the experience of my own anger, frustration and inability to act. Then I began reflecting on what it meant. Lottie Barkan was the victim of a diseased and fractured culture. This deep seated cultural malaise was so strong that the nursing home exacerbated my grandmother's illness and effected everyone around her.

Our society has pursued youth and denied a meaningful role for elders at the same time that institutions such as nursing homes and regulatory agencies have put their own agendas way above the individual and collective needs of elders. No wonder nursing homes had evolved into frightening, sterile environments where the souls of most people who touched them were degraded and crippled. They were not anchored in a meaningful reality.

The lives of the elders in the nursing home had very little meaning as physical, mental, emotional and spiritual disease increasingly provided the context through which the world related to them. There was no venue for them to be potent in the environment in which they lived, to engage the contemporary world around them, and to collectively build an active present tense that draws from the past and builds towards the future. Perhaps the greatest insult of all, was that when someone died, she was wheeled out the back door with no mention, lest it "upset the old people." This failure to even minimally recognize a person's death rendered as meaningless the experience of one's life in the elder care setting.

It was these recollections that stayed with me to ultimately influence the conceptualization and implementation of the Regenerative Community meetings as vehicle for learning, growth and connection among the elders.

COMMUNITY MEETING IS THE REFERENCE POINT FOR THE LIVE OAK CULTURE

Although the Live Oak Regenerative Community is a complex organism that can be encountered at an almost unlimited number of points, at the Live Oak Living Center the central organizing venue is the Live Oak community meeting. The shared cultural context, the underlying environmental reality, and the community memory are consciously cultivated at the community meeting.

There is a mysterious ripple effect that emanates from the community meeting, bringing the binding force of goodness, compassion and joy to the concentric circle of those who touch it, whether they be workers on the night shift who never see a community meeting, family members, state inspectors or visiting celebrities.

Betty Friedan Meets the Live Oak Elders

Betty Friedan is the pioneering change maker who many say catalyzed the women's movement with her landmark book, *The Feminine Mystique* (1963). With her book *Fountain of Age* (1993), she sets out to catalyze a similar change in the culture of aging, challenging the way we think about ourselves as we grow older and the way society thinks about aging.

When she visited the community meeting at the Live Oak Living Center, it was with a sense of "dread" driven by the experience of her mother's death in a skilled nursing facility. She wrote in *Fountain of Age*:

> I admit my overwhelming dread and prejudice against nursing homes. In ten years of research, no data has emerged to counteract my impression of nursing homes as death sentences, the final internment from which there is no exit but death. In some research I have seen, no matter what their condition upon entering, men or women tended to die within six months of a nursing home. Even if they were not dying or in any state of terminal disease when they entered . . . something happened, as a result of being put in a nursing home that led to death. Of 'no apparent cause' as they said of my mother. She died in her sleep 'of old age'; she was ninety. I think she had no wish to live any longer, in the nursing home: no bonds, no people she cared about, no purpose to her days. (Friedan, 1993)

When I picked her up at her hotel to drive her to Live Oak, Betty reiterated her passionately articulated misgivings about nursing homes. The institution, itself, was so misconceived that she had no expectations of finding anything that would challenge her negative assumptions. "You understand," she said, "that no matter what I find, I will report it accurately and my coming to Live Oaks (as she called it even in her book) may not be a gift to you."

Yet, even with that preamble, in *Fountain of Age* she described her experience at the Live Oak Living Center fairly and positively:

> I sat in on the daily community council meeting at the Live Oaks in the sunny atrium . . . The residents and staff were dressed in diverse summer garb, no uniforms. They did some exercises together, discussed what

was going on in the community and also the national politics and developments in the world. Told that I was going to visit, they had been discussing women's issues.

Perhaps it was the sunshine, but despite canes and walkers, Laura in her hot pink slacks, Harriet with bright red sandals, Helen in a blue-and-white checked slack suit did not look old and sick like the residents of other nursing homes I had interviewed. Helen's daughter who was visiting, told me that her mother's walking over to meet me was new to her. The doctor told her after her stroke that there was no hope she'd ever walk again; now she's recovered most of her balance. Anna in a striped pant suit strutting up to me was ninety-four. Four years ago when she came in with diabetes, she had to use a walker.

They were interested in hearing about the women's movement. 'Women felt that they deserved to be known for who they really are,' I told them. As prejudiced as society was about women, its view of elders is even more distorted. They have to see elders not just as sick old people. They nodded their heads with no less intensity than the students I had spoken to at Stanford the night before. One of the women told me she didn't agree with women's lib and one of the male minority said it should have happened a long time ago. They all acted as if their opinions still counted, and, in one way or another, with every issued raised, seemed to ask: What can we do as elders, here, now, to make a difference.

Ken, a man in a green lumber jacket and plaid shirt, was teased about his crush on Dolly Parton. He was eighty-four when he came to Live Oaks from a nursing home where got very disabled. 'I was ready to give up the ghost. I was hearing Gabriel's horn, not long for this world. Now, it seems I'm getting my strength back.' He said men should take a more active part in the women's movement, so it won't be a cat-dog fight, women versus men. I agreed. And they got into a big argument about whether there could be a woman president, and why women lived so much longer than men . . . (Friedan, 1993)

A Community for Everyone

What Betty Friedan didn't mention, perhaps because it wasn't so obvious, was that most of the people in the community meeting she attended were in various stages of cognitive loss. By design, at Live Oak our people who are cognitively impaired are not isolated from those who are cognitively integrated. Our culture makes no distinction based on a professional definition of capacity and participants include the full range of residents within the environment.

The community meeting is for all residents. No one is forced to participate, all are encouraged. There is something about the authenticity of the experience at community meeting that sets a norm to which virtually every participant seems to adhere. Although it is routine for people suffering from Alzheimer's and related disorders to attend, calling out, shouting and disruption seldom occur.

Weaving a Tapestry Through Time

Perhaps one of the greatest institutionally induced ailments is that our relationship to time becomes distorted. In institutional life where there is little that is positive in the present tense to grab one's attention, there is a tendency to languish in the past with little or no looking forward to the future. This is not healthy reminiscence. Individual and collective torpor is experienced in the environment as people's worlds contract and they are not aware of one another, of visitors and changes.

In the regenerative community, time is consciously recontextualized for individuals and the community. The community meeting occurs at a point in time and space that is held sacred and involves constant sharing, day in and day out, each day building upon the next, drawing from the past and planning the future. A healthy relationship to time is a key concept in the Live Oak Ethos that was presented at the first community meeting at the old Jewish home in 1977: "Live in the present, draw from the past and prepare for the future."

People are alive in time as they connect to their individual and collective histories, and move constantly towards their future. In this rich stew, a cultural life, a collective memory, emerges as a living heritage and communal legacy.

A Learning Environment

Repetition may just be the mother of invention as a foundation is established for an often deep and meaningful experience. Almost five thousand times over the course of the last 16 years at the Live Oak Living Center, each day has begun with a community meeting as a parade of residents, family members, staff members and a constant flow of visitors have gathered together to weave the heart of the culture that is redefining the eldercare experience for all those who are connected. The same songs are sung again and again, perhaps thousands of times. The same exercises are repeated almost daily, again thousands of times. The same jokes are oft repeated as are the same comments by residents with broken cognitive synapses who have no memory of what was said two minutes ago.

Although each community meeting follows its own flow and its own unfolding, the structural design for the community meeting is as follows:(1) Welcoming ritual and song; (2) News of the world; (3) News of the Home; (4) Discussion of the day; and (5) Closing song. The news of the world provides an opportunity to discuss everything from presidential scandal to latest developments in science and technology. The news of the home provides an opportunity to welcome new members, to share "gossip," to offer prayers for elders who are sick and to remember residents who have recently died. The discussion of the day focuses on themes that range from human cloning to aspects of the news that capture the imagination of residents. It also provides the opportunity for special events such as meetings with local politicians running for political office.

One of our fundamental assumptions that defines the Live Oak Regenerative Community is that everyone is capable of learning and growth at all life stages. Any other assumption limits people and imprisons them in a box. The elder who dropped out of school 65 years ago during the great depression, learns about such modern phenomena as human cloning and then takes a position on it as the residents share and sometimes ardently debate opinions and values. The woman with Alzheimer's disease who clinically may be considered cognitively dysfunctional, sings a song that she never heard before coming to Live Oak with familiarity or lights up at the sight of a person she knows for only a few weeks.

First Contact: It's Not My Grandma's Nursing Home

There is a persistent evangelism for life that lifts the spirit yet is not afraid to encounter sadness and despair in a way that is always respectful. On one recent day, Elizabeth Smith (not her name) was escorted to the community meeting by a nursing assistant on the day after she came to the home. A clear and articulate woman, she was invited to tell the 35 or so elders gathered in the room who she is and from where she had come. She spoke of her demoralization about being in a nursing home.

"I never thought it would come to this," she said in a voice filled with sadness and resignation.

A few other residents, shared their own first day experience. Then, Cleta Shelton, the community developer (this role is explained later) with a passionate respect for elders, who is an activity professional, a former certified nursing assistant, and a minister in her church said, "Elizabeth, every time a new person comes to our community, we sing our *resident rights song* to them. It's our way of letting you know that this is a place where we respect your rights. Do you mind if we sing to you?"

"Okay," said Elizabeth tentatively, apparently not knowing what to expect. "I guess that will be all right."

The *Live Oak Resident Rights Song* was collectively written by a group of 20 residents in response to the question: "What is the best way to teach new members of the community that they have rights?" The federal mandate of resident rights in every nursing home throughout the land is one of the great victories in the cultural revolution. However, reading each resident her rights is a legalistic experience that does not sufficiently convey the good news.

So now the residents sing their Resident Rights Song, which borrows its tune from the "Battle Hymn of the Republic," to new staff members and residents alike. As the residents began to sing to Elizabeth Smith, a number of people who had been seemingly nodding off perked up and began to sing the words, chant the melody or clap their hands.

Chorus
Glory, Glory Hallelujah.
Glory, Glory Hallelujah.
Glory, Glory Hallelujah.
Our rights go marching on.

We have the right to worship and to pray just as we please,
We have the right to raise our own flags way up in the breeze,
We have the right to watch the clouds and sit under the trees,
Our rights go marching on.

We have the right to greet our friends and the right to entertain,
We can recommend new changes and it's our right to complain,
We're entitled to our privacy and a room that has our name,
Our rights go marching on.

Our bodies are our own from our heads down to our toes,
When we ask about our meds, don't you treat us like your foes.
We are a group of elders who have the right to know,
Our rights go marching on.

Orienting New Staff at Community Meeting

A few minutes later, the director of staff development at the Live Oak Living Center dropped in to introduce a new staff member to the resident community. As a pioneering nurse-educator she has spent the last 40 years battling the stereotypes of aging among nurses and others who work in nursing homes. On this day, Joyce Terry explained to Charanjit, the new staff member, that at Live Oak we are all part of the same community. The new CNA, who not too long before had lived in the Punjabi region of India, stood in the middle of the circle of residents as they sang to her about their rights, letting her know the expectations of the resident community in the kindest possible way. Then community members asked her such questions as where she had come from, who was in her family, and how long she had been in the United States?

Community meeting is one of many vehicles through which our values and beliefs within Live Oak are communicated directly to new staff members. The same values about the specialness of each resident and her or his tradition are applied to the workers and conveyed in the orientation process. Much consciousness and effort goes into building a culture that welcomes everyone and validates their experience and their origins. Staff members learn from their earliest experience with the residents that this is a place where elders are valued and where everyone's culture is honored and respected. When people who come from far away places are invited to share the details of their own cultures, the community's living commitment to diversity and inclusiveness is given expression in the rituals of daily life.

The Community Developer Nurtures the Embers of the Culture

The Live Oak Regenerative Community culture is consciously cultivated by people who take responsibility to be *community developers*. The community developer facilitates change and renewal, nurtures the embers of the community, fans its flames and keeps it growing by helping its participants to be all they can be and to create a shared future together.

The community developer is an evangelist for life and a mediator of the shared reality. She or he holds the vision and serves the values, working assiduously to keep these alive in the heart of a system that for a myriad of reasons can be dysfunctional and counter productive to the values of the Live Oak Regenerative Community culture.

In the early and most difficult days of our work as community developers, we had no empirical evidence that we were on the right track. All we had was our belief that the regenerative community would work and the determination to cleave to that belief as we stood each day in the middle of the circle of residents. We learned to rely heavily on our own emerging Live Oak folk wisdom and from this a definition and methodology for the community developer began to coalesce.

The number of community developers in each setting varies. At the Live Oak Living Center the activity professionals are the community developers and in recent years each activity director has trained and coached successors and assistants. The role of community developer does not represent a separate salary line but is another role added to the job description.

The Community Developer's Role

Role is a key concept in the lore of the Regenerative Community: we spread the values of the program by role modeling their application and by publicly acknowledging the elders who (themselves are) role models or living examples of what the community stands for; a major goal of the Regenerative Community is to help elders within institutions establish positive and active roles for themselves; the (Live Oak) ethos teaches that the role we have is the role we choose.

As Shakespeare wrote, each of us plays many roles in our time. This is also true in our professional job functions. The role of the community developer is an added part of the professional repertoire. Thus you need to begin thinking of yourselves not only as administrators, nursing directors, and activity directors (etc.), but also as community developers.

The first step in taking on a new role is to have both an image of the role and of yourself within it. The primary function of the community developer is to facilitate and nurture the development of an active and current life among the residents of your homes. Functionally as the community developer goes about the business of weaving a community among the residents, he acts in five major capacities. These are Teacher, Leader, Participant, Advocate, and Learner.

Teacher: The community developer teaches the Live Oak Lore to the community.

Leader: Another major goal of the Regenerative Community is to bring the resident to a point where they are making their own decisions about their communal lives. Outside leadership is required to help them assume this responsibility. In her leadership capacity, the regenerative community developer will help the community formulate its programmatic and organizational directions. An important aspect of leadership in the Regenerative Community is assuring that each community member is heard and that stronger residents do not dominate those who are less connected, strong or articulate.

Participant: The community developer is also a member of the community he is developing. He is not separated from the community by professional role. He shares his own experiences and he, too, grows and develops through his participation.

Advocate: Particularly in the early days of Regenerative Community building, the community developer is an advocate for the residents. In this capacity, the community developer helps staff, family members, physicians, and others to better understand the world as residents are experiencing it.

Learner: The community developer is constantly learning from the performance of her role. She is refining her skills, developing new insights, and expanding the lore. She is also learning directly from the residents who are providing constant feedback and who are sharing the experiences of their lifetimes.

There are a number of personal traits or qualities that contribute effectively to the performance of the community developer. Foremost among these are: *commitment; vision; caring; genuineness;* and *humor.*

In varying degrees, these qualities already exist within everyone. Simply by remaining aware of them as we perform the functions of the community developer, they will grow within. (Barkan and Barkan, 1981)

ACTION CONCEPTS FOR EFFECTIVE CHANGE MAKING

A number of action concepts make us effective agents of change. Radical in their simplicity, they enable us to transcend our own conditioning and emotional responses and to be responsive to virtually any situation, whether walking rounds, dealing with conflict or working with residents, staff members, family members or state surveyors. Some of these action concepts are described below.

- Center program development in the in-between space where no one else has turf that they are protecting.
- Stay focused on the future.
- Keep the focus on what's well within each individual and within the group.
- Always be on duty to champion the good.
- Constantly strive to be kind.
- Keep a sense of humor.
- Find a way to positively acknowledge the valuable kernel of truth at the heart of whatever a person is saying, no matter how negatively it might have been expressed.
- Welcome each person as if he is the most important person in the world.
- Help each person to be known to herself and to others.

- Give over our blessings as if our blessings do have the power to heal and renew.
- Take each person's concerns seriously.
- Avoid taking sides.
- Avoid getting bogged down in defending a position, even if you may be right.
- Make no one bad.
- Constantly expand the middle ground so that everyone has a place in the community.
- Be a cultural translator, honoring the traditions of all participants and seeking to find common ground among them.

Although, at first glance, the role of community developer may appear challenging, any one with the intention to assume the role and with the willingness to commit to a path of learning and growing can be an effective community developer. The main source of the community developer's capability lies within and comes from each individual's unique configuration of talents, experience, personal legacy and beliefs. Thus there is no cookie cutter mold for a community developer. Within the context of the regenerative community and what it stands for, the role can be adapted to our individual personality, style and connection to meaning.

Becoming Champions of Culture Change: A Mastery Path

Virtually all spiritual traditions have mastery paths. However, the universal places where commerce, service, science and governance meet are generally devoid of such paths which provide a cultural context for each person's own individual journey towards wisdom, well being and enlightenment and society's collective journey towards wholeness and prosperity.

A weekly seminar has been initiated at the Live Oak Living Center to develop a mastery path as the next evolutionary stage of the community developer's role. A simple methodology to better understand and take responsibility for the cultural environment in which we operate is being tested so that we can be more accountable, take greater responsibility, foster hope for the future, consciously learn together and create a more joyful and forgiving environment. We are working to cultivate such personal qualities as vision, consciousness, willingness to yield, generosity, responsibility, humor, pardon and optimism. We are developing a "Way of Quality" as an action path that includes such attributes as being a friend to everyone, modeling our beliefs, facilitating communications, resisting the urge to judge and taking time to grow and learn.

Initially the seminars are for members of the management and multidisciplinary leadership teams, but ultimately we intend to initiate all staff members, residents and family members who are willing to participate so that everyone in the community is involved in building a new culture of aging.

A VISION FOR THE FUTURE

For years now, each time I speak about elder care, I invite the people in the audience to reach over and shake the hands of the potential nursing home resident sitting next to us. When I first began this work of Regenerative Community development 25 years ago, I was a relatively young man in my mid-thirties. Among my friends, I was virtually the only one thinking about the potential impact we may have on the future of aging.

Today there is a vast cohort of us that, ready or not, is inexorably moving towards our own old age. Each year, the possibility gets closer and more real as we are aging in place and among our friends, our siblings, our partners and our parents the specter of aging becomes more prominent. There are elders we serve at the Live Oak Living Center who are my age.

If we have the gift of years, we are the ones who will be the elders of the people. We have the potential to craft and define the role in a way that has never consciously occurred before on such a large scale. We can in the years that remain for us, create a tradition of the *millennial elders*, taking responsibility for our own conscious evolution and for the lives of those who will come after us.

At Live Oak Institute we have long been germinating the concept of the Live Oak Elders Guild, a multi-generational communal organization through which we will enter a path of mastery and learn together to create a legacy for future generations that will heal the excesses of our past. Now, perhaps because we don't only work with elders, but are emerging elders in our own lives and in our communities, we are ready to make the Elders Guild a reality.

As we envision it at Live Oak, there are three key foundations for the Elders Guild:

- *The guild community* provides the backdrop for the members and our families to continually celebrate of our lives, our passages and our connection to one another, even as we may move from locale to another.
- *The mastery path* through which we: establish repositories of our elder wisdom and lore; involve ourselves in learning, growing and developing as we learn to be ever more effective, more joyful and more adept in our internal lives and in our relationship to those with whom we are most

connected; and progress on an acknowledged path of mastery for our own sakes and for the sake of society which urgently needs to know the masters among us as models and resources.

* *Service* through which we work together to leave our individual and collective legacy to make the world a better place for our grandchildren and their grandchildren. As we envision it, legacy is consciously crafted from all of our resources, experiential, social and financial and it is the place where our wisdom and mastery is applied in our own families, our communities and in far away places that call out to our hearts.

Our vision is that the Elders Guild will take root in all communities, Muslim, Christian, Jewish, Sikh, Hindu, Buddhist, atheist, European, Arab, African, Asian, and Latin. Wherever we go we can come to Elders Guild communities that share common rituals, common traditions and common ways of helping us to be at home with one another. The idea is that we can take this pioneer culture which has been effectively established in the nursing home and make it at home throughout the world, transforming the role of elder in powerful and meaningful ways.

REFERENCES

Barkan, B. (1977). *The Live Oak Definition of An Elder*, published as a poster by Live Oak Institute.

Barkan, B. (1979). *The Live Oak Regenerative Community*, Proceedings of the Syposium, Environments for Humanized Health Care, Berkeley, CA, 139-141.

Barkan, D. and Barkan, B. (1981). *Live Oak Regenerative Community Training Program: Learners Journal*, Oakland, CA, Live Oak Institute, 48-49.

Cohn, J., and Boldac, M. (1982). *An Evaluation of the Live Oak Program in Three Bay Area Nursing Homes*, Andrus Gerontology Center, University of Southern California, submitted to the Luke B. Hancock Foundation, 33.

Cohn, J., and Bolduc, M. (1985). *Final Report: Evaluation of Live Oak Institute*, Andrus Gerontology Center, University of Southern California, submitted to the Luke B. Hancock Foundation, 20.

Friedan, B. (1993). *The Fountain of Age*, NYC, NY, Simon and Schuster, 522-523.

McConnell, S.R., Cohn, J., and Kobata, F. (1979). *An Evaluation of Selected Components of the Live Oak Project*, Andrus Gerontology Center, University of Southern California, submitted to the Evelyn and Walter A. Haas, Jr. Fund, 44-45.

Thomas, W., MD. (2002). Telephone conversation with the author.

SECTION 3
CASE STUDIES:
IMPLEMENTING CHANGE

Teresian House–
Using the Environment
to Support Cultural Change

James S. Brennan
Sister Patricia Brancaccio
Sister Pauline Brecanier

SUMMARY. This case study describes the nearly 10 year culture change program at Teresian House, a 300 bed, faith-based facility in Albany, New York. Building on the mission of the Carmelite Sisters for the Aged and Infirm, a series of simple environmental changes prepared the facility for operational culture change. The problems and challenges which emerged, and the responses, are discussed. The article outlines

James S. Brennan is a freelance writer.

Sister Patricia Brancaccio, OCarm, MSW, is Social Work Coordinator, and Sister Pauline Brecanier, OCarm, is Administrator, both at Teresian House.

Address correspondence to: Sister Patricia Brancaccio, OCarm, Teresian House, 200 Washington Avenue Extension, Albany, NY 12203 (E-mail: info@teresianhouse.com).

[Haworth co-indexing entry note]: "Teresian House–Using the Environment to Support Cultural Change." Brennan, James S., Sister Patricia Brancaccio, and Sister Pauline Brecanier. Co-published simultaneously in *Journal of Social Work in Long-Term Care* (The Haworth Social Work Practice Press, an imprint of The Haworth Press, Inc.) Vol. 2, No. 3/4, 2003, pp. 223-231; and: *Culture Change in Long-Term Care* (ed: Audrey S. Weiner, and Judah L. Ronch) The Haworth Social Work Practice Press, an imprint of The Haworth Press, Inc., 2003, pp. 223-231. Single or multiple copies of this article are available for a fee from The Haworth Document Delivery Service [1-800-HAWORTH, 9:00 a.m. - 5:00 p.m. (EST). E-mail address: docdelivery@haworthpress.com].

10.1300/J181v2n03_01

specific environmental factors and their value to the nursing home residents in their physical, psycho-social, and spiritual health. The community's response to the new setting is also addressed. *[Article copies available for a fee from The Haworth Document Delivery Service: 1-800-HAWORTH. E-mail address: <docdelivery@haworthpress.com> Website: <http://www.HaworthPress.com> © 2003 by The Haworth Press, Inc. All rights reserved.]*

KEYWORDS. Elder care, environment, nursing home, transformation

INTRODUCTION

A recent *New York Times* editorial (1999) noted both the problem and the Teresian House's effort to solve it:

> The Teresian Home (House) had decided to end the tyranny of structure and schedule that herds old people through the day in nursing homes across the country: up at 6:30AM . . . back in bed by 8, two to a room, on long hallways . . . Rightly or wrongly, nursing homes have come to have a terrible reputation among the old. No one wants to end up there . . . some real, caring changes could do them a world of good.

It was precisely what the Teresian House Administrator had seen a dozen years earlier.

Sister Pauline Brecanier, OCarm, was appointed to lead Teresian House in 1987. The 300-bed, not-for-profit nursing home had opened in Albany, New York in 1974. Sponsored by the Roman Catholic Diocese of Albany and managed by the Carmelite Sisters for the Aged and Infirm, it originally cared for the well-elderly. It emphasized preventative health services, and sought to sustain the residents' total well-being and independence. Its original population was generally in their mid to upper 70s, ambulatory and independent. The home itself was the traditional hospital-like design. Six floors, each with two long hallways, separated by a nursing station. The rooms were a mixture of single and double beds. All residents followed the same schedule. There was a uniform wake-up in the morning and lights-out at night. Medicines were dispensed on schedule. The nursing home formatted the day, and the residents complied. The conformity produced efficiency, but it conflicted with Sister Pauline's vision of the Carmelite mission. She saw a facility as more home-like, and less institutional, and she agreed with the residents' desire for more say in their care.

THE CARMELITE MISSION

The Carmelite Sisters for the Aged and Infirm was founded in 1929 by Mother Mary Angeline Teresa. Profoundly influenced by her elderly grandfather in her native Northern Ireland, she was struck by how the old were generally viewed as lonely, hungry and cold (Pastva, 2000). Entering the Little Sisters of the Poor as a teenager enabled her to relate to those leaving their family, belongings and independence to live a common life (Pastva, 2000). That understanding would ultimately define the Carmelite Sisters' mission of responding to the individual person, not just his or her malady. Meeting the physical and medical requirements was certainly important, but responding to the spiritual, emotional and social needs of the individual was equally valued. This resident-centered philosophy is the foundation of each of the 25 homes the Carmelites operate. But whereas they incorporated their style of care into the traditional nursing home setting, Sister Pauline sought to change that setting. She believed the nursing home should look and function as any family home would. The transformation she engineered was interactive and gradual, yet a decade later is considered frame-breaking.

THE WORK BEGINS

The initial changes, begun in the late '80s, were cosmetic. The plastic and metal waiting room style seats in the lobby were replaced by upholstered sofas and chairs. Painted walls were wallpapered and pictures were hung. Tile and linoleum floors were carpeted. The double doors on the ladies first floor restroom were taken down, and replaced by a privacy wall, more easily navigable by wheelchairs and walkers. These changes served as metaphors of things to come, physically, organizationally and psycho-spiritually. Teresian House started to look and, most importantly, feel like a home. The remodeling began on the first floor, and continued to the residential floors above as funding would allow. Projects were not begun until financing was in place. As a result, the makeover was generally not time constrained, which allowed for simultaneous work on several fronts.

Another early fundamental change targeted the resident and employee handbooks. The long list of must-do's and cannot-do's was far too negative. While a re-write did not appreciably change the rules and regulations, it did make them more palatable and people friendly. It was an important step in changing the culture from doing things the nursing home's way, to doing them in a way that better met the needs of both residents and staff.

Those needs were themselves changing. The nursing home's well-elderly of the mid '70s had given way to a more mixed population in the '80s and '90s; some assisted living, others requiring more skilled care. The number of residents with dementia had been growing. Today, the average age of the residents has risen to 87 years. The Teresian House case mix index (CMI) is 0.89. In relative terms in New York State parlance, the population is less dependent than the "average" population in the State. The payor mix is 29% private, 69% Medicaid, and 2% Medicare.

PUTTING THE PLAN INTO MOTION

The operational overhaul began in earnest in 1991 with a detailed study of the nursing home's strategic plan, including the physical layout of the building, the daily programs and policies, and the role of the staff and residents (Gould, 2001). It included interviews with staff, residents, and their families to gauge attitudes toward the facility, and to solicit ideas for improvements and new directions. Sister Pauline wrote a vision statement, and encouraged employees to do likewise. Once the input was assimilated, goals were formalized and priorities set.

Dementia care was the first to be addressed. The program that was designed and implemented over the ensuing years for the dementia residents was one that would radically change the care delivery system. Staff was given specialty training to better recognize and provide for the needs of the resident with dementia. Team approaches to care giving were implemented, and physical changes were made; for instance, residents with dementia were given their own dining room to minimize distractions. This individualized care delivery system was to change the way care was delivered to all Teresian House residents (Gould, 2001).

To facilitate the new system, the nursing home's traditional top-down organizational chart was redesigned to one more resident-centric. All departments and services were directly linked to the resident. Some departments were eliminated, and virtually every employee's duties became more global, as family-style elder care demanded everyone "pitch in" and work together. So, the centralized nurse's stations were removed, and each employee's work space was incorporated into the resident's living area. It allowed for far greater interaction, and for the family concept to flourish.

A key component was the organizing of the staff into 7 teams, each headed by a Resident-centered Care Coordinator (RCC). The RCC is a leadership position created to replace the traditional concept of an RN unit manager. Candidates were solicited from the staff to enter a 16 week training program developed by the Teresian House administration. Health and human service backgrounds were preferred of the candidates, but not required. Eighteen applicants responded.

The training program centered around a series of workshops and presentations on disciplines ranging from nursing, social services and dietary, to financing, human resources and pastoral ministry. They were typically directed by Teresian House management, though there were some instances in which outside experts were brought in; one example was a two-part seminar on "keeping cool while managing difficult people." Candidates also worked on a series of projects involving budgeting, staffing and supplies. They were graded on a points system, and interviewed post-training by the Administrator, two Assistant Administrators, and the Director of Nursing. The top seven were chosen. They were professionals from nursing, social work, dietary and activities, heading teams of nurses, social workers, activities coordinators, housekeepers and resident assistants.

A NEW ADDITION

All the while, the physical layout of Teresian House was evolving. As the cosmetic rehabbing continued, a new $13.2 million, 100 bed addition was opened in 1998, divided approximately equally between the more independent residents, and those with dementia. It also included two respite rooms. Unlike the traditional hospital wing, this unit had two figure-eight type floors with a series of 12 or 13 bed "clusters," each with its own kitchen and dining room. It provided residents with their own small neighborhood with room for wandering. These units also allowed the residents to remain close to their rooms, and for the staff to remain close to them. It also provided smaller social groups that would become like extended families (Noell, 1995).

Moving the independent and dementia residents into the new space freed their rooms in the main building, and allowed for a major renovation there. The neighborhood concept was implemented, and all double rooms were converted to singles, resulting in 300 private rooms facility-wide, each with its own bath. The number of residents per floor was reduced from 60 to 40. Kitchens and dining rooms were put in the neighborhoods, as was a family room with TV and comfortable furniture. Each floor included a washer and dryer so residents could have their laundry done individually. Teresian House was now a community of 28 neighborhoods, with 14 kitchen/dining areas. It was part of a new breed of nursing homes providing flexibility and diversity, that are homey, efficient and economical (Noell, 1995). Yet, it was its own model; a unique combination of philosophy, ideas and designs consistent with the mission of the Carmelite Sisters.

CARING FOR THE WHOLE PERSON

While the physical and organizational remaking of Teresian House was extensive, it was just a part of the new design of resident care. The spiritual and psycho-social well being of the individual residents was also addressed to a much greater degree. The administration had formal meetings with residents and their families to advise them of the planned changes and to seek their input. They were shown blueprints. They were invited to, and updated on, weekly floor meetings. Their suggestions were solicited and acted upon. The residents wanted, and consequently enjoyed, more autonomy and greater voice in their lives. This is when the structured wake-up and bed times disappeared. Residents could eat in their neighborhood kitchen when they wanted to, and the often arduous trip to the elevator and down to the first floor dining hall was eliminated. Activities were provided both in and outside the building to meet their requests.

A pre-admission assessment form was designed to determine a prospective resident's likes and dislikes, habits and routines, so a daily schedule could be created with, and for, each individual.

A pastoral team administers to both the Catholic and non-Catholic residents. Time and space are made for residents and staff to grieve for those who die. Funerals are held on-site when desired, and staff is given time to attend off-site funerals and wakes. A cocktail/coffee shop has become so popular with residents and their families that reservations are now being requested. There is a small country store in the building, and a beauty parlor with three full-time beauticians, and a child care center that allows residents to interact with children when, and if, they desire (Evangelist, 1999). To the extent possible, anything a person did before living at Teresian House, they can do while living at Teresian House. Even their pets are welcomed visitors, though not allowed permanently. However, the nursing home does have three house cats for the residents' pleasure.

THE STAFF STRUGGLES

While the residents welcomed the new way of life at Teresian House, the staff was much less accepting. The 350 employees include an administration and clerical staff of about 50, some 80 professionals and technicians, and 220 service workers. Their workplace had been revolutionized, and it was unsettling. A new way of doing things meant old routines disappeared, and in many cases co-workers changed. Some employees even wondered if they would have a job after all the transitional dust settled. The biggest concern, though, involved working as a family, rather than a business.

The family philosophy meant everyone helping wherever needed. As a result, a majority of the day-to-day tasks at Teresian House became global. Anyone could, and should, do whatever needed to be done, except where professional expertise was required. Only a nurse could dispense medicine, but anyone could sit with the dying. If a housekeeper was engaged with a resident, someone else should empty the trash. A social worker could answer a call bell and make a resident a snack in the neighborhood kitchen, rather than wait from someone from dietary to become available. The system worked, but it was difficult for some staff to accept. They were used to working in a department, with its own agenda and rules and regulations. The professionals on staff had never been asked to do anything other than that for which they had been trained.

Some of the residents, who benefited from these changes, had concerns. They felt it was beneath their caregivers to make them wait on tables and do dishes. The caregivers agreed, particularly the social workers. While there were some defections of employees not interested in global duties, the turnover among social workers was total. Though the number of fulltime social workers was increased from 4 to 7, all eventually departed. In fact, that staff has turned over about two-and-a-half times since 1998, 17 departures in all.

Sister Pauline concedes the social workers just could not get on board with the changes. Exit interviews revealed various reasons for leaving, but complaints over kitchen duty and feelings of being unappreciated were recurring themes, as was the belief they were not doing what they were trained to do. The nursing turnover since '98 was not as radical. It peaked at 46% in 1999, the same year the overall facility turnover peaked at 56%. Nursing departures have declined in the two years since, to 37% in 2000 and 25% in 2001.

COST MANAGEMENT

The cost of the two-story addition and the retro-fitting of the main building approached $25 million. Most of the funding was secured when the New York State Dormitory Authority accepted the Teresian House's Certificate of Need and agreed to finance the project. A Capital Campaign raised the 10% in private equity the State Department of Health required be reinvested in the project. Concurrently, the Teresian House Foundation was begun to oversee and administer the charitable donations including planned giving, memorials, fundraisers, and the annual appeal.

The operational changes brought some marginal increases in expenses. The dietary budget rose initially, but then declined and leveled off as needs became clearer. Payroll actually had a net decline. Fulltime additions in Social Services and Activities were offset by reductions in Dietary and Laundry. The operating budget has kept pace with inflation, rising from $9.1 million in 1990 to $13.1 million in 2001.

FINE TUNING

Today, Teresian House residents are seemingly better able to cope with their frailties. They have more control over their own care and lives, and are now, with few exceptions, allowed to age in one place without fear of being moved when their abilities diminish (Gould, 2001). Their satisfaction, and that of their families and the staff, was documented in a 2001 Teresian House Managerial Survey. Ordinal data were collected in the areas of residents' environment, facility operations and medical care provided. The residents, their families, and the staff were in complete agreement in ranking issues regarding resident environment, each listing resident's rights, positive attitudes, home atmosphere, family rights and problem solving #1 through #5, respectively.

Rankings for facility operations saw families and staff rate a strong administration #1, whereas residents listed that #4. They ranked hot food the top priority. The three groups agreed on the #2 choice, clean rooms.

Medical care value rankings again saw unanimity in the #1 selection, prompt attention. Families and staff rated adequate staffing #2. Residents ranked it #4. Their #2 priority was having their call bells answered promptly. On a broader scale, the success of the transition is marked, in part, by a lack of changes in State survey results. A key element to that was keeping the Department of Health appraised of each step in the process. It ensured they were not surprised at the sight of something new.

Still, the new culture is a work in progress. It was easy for employees to see improvements when the new addition was built or the interior was remodeled. It is more difficult to see the successes now that the culture has itself changed. The administration recognized the need for new incentives to reward outstanding work to augment the employee recognition programs that have always been a part of Teresian House operations. Savings bonds, parking privileges, etc., are visible signs for the staff to see that their work is noted and appreciated. Though residents may nominate an employee for recognition, selections are made by management, or in the case of employee of the month, by peer vote.

As noted earlier, social workers had difficulty with so many of their individual duties being assumed by the team. Their complaints were recognized, and a restructuring put them back in charge of coordinating care relating to family and social issues. They are now the link between the residents and the psychiatrist, psychologist and medical personnel.

Not all challenges have a ready solution. More staffing is always welcomed, but not always financially feasible. Less obvious, but equally important, are the attitudes, philosophies and relationships that need to be in line for the optimum delivery of individualized care. The caregiver needs philosophical skills as well as technical skills. He or she needs to know the value of listening skills and problem solving ability. Individualized care is more demanding.

It is also the new culture of elder care. The Pioneer Network, of which the Administrator is a board member, calls it "life affirming, satisfying, humane and meaningful." Teresian House has always had a high end reputation for quality in the Albany and Capital District area of New York, and now it may be higher. The House receives an ever-increasing number of inquiries from people in other nursing homes who have heard of the neighborhood concept. Applications are up, from 472 in 1998 to 590 in 2000 and 588 in 2001. There appear to be more requests for tours from prospective residents and administrators from other nursing homes, though the numbers are not documented. The Teresian House way of looking at aging the in 21st Century is drawing notice. It has established a culture of respect for seniors, and for the place in which they live. Teresian House is not just keeping its residents alive, it is keeping them living.

REFERENCES

Gould, M.O. (2001 Nov/Dec). Resident centered care. *Health Progress*, p. 56-58, 72.

Noell, E. (1995). Design in nursing homes: Environment as a silent partner in caregiving. *Generations 19*(4), p. 14.

Pastva, L. (2000). *The Carmelite Sisters for the Aged and Infirm*. Strasbourg, France: Editions du Signe.

Daycare center to unite children and family. (1999, September 9). *The Evangelist*.

A better way to treat the old. (1999, October 11). *The New York Times*.

Center for Nursing and Rehabilitation–
Culture Change in an Urban Environment

Clari Gilbert
Gails Bridges

SUMMARY. Imagine a nursing home where the waiting rooms look like comfortable, homey living rooms; the residents' rooms become "suites"; the bathrooms are referred to as "spas" and the reception area is staffed by a "concierge." A place where each resident determines his/her own schedule based upon individual preferences rather than following a routine set by the nursing home. A place which liberates and empowers residents, staff and families to build relationships. This article describes the Center for Nursing and Rehabilitation in Brooklyn, New York, an urban facility with 320 residents and a 564-person staff, and its journey toward culture change, moving from "Units" to "Neighborhoods." This change in paradigm is

---

Clari Gilbert, MA, is Senior Vice President of Operations, CNR Health Care Network. She is a licensed nursing home administrator and has held various positions in long-term care for the past 20 years.

Gails Bridges, CSW, is the Director of the CNR Community Resource Center. Previously she was Director of Penthouse Gardens and prior to that its Director of Social Work. She has been in long-term care for more than 20 years.

Address correspondence to: Clari Gilbert, MA, Senior Vice President of Operations, CNR Health Care Network, 520 Prospect Place, Brooklyn, NY 11238 (E-mail: Cgilbert@cnrhealthcare.org).

[Haworth co-indexing entry note]: "Center for Nursing and Rehabilitation–Culture Change in an Urban Environment." Gilbert, Clari, and Gails Bridges. Co-published simultaneously in *Journal of Social Work in Long-Term Care* (The Haworth Social Work Practice Press, an imprint of The Haworth Press, Inc.) Vol. 2, No. 3/4, 2003, pp. 233-243; and: *Culture Change in Long-Term Care* (ed: Audrey S. Weiner, and Judah L. Ronch) The Haworth Social Work Practice Press, an imprint of The Haworth Press, Inc., 2003, pp. 233-243. Single or multiple copies of this article are available for a fee from The Haworth Document Delivery Service [1-800-HAWORTH, 9:00 a.m. - 5:00 p.m. (EST). E-mail address: docdelivery@haworthpress.com].

http://www.haworthpress.com/store/product.asp?sku=J181
10.1300/J181v2n03_02

guided by the values and principles of integration, creativity and com-
passion. *[Article copies available for a fee from The Haworth Document Delivery
Service: 1-800-HAWORTH. E-mail address: <docdelivery@haworthpress.com>
Website: <http://www.HaworthPress.com> © 2003 by The Haworth Press, Inc.
All rights reserved.]*

KEYWORDS. Culture change, integration, creativity, compassion, neighborhoods, innovation, skilled nursing

INTRODUCTION

The Center for Nursing and Rehabilitation is a division of the CNR Health Care Network, a voluntary, non-profit organization that also serves the community through a variety of home care and adult day care programs, a hospice program and a Short Term In-residence Rehabilitation and Subacute Care program. At the very heart of the Network is the nursing home, which opened in the summer of 1978, and has been a window in a medically deprived community leading to the development of outreach programs to serve health care needs of the elderly.

Located in Crown Heights, Brooklyn, New York, the Center for Nursing and Rehabilitation is a 320-bed skilled nursing facility having four resident care floors with 80 beds on each floor. Traditionally, in addition to nursing and medical care, a complete range of health services have been provided to residents including physical, occupational and speech therapy; therapeutic recreation; social work; ophthalmology; dental care and short-term rehabilitation. Approximately seventy-eight percent (78%) of the residents are over age sixty-five (65). All reflect the ethnic diversity of neighboring Brooklyn communities which include native African Americans, Caribbeans, Haitians and Caucasians. The majority of the 564 employees live in the surrounding communities and also reflect the diversity of Brooklyn's neighborhoods. Approximately 90% of the staff have been employed for more than 5 years, and 85% are members of local 1199, New York Health and Human Services Union.

Prior to the beginning of this change program in December, 1999, each floor of the Center for Nursing and Rehabilitation operated under the auspices of Directors/Department Heads according to the traditional medical model. The main objective in seeking fundamental change was to establish a warmer, more friendly, resident-centered environment in which all staff, residents and families are mutually interactive in providing and receiving care and services, thus promoting better quality of life and increased satisfaction for everyone involved.

The concept of resident-directed care was first introduced to the Center in 1997 during social work month by one of its pioneers, Catherine Unsino, CSW. The concept heightened our awareness of the need for a new approach to increased resident involvement in their care. The senior Vice President of Operations made a field trip to Providence, Mount St. Vincent Home in Seattle, Washington, which had been operating successfully within this resident-directed framework for ten years, in order to observe the program first hand.

MODELS FOR CHANGE

Before determining a specific model of resident-directed care, a team of administrative staff looked carefully at the various models in place in other institutions. One concept that is gaining strength throughout the country is that of physically redesigning the nursing home into households with the individual resident rooms as bedrooms opening off a common area that includes a living room, dining room and kitchen. A challenge for CNR was how to create a similar environment without losing resident bedroom space. While this popular household concept is an attractive alternative to the status quo and works well in suburban and rural areas such as Fairport Baptist Home in Rochester, NY and Teresian House in Albany, NY, it requires more land space for building expansion or decertifying beds, which is not financially feasible for CNR. For instance, a two-bedded room at CNR is 12 ft. by 22 ft. and the corridors running outside them are 8 ft. wide. Even making bedrooms a little smaller and absorbing the corridors would not create adequate footage in which to add living and dining rooms and kitchens and it is questionable whether the entire redesign would receive regulatory approval. Additionally, renovations of this extent would require gutting of the existing facility and be prohibitively expensive. A significant question is, "Where would the residents be housed and cared for during any major physical renovation?"

These pressing issues became moot the more thought was given to the residents and the way in which they are accustomed to living. Actually, most New York City dwellers do not live in large houses but, rather, in small apartments. What New York does have, however, are neighborhoods. Brooklyn, in particular, is known by its neighborhoods. In fact Brooklyn has more than 25 distinct neighborhoods, such as Carroll Gardens, Brooklyn Heights, Bedford Stuyvesant, Crown Heights, and Park Slope, to name a few.

Brooklynites come together in their neighborhoods for socialization and companionship and then return to their personal spaces. In view of this lifestyle and the space limitations at the Center, The Neighborhood Concept, a model that originated in the Anchorage Pioneers' Home in Anchorage, Alaska, in which the nursing home units are transformed, through organizational and limited physical restructuring, into neighborhoods, was the logical one for CNR to pursue (Glickstein & Brundige, 1998).

THE CHARACTERISTICS OF CULTURAL CHANGE

Various configurations for the delivery of nursing care have evolved within the rapidly changing health care industry. These changes have paralleled major economic, societal, and demographic trends. The rise of consumerism, with its emphasis on resident involvement, and the change in societal values and expectations all contribute to the multifaceted nature of care delivery systems. The functional model, a task oriented approach, involved the use of a variety of personnel. It was regarded as a highly efficient, regimented system and was designed to take advantage of different levels of caregiver skill. In functional care the nurse was required to organize and manage a number of given tasks within a certain time (Poulin, 1985; Stevens, 1985).

The issue associated with the functional approach in nursing care delivery was the fragmentation that occurred when meeting the needs of both patients and staff. Components of patient care that were not addressed raised the frustration levels of both the caregiver and the patient. The sole reliance on regimented tasks was one of the functional model's major drawbacks and resulted in dissatisfaction for both the patient and the nurse (Poulin, 1985; Stevens, 1985).

In a resident-directed care culture, residents are offered choices, make decisions and staff are encouraged to meet their desired needs (Glickstein & Brundige, 1998). Rather than float, staff are consistently assigned to the same neighborhood team, and instead of knowing residents only by diagnosis, they develop personal relationships with each resident in the neighborhoods. Instead of being rigidly structured, activities are spontaneous and around the clock, and care is individualized in such a way as to nurture the human spirit. Both staff and residents function as members of the neighborhood team.

By having staff view and treat the resident as an independent, responsible and valued member of the neighborhood, we transform not only the institution's culture but also enhance the resident's feelings of self-efficacy. As the resident begins to cope actively with, rather than passively submit to the environment, it is hoped he/she experiences feelings of increased belonging, self worth and dignity.

Even though in 2 years time CNR's culture change effort was well underway it was nonetheless important to understand the residents' perceptions of the culture during this change process. Thus at the end of 2001 a quality of life survey was conducted.

Differing from standard satisfaction questionnaires routinely used at the Center and by other in-residence health care institutions, the survey instrument was designed to probe feelings, asking about loneliness, pain, anxiety, fear, personal relationships with staff, etc. To make sure the responses would reflect only the thinking of the residents, two graduate students who had no prior relationship with Center were hired to assist those who required help in completing the questionnaire. They were instructed not to press unduly for answers nor record their own assumptions of what a resident might be trying to express.

Eighty-four residents responded to the survey representing one-third of Center's population in-house at the time, excluding those who, by reason of their disabilities, would not be capable of participating (see Table 1).

CREATING NEIGHBORHOOD CARE TEAMS

The first–and perhaps most difficult–step towards achieving the objective was the reorganization of the entire facility. Theoretically, we could have kept the table of organization intact and simply added personnel as Neighborhood Directors, but that would have proven costly and counter productive. Consequently, the discrete departments were eliminated (except for the Department of Nursing, which is mandated by New York State regulations), and all staff–social workers, nurses, certified nursing assistants, dietitians, etc.–were absorbed into neighborhood teams. The Director of Nursing became the Director of Clinical Services. Every team member reports to a Neighborhood Director who overseas the neighborhood's function: staffing, budgeting, purchasing, hiring, education and program development. The Neighborhood Director's role is a most critical one in successfully implementing a resident-directed and supportive system of care. A Neighborhood Director must be professionally endowed with attributes of a skillful manager, team builder, motivator and committed to the concept of "Resident-directed" care. The table of organization was turned upside down so that the residents are on top.

Natural resistance to change would most likely have resulted in staff continuing to operate as they always had, i.e., looking to their department heads for direction, had we simply added on to the old structure. Consequently, without the departmental framework in which to function, staff have nowhere to look for leadership or collegiality but to the team.

TABLE 1. Resident Satisfaction Responses

Questions	Positive Responses
Does staff seem to care about whether or not you are happy?	89%
On the floor where I live, the staff is kind	99%
My neighborhood is like home to me	85%
My special needs are met	91%
Since the Neighborhoods were developed, my care is better	89%
Staff members treat me with respect	97%
Nothing stops me from going to every activity I want to join	95%

The next step was to appoint directors for the neighborhood care teams. After soliciting candidates internally and with careful consideration, the Director of Social Work Department, the Director of Rehabilitation, the Associate Director of nursing, and a charge nurse were appointed. These selections were made by administrative staff. These are all valued members of the staff whom we did not want to lose in the reorganization. Neighborhood Directors report directly to the Administrator and are responsible for managing budgets, staffing and implementing performance improvement programs in addition to overseeing the four neighborhood teams, which include health professionals from all disciplines, as well as residents and their families.

All staff on all shifts became part of their respective neighborhood teams, with Neighborhood Directors having 24-hour responsibility for the management of residents and staff in their respective neighborhoods. This blurred the differentiation between day, evening and night shifts and, along with it, the tendency to think in terms of "This is the next shift's job." Departmental offices were eliminated. "Team Rooms," where team members share space and, consequently, information, were created. Finally, to further foster the team mind-set, separate uniforms that define roles were eliminated. Now everyone, regardless of function, dresses in the same manner, in multi-colored tops and matching pants or skirts, with only name badges to identify an individual as an RN, LPN or CNA.

DEVELOPING NEIGHBORHOOD ENVIRONMENTS

As the neighborhood care teams were formed, the two units on each floor were combined into a single, distinct neighborhood. Families, residents, and staff in each neighborhood joined together in suggesting and voting on names for their neighborhoods, ultimately settling on Hope Gardens, Pleasantville,

Park Haven and Penthouse Gardens. Physical changes designed to create a more home-like environment occurred including the remodeling of its seating. Decorations were added such as wallpaper, wall sconces, pictures and plants. One neighborhood added a fish tank with tropical fish, another birds in cages. Each neighborhood had decorating teams who met to discuss decorative ideas. There was no set budget; once ideas were finalized all areas were discussed with and approved by the administration.

Residents' rooms are now referred to as suites, the common bathing rooms are called neighborhood spas and the dining rooms have been given names such as Penthouse Gardens Diner. These were all ideas from the decorating teams which consisted of Certified Nursing Assistants, licensed staff, social workers, recreation therapists and the Neighborhood Director.

With cooperation from the kitchen and dietary staffs, some residents are now served meals restaurant style in their neighborhood dining rooms. Tables are set with linen tablecloths and napkins, and there is a vase of flowers on each table.

The plan is to enlarge the neighborhood pantries to include snack foods and even equip them so that residents who prefer to sleep late can have breakfast at their leisure. The aim is to encourage residents to live according to their own schedules, as they would at home, rather than rising, eating and going to bed when *we* say they should.

Other homelike amenities include an aviary, aquarium and our resident cat, Kittin, who wanders from one neighborhood to another and is fed and gently cared for by the residents, helping to connect the human spirit with a favorite pet. Building upon the Eden Alternative (Thomas, 1999) with its emphasis on vibrant gardens, a mobile garden cart has been created to allow residents to interact with the earth by planting their favorite herbs.

RESIDENT/FAMILY/STAFF INTERACTION

Each neighborhood has a core "council" of staff and residents that provides neighborhood oversight, assisting in designing programs and activities and in general contributing to neighborhood leadership. The councils each elect a neighborhood captain who, with the assistance of the social worker, serves as council leader.

Neighborhood Directors meet monthly with residents, families and staff to encourage meaningful communication and social interaction. Such meetings also serve as excellent forums for sharing neighborhood-related information and ideas, acknowledging achievements, problem solving and quality improvement.

Family members have become much more involved than they were in the traditional culture. For example, where, in the past, only 5 to 15 family members attended the house-wide monthly family council meetings, there are now on average 25-30 family members present for each neighborhood meeting.

Family members volunteer in the neighborhoods, assisting with feeding and providing friendly visits to residents who do not have frequent visitors. All volunteers are trained in appropriate feeding techniques. They also assist in the production of neighborhood newsletters, which are mailed to all families. There have been a number of studies showing the value of such networks in which neighbors and kin provide support that might ordinarily have to be provided by professionals (Antonucci, 1990; Biegel et al., 1984).

COSTS

The budget for this first phase of the project was a total of $40,000. Of this, $18,250 was spent on training resources such as off-site visits to other facilities, consultants, seminars, workshops, books, videos and equipment. Another $5,000 was spent to provide training of volunteers in feeding techniques, friendly visitation and transporting residents. The remainder of the budget went to environmental design and construction and to programs such as the aviary in one neighborhood and the mobile garden cart, and the purchasing of computers with Internet access for our residents.

THE CHALLENGES

Implementing change is not easy. In that regard, the four new Neighborhood Directors faced a unique challenge. Each was now in a position of having to make decisions in areas other than their formal expertise. For example, the former director of Social Work had responsibility not only for the social work services in her neighborhood, but for nursing, therapeutic recreation and every other aspect of resident care, as well. The loss of discipline identity and perceived loss of status as a department head, as well as the lack of Medical/Nursing knowledge, made for some uncomfortable feelings, fears and challenges. However, with the support of clinicians within her team, the comprehensive training, and assurances of confidence in her ability to do the job from the Administration, she and all Neighborhood Directors became competent and comfortable in their roles.

Another challenge arose out of implementation of a feeding/dining program, which required cross training of staff. Some professional staff were apprehensive about loss of role identification and image perception; many staff feared they would have to be involved in all aspects of hands-on care; two social workers resigned, and returned a few months later.

To address this, many meetings were held for information sharing, discussions and alignment of teams. A series of educational programs designed to promote understanding of the concept and philosophy of resident-directed care, including a seven-week comprehensive management-training program for Neighborhood Directors and managers, were held.

Safety Awareness Training programs including a safety carnival, guest speakers and skits performed by the residents, among other features, further helped to educate the staff and reassure them about their abilities. We observed that as the training continued, some non-nursing staff who, in the past were reluctant to assist in care, began to willingly engage themselves in resident care issues.

CONTINUING SUPPORT

In the December, 2001 resident satisfaction survey among the areas for improvement is the need for staff to offer choices to the residents. A total of 55% of the residents stated that they are given choices about time for bathing and bedtime, and 83% are given choices about the food they can order. Therefore there is a need to continually communicate to staff our core values and to align these values with care practices on a daily basis. Without some method of identifying gaps between values and behaviors, such concepts as creativity, compassion, caring and nurturing the human spirit constitute nothing more than a wish list.

A revised mandatory in-service training program created by the Director of Staff Development was implemented to help staff members perform in the spirit of the principles and core values adopted by the neighborhoods, as well as to support the goals established by the administration. An important aspect of the educational effort is behavior modeling. Telling staff to encourage residents to exercise independence and choice will not have any clear meaning unless all staff demonstrate what these behaviors look like. Some staff have demonstrated the inability to be empathetic, or to reflect the feeling another person expresses. Further training in sensitivity and communication techniques are necessary to address this issue.

A computer program for both staff and residents has emerged, and we are developing programs to upgrade the computer skills of Neighborhood Directors and clinical associates. Some of our residents already have computer skills and the addition of computers complete with Internet and email access will add further dimension to their daily activities.

EVALUATIONS AND REFINEMENTS

The cultural change, which began in December, 1999 is still in the embryonic stage. Inevitably, mistakes were made that had to be corrected. For example, the assumption that one person, regardless of her competence, could function successfully as a Neighborhood Director and still oversee the Rehabilitation Department was erroneous. At CNR, rehabilitation is too essential a service to be left to a part-time head, and eventually, a change was made. The Neighborhood Management team, comprising of Administrators and Neighborhood Directors, is continually assessing areas of deficiencies that can inevitably erode the foundation that has been laid.

The pursuit of quality requires a solid program for measuring customer satisfaction. Such a program will be added at CNR to include informational data collected through periodic interviews with staff, residents and families; neighborhood reports and staff performance data, and reports on the effectiveness of project design implementation. A Customer Satisfaction Index is being established and monitored on an ongoing basis, with focus groups, surveys and resident/family interviews serving as a backbone to this program.

Performance measurements and data collection will also focus on processes and practices that could be perceived as high risk, high volume or problem prone. Monitoring of clinical practice, in conjunction with established quality indicators, through clinical observation and the MDS 2.0 Assessment tool, is carried out at least quarterly. Relevant data such as presence of nosocomial pressure ulcers, frequency of resident falls and injuries, unplanned weight loss and rates of complaints per neighborhood are collected on a monthly basis.

Resident/family questionnaires and interviews are being done to address quality of life issues, degree of satisfaction with the neighborhood, degree of resident participation and involvement in care planning and neighborhood activities and similar issues. The questionnaire is designed with input from management and from each neighborhood and is done annually, the first in December, 2001.

NEXT STEPS

The renovation of kitchens, and new dining rooms and living rooms in each neighborhood has begun in order to provide greater and more comfortable, homelike common space. These changes to the physical plant help to further feelings of independence simply by increasing the residents' choices of where to go and when, as well as to facilitate socialization and the feeling of living in a neighborhood. The need for research and quantifiable data is indicated in order to give credence to this concept.

This time of constant change dictates that attention be paid not only to improving the present process but, also, to designing for the unknown future, to simultaneously maintain the dual strategies of improvement and innovation (Blanchard & Waghorn, 1977). Such an approach is viewed as critical to help CNR to adapt to changes before a crisis develops.

By continually reviewing and re-evaluating processes, changes will be made to enhance the resident-directed care approach. With this commitment, the permanency of this new culture can be achieved, maintained and serve as a model for other urban nursing facilities.

REFERENCES

Antonucci, T.C. (1990). *Social supports and social relationships.* In Binstock, R.H., & George, L.K. (Eds.), *Handbook of aging and the social sciences.* Third Edition. San Diego, Academic Press.

Biegel, D.E., Shore, B.R. & Gordon, E. (1984). *Building support networks for the elderly.* Sage, Beverly Hills.

Blanchard, Ken & Waghorn, T. (1977). *Mission Possible: Becoming a world-class organization while there's still time.* McGraw-Hill.

Cohen, E.L. & Cesta, T.G. *Your Nursing care management: From concept to evaluation,* Mosby–Yearbook, Inc. St. Louis, MO, 22-28.

Glickstein, J. & Brundige, L.C. (1998). *Reengineering for a successful future: The Anchorage Pioneer's Home Project. Focus on geriatric care and rehabilitation,* 12(4), 1-11.

Poulin, M. (1985). Configuration of nursing practice. In American Nurse's Association (Ed.), *Issues in professional nursing practice* (pp. 1-14). Kansas City, MO: The Association.

Stevens, B.J. (1985). *The nurse as executive* (pp. 105-137). Rockville, MD: Aspen Publication.

Thomas, W.H. (1999). *The Eden Alternative Handbook: The art of building human habitats.* NY: Summerhill Company.

Triandis, H.C. (1972). *The analysis of subjective culture.* New York: Wiley.

The Providence
Mount St. Vincent Experience

Charlene K. Boyd

SUMMARY. In 1991, a strategic planning team at a senior-living care facility in Seattle, Washington, began a process of organizational and cultural change. The process transformed both the philosophy and model of care, as well as the physical environment of Providence Mount St. Vincent. In 1998, a *New York Times* writer described the results she observed within and around the nearly 300,000-square-foot building constructed in 1924: The Mount, as those who live there call it, is widely regarded to be what many Americans consider an impossibility–a good nursing home. That is to say, in an industry freighted with the dread of old age, disability and loneliness, and periodically tainted by scandal and abuse, The Mount has found ways to be a home to people who can no longer care for themselves, to provide a sense of community in a place

Charlene K. Boyd has served as Administrator of Providence Mount St. Vincent–a Providence Health System senior-living care facility established by the Sisters of Providence–since 1996. She was a key member of the facility's 1991 strategic planning team and subsequently became a founding board member for the Pioneer Network–a national organization leading the culture change movement for the long-term care industry. Her career in long-term care began during the 1970s in occupational therapy.

Address correspondence to: Charlene K. Boyd, Providence Mount St. Vincent, 4831 35th Avenue SW, Seattle, WA 98126-2799 (E-mail: cboyd@providence.org); <Website: www.providence.org/themount>.

[Haworth co-indexing entry note]: "The Providence Mount St. Vincent Experience." Boyd, Charlene K. Co-published simultaneously in *Journal of Social Work in Long-Term Care* (The Haworth Social Work Practice Press, an imprint of The Haworth Press, Inc.) Vol. 2, No. 3/4, 2003, pp. 245-268; and: *Culture Change in Long-Term Care* (ed: Audrey S. Weiner, and Judah L. Ronch) The Haworth Social Work Practice Press, an imprint of The Haworth Press, Inc., 2003, pp. 245-268. Single or multiple copies of this article are available for a fee from The Haworth Document Delivery Service [1-800-HAWORTH, 9:00 a.m. - 5:00 p.m. (EST). E-mail address: docdelivery@haworthpress.com].

where no one wants to be, to be a community that is more about living than about dying.

Prior to the change process, The Mount maintained a traditional, medical model of operations designed to achieve staff efficiencies and meet residents' medical needs within a mission of compassionate care. Studies to measure residents' daily levels of activity and engagement helped determine quality of life within a medical model setting. In a typical U.S. nursing home, residents spend 25-35 percent of their day engaged in some activity.

Based on a series of behavioral studies at The Mount in the early 1990s conducted with approximately 1,400 observations of resident activity, a typical waking day in the life of a nursing home resident included engaging in any type of activity for 32 percent of the time. After The Mount's strategic planning team introduced a "neighborhood" concept for people receiving nursing care, the measure of engagement jumped from 32 to 42 percent and the death curve reversed and improved by 83 percent.

For the past five years, The Mount has worked with and through a national group called the Pioneer Network to serve as a culture change resource and learning laboratory for other senior-living care providers around the country. This article describes the journey and outcomes of culture change in this facility. *[Article copies available for a fee from The Haworth Document Delivery Service: 1-800-HAWORTH. E-mail address: <docdelivery@haworthpress.com> Website: <http://www.HaworthPress.com> © 2003 by The Haworth Press, Inc. All rights reserved.]*

KEYWORDS. Long-term care, geriatric care, culture change, resident-directed philosophy/social model, senior living, nursing home, assisted living

INTRODUCTION

In 1924, a small group of Sisters from the Daughters of Charity Servants of the Poor (a religious congregation now known as "Sisters of Providence") established St. Vincent's Home for the Aged in Seattle, Washington, to care for aging, indigent men and women. With the help of a wealthy philanthropist, the Sisters erected a five-story brick building surrounded by gardens atop a West Seattle hill with panoramic views of waterways and mountain ranges. The setting was thought to be therapeutic and healing in its own right. For 40 years, the facility operated with a mission of compassion to promote the physical and spiritual well being of adults who could no longer care for themselves.

Once federal and state governments began providing health care insurance (Medicare and Medicaid) in the mid-1960s, the facility adopted a medical model for operations focusing on staff efficiencies and residents' medical needs to meet the arduous reporting requirements necessary for reimbursement. While the facility maintained high standards of care, large-scale, centralized systems supported a sterile, institutional setting. By the late 1980s, an outdated building interior prompted the Sisters to consider major changes.

In 1991, a strategic planning team–consisting of a new facility administrator, an assistant administrator, a psychologist/researcher, two architects, two nursing managers, a physical therapist and a social worker–decided to move beyond financial, structural, programmatic and marketing issues to embrace what it viewed as a grand vision: a community directed by its residents. The team aimed to provide care based on a social or community model; to create a place where people wanted to live, rather than where people came to die (Vision, 1994).

So began a journey that continues today. While still a work in progress, Providence Mount St. Vincent has been cited as a national leader in culture change for its philosophy of compassionate, resident-directed care. According to a *New York Times* writer who spent several weeks at the facility in 1998:

> The Mount, as those who live there call it, is widely regarded to be what many Americans consider an impossibility: a good nursing home. That is to say, in an industry freighted with the dread of old age, disability and loneliness, and periodically tainted by scandal and abuse, The Mount has found ways to be a home to people who can no longer care for themselves, to provide a sense of community in a place where no one wants to be, to be a community that is more about living than about dying. (Rimer, 1998)

As described in a 1999 *Seattle Times* article, what The Mount is doing seems like simple common sense; but it's considered at the forefront of a revolution in the nursing home industry (King, 1999). Owned and operated by the Sisters of Providence and the Providence Health System, The Mount is home to more than 400 adults during their transition from independence to increasing reliance on the support of others. Residents range in age from 29 to 103, with an average age of 89 years. Additionally, The Mount provides management services for other long-term care providers including a nearby Vashon Island senior-living care center.

Programs and services offered by The Mount include ten 23-bed "neighbor-hoods" with skilled nursing services; a 20-bed, short-term, sub-acute medical rehabilitation unit; 112 studio and one-bedroom apartments with assisted living services; an adult day health program; physical, occupational and recreational therapeutic services for both residents and the broader community; a licensed childcare center serving 125 children ages 6 weeks to 5 years; an off-site adult family home for people with dementia who prefer a small, structured program; and a clinic for optometry, podiatry, dental, audiology, medical, acupuncture and massage. Most of these programs and services emerged or took their current form following the 1991 strategic planning process.

In 2001, The Mount's employees numbered 476 and the cost to operate the facility was $20 million. Occupancy for most programs–including the skilled nursing neighborhoods, assisted living apartments, adult family home, and childcare center is 100 percent or greater (i.e., wait lists). The Mount operates under contracts with the Service Employees International Union (SEIU) and the International Union of Operating Engineers. Nearly all of the facility's direct-care staff are covered by the SEIU contract.

CHANGE MODEL AND THEORETIC FRAMEWORK

The 1991 strategic planning team was convened by a new administrator who joined The Mount in late 1990 bringing experience in both the regulatory and direct-care sides of the long-term care coin. The Sisters had hired the new leader four years earlier to build a nursing facility in Alaska for the Cook Inlet Native Corporation to be named the Mary Conrad Center. At approximately the same time, in 1987, nursing-home reform legislation known as OBRA (Omnibus Budget Reconciliation Act) mandated landmark changes in the long-term care industry. The law, paraphrased, stated that residents come first and must be afforded the potential to live each day as though they are in a true home.

The Alaska project was an opportunity to incorporate new concepts inspired by OBRA–to determine if a nursing facility could be a "home" in the true sense and the residents could have a real say in the services they received. The opening of the Mary Conrad Center in Anchorage was difficult and very costly. The facility lost $1.5 million its first year. Leaders deliberately staffed the 90-bed facility with people experienced in community-based organizations and the hospitality industry. These new staff, who had no medical-model training in skilled nursing, found it natural to identify and build on residents' strengths.

The second year the facility had $100,000 surplus. Ultimately, the new Mary Conrad Center did not resemble a traditional nursing home: It provided a novel "neighborhood concept" for a long-term care facility and residents enjoyed simple pleasures such as access to a kitchen and snacks at all times (Ogden, 2001). The project ultimately received a number of national awards for architectural and operational innovation (*Contemporary Long Term Care*, 1991).

The Mount's new administrator brought the best of this Alaska experience including a psychologist/researcher who became a key factor in The Mount's education about the community model of care, putting residents first and building a system that helps direct-care staff feel and be empowered. The Mount's team soon connected with two local architects who wanted to change the physical environment to create a more homelike environment.

THE MOUNT'S CHANGE

Original Culture

For at least 30 years, from the mid 1960s to the early 1990s, The Mount operated similar to a hospital. Many systems (i.e., laundry and food delivery) had developed in response to federal and state regulations. The Sisters' tradition of providing compassionate care, spiritual ministry and quality of life existed within an environment driven by regulators and medical charts. During the 1991 strategic planning process, one nursing manager noted that her hope for The Mount was to provide more than a supportive and medically safe passage to death (Scheer, 2001).

The recollections of a nursing unit manager who joined The Mount in 1979 as a nursing assistant give an indication of the old culture:

> direct-care staff wore uniforms; people living in apartments hid serious health problems or incontinence for fear of being moved to the facility's nursing home; and people suppressed the grieving process to protect other apartment residents, nursing home residents and family members. (Jennings, 2001)

Centralized departments were designed for economies of scale. For example, The Mount used 450-pound commercial clothes washers the size of a small car. To ensure operational efficiency, the equipment was located in a laundry room in the lowest level of the building. Similarly, The Mount's kitchen produced 1,700 meals a day. For a nursing home resident, breakfast arrived off the tray at 6 a.m. so s/he had to eat on schedule rather than when s/he was hungry. The system had little room for personal needs and preferences. Subsequently, about 40 percent of the food was returned uneaten.

Structurally, the building had been remodeled in the '60s. Apartments were added with healthy retirees in mind–people in their 60s. Sterile corridors–as long as football fields–and cold, hard surfaces were reminiscent of sterile hospitals. Floor, wall and ceiling materials were designed for durability and ease of maintenance. Spaces felt tight; apartment residents, nursing home residents and equipment crowded the hallways.

Nursing Home

Based on a series of behavioral studies at The Mount in the early 1990s conducted with approximately 1,400 observations of resident activity, a typical waking day in the life of a nursing home resident included engaging in any type of activity for 32 percent of the time; either napping or sitting idle for 68 percent; and interacting with another person for seven percent (Fey, 1995; Richardson et al., 1997).

During community meetings involving residents, family members and staff, residents expressed that they felt well cared for, but at the same time frequently felt bored, lonely or that they no longer held any control over their lives. Administrators, staff and even family members mostly shrugged, feeling at a loss to affect change over what was seen at the time as a necessary condition.

Staff positions were often separated by task so that many employees carried out specific duties. A bath aide, for example, bathed residents exclusively. Baths were available when the bath aide was working, rather than when the resident wanted a bath. Task-driven routines made it seem easier for staff to ensure that residents had eaten and gone to the restroom. Hospital-like language prevailed: "patient," "ward," "floor," and "unit." A hierarchical structure segregated management and frontline staff.

The building had four floors of nursing units with the typical unit consisting of 56 beds along a double-loaded corridor approximately 300 feet long. A small dining and activity space was centrally located with utility rooms at each end of the long hallway. The dining room was not large enough to serve 56 people at once, so residents ate in shifts. Typically, the hallways would become clogged with food carts and people waiting to eat.

Most staff time was structured around the delivery of care according to the medical model. There was little time available for social interaction between nursing home residents and staff. Due to the interior building layout, a portion of staff time was spent simply moving between spaces. A large separation existed between the area where one would find residents and the area where staff activities occurred. Interaction was more likely to occur when residents were "parked" in the corridor, in front of their rooms, and near elevators or staff spaces.

New Social or Community Culture

The goal of the 1991 planning process was a new model that would allow The Mount to provide care that is more directed by residents' preferences and needs and places high value on human interaction. Under the new model, staff honor residents' deep, healthy desire to retain control over their lives. "Resident-directed care" places residents in a primary role as participants in developing their individual care plans. As much as possible, residents choose their own daily routines and the services they wish to receive.

Residents in both assisted living and nursing neighborhoods have opportunities to be active and involved most of their waking day and to form warm relationships with resident assistants and other staff. The flexible care residents receive allows them to feel comfortable and remain in their own apartments or rooms as their needs increase.

All departments function in small, multi-functional teams that directly serve residents, so that the residents' perspective is always top-of-mind. Staff place supreme value on listening and knowing resident backgrounds and personal preferences, while helping them with concerns related to their health and wellbeing. Understanding individual needs, learning, and collaboration are the ingredients that create each plan of care; a plan that is fluid and evolves with changing needs and wishes, and continued sharing and listening. Language used by staff gives power and respect to residents who live in apartments or neighborhoods (rather than "floors," "wards" or "units").

Both staff and family members are committed to supporting resident independence. Tasks in both the nursing neighborhoods and the assisted living apartments are shared by a variety of staff members in an environment that caters to residents holistically. The position of resident assistant (RA)–formerly known as a "patient aide" or "nursing assistant"–has components of being a caregiver, a neighbor, and a surrogate family member. RAs receive special training in the resident-directed philosophy and communicating in relationships. The ability to communicate and listen is most important for an RA. They recognize residents' healthy need for variety each day and provide much more than a "chore service." If a resident invites them to have lunch or listen to a story, they can accept. RAs see their job as a series of connected, meaningful engagements and feel valued and respected.

RAs, who come to know residents in the complex way of family members, work closely with their team nurses who hone in on specialized physical problems. Physicians and nurses believe that medicine does not need to control residents' lives. Family members play a key role in developing resident care plans and participate in neighborhood and recreational activities. They build warm relationships with staff members and other residents.

New Assisted Living Apartments

Apartments are suitable and accessible for an older, more frail population. All residents pay one fee and receive however many or few services they need or desire based on a negotiated service plan. As long as the assisted living program is able to meet their needs, residents move from their apartment only if they choose to do so themselves.

New Nursing Neighborhoods

Ten neighborhoods are home to 20-24 residents. Each neighborhood has a shared staff of about 18 people including: a neighborhood coordinator, resident assistants, recreational therapists, food and nutrition workers, a social worker, nurse, spiritual care worker and housekeeper. All staff routinely multi-task to help residents with any need including going to the restroom, brewing coffee, doing laundry, fixing a sandwich, and eating. This kind of highly capable staff that shares tasks supports resident independence and choice.

As envisioned by The Mount's contracted architects and the strategic planning team, neighborhoods feature a light, spacious kitchen with round tables and all the usual home supplies, from tablecloths to tea kettles. Residents wake when they prefer and ask the neighborhood host (or food and nutrition worker) to prepare their food. Lunches and dinners are prepared in the central kitchen, but brought up to each neighborhood and placed in steam trays so tempting smells can drift through the rooms. Residents' favorite snacks and drinks are stocked in the kitchen and available at any time. If a resident craves ice cream at midnight, toast at 3 a.m. or a banana and cookies in the afternoon, s/he can have it.

At the far end of the kitchen space is the open care station for social workers, nurses and other staff. A laundry room is available for each neighborhood. Residents who enjoy folding warm clothes may do their own laundry. Each neighborhood has access to a solarium that brings a sense of the outdoors to less mobile residents. Solariums are designed as a green house, a game room and library, and an intergenerational classroom complete with an aviary. The intergenerational classroom on the third floor, a permanent space for preschool children enrolled in The Mount's Intergenerational Learning Center, is a common area where residents spend time talking or playing with the children.

Each neighborhood has a distinct personality. Differences in style and color help orient residents who visit other neighborhoods. Details were chosen by the architects and strategic planning team for their warmth to create comforting surroundings conducive to familiar, pleasant domestic routines–making soup, playing cards, or reading at the kitchen table. The team aimed to create an environment where people could find multiple inviting settings for unscheduled, relaxed conversation and contact.

TIMEFRAME AND SUSTAINABLE CHANGE

The change process at The Mount has encompassed more than a decade to date and will continue indefinitely. The Mount's physical environment was transformed in about the first three years. Challenges arose at each juncture. In facing and working through the challenges together, everyone involved created an operational foundation for sustainable change. The new culture of care began to take root by 1994. Resident-directed care has become more and more visible through transformation in perspectives for both staff and residents.

In the spirit of pioneers, The Mount's care providers, recipients and stakeholders have proven steadfast in the ongoing journey. From many perspectives–among them residents, family members, staff, the local community and other providers across the country–the new culture is firmly rooted at The Mount. Sisters and administrative leaders work to ensure that the tradition of compassionate care continues and the community model and resident-directed philosophy outlive the tenure of any individual.

PROCESS

To launch the process, the strategic planning team conducted a series of meetings with stakeholder groups. No group felt strongly that The Mount was "broken" or needed change, according to most standards. Residents receiving all levels of care wanted to "age in place" as much as possible, but the team experienced difficulty at first in achieving consensus among stakeholders to move forward. The idea of placing more control with nursing home residents, especially, tested established belief systems. Chart 1 describes the goals of the strategic planning team.

Chart 2 details the specific goals of resident directed care.

CHART 1

In 1992, The Mount's strategic planning team adopted the term "resident-directed care" to describe the new philosophy and began meeting weekly. The team outlined specific goals and objectives in the three-year plan:

- Begin a process of change to allow residents more choice and control over their care and their lives;
- Support aging in place for the residents living in the apartments as an alternative to the nursing center;
- Renovate the nursing center to accommodate a more home-like residential environment;
- Expand the rehabilitation services to meet the needs of both the facility and the community;
- Decentralize decision making in order to expedite problem solving among staff and residents as well as allowing the nurses more time to provide clinical care; and
- Implement systems to improve employee recruitment and retention.

CHART 2. Resident-Directed Care Goals

- Improve resident satisfaction and quality of life

- Improve resident function and health status

- Improve staff efficiency and productivity

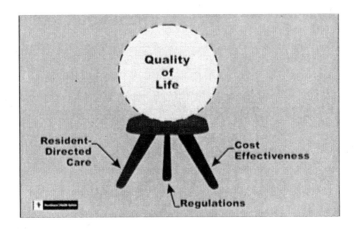

Team members presented the concept of re-introducing residents to a set of familiar and meaningful activities of daily life in order to increase activity levels. For example, residents who enjoy folding warm clothes may like to do their own laundry, or at least help staff. Likewise, meal planning and preparation had been a central focus in the lives of so many residents prior to entering the institutional setting. These daily processes provided satisfaction and filled a portion of their day. The new vision for The Mount would help bring opportunities for residents to participate in, or to at least see and/or smell more regularly, their own laundry and food preparation each day.

Of course, centralized service systems could not be changed overnight. Drawing upon lessons learned from a site visit to Minnesota, the team incorporated portable steam tables on each floor. At the suggestion of a resident assistant, the team had sent representatives for a tour of St. Benedict's Senior Community in St. Cloud, Minnesota, where staff used open work stations and steam tables on floors. With steam tables keeping food available for longer periods, staff found themselves able to accommodate resident preferences for meal times.

As one system began to change, other systems were affected. The volume of resistance among stakeholders decreased as anecdotal "proof" of positive outcomes traveled through the facility grapevine. For example, stories of previously inactive residents included the woman who began using utensils again to eat, the man who returned to his love of playing piano, a man who painted a cabinet in his room, and the man who enjoyed the taste of his favorite bacon again.

Assisted Living Apartments

The needs and profiles of The Mount's apartment residents had changed by the time the 1991 strategic planning process began. The apartments were now homes for more frail, older adults in their 80s who needed assistance with daily living: dressing; reminders to take medications; physical therapy; bathing; and personal care. Calling on the "form follows function" theory of American architect Louis Sullivan (1856-1924), The Mount's strategic planning team introduced a change in the care-giving function while simultaneously offering a plan to change the physical environment in a manner that would embrace that new function.

The new care philosophy was first introduced to the residents of The Mount's apartments through an assisted living program called "Hand in Hand." Along with family members and staff, each resident (even the frail and those with dementia as long as the program was able to meet care needs) helped to determine how much assistance he or she needed. Both the staff and family members had difficulty seeing the changes as beneficial–they had been institutionalized, and were comfortable with that "lifestyle" (Ogden, 2001).

Slowly and surely, the strategic planning team faced the challenge of getting the residents to take charge of their lives.

Assisted living residents took to the change immediately. With many RAs who had no background in medical model long-term care, they received and implemented training easily. The program had its initial difficulties, however. For instance, the costs of assisted-living services were built into apartment living as part of the rent, rather than having services negotiated on a financial basis. This way, residents were not afraid to ask for extra help if they needed it, worrying that they could not afford it and making do while growing more and more isolated. Services are now available to all residents if and when they need them. If a resident requires intensified help in his or her apartment for several weeks (on a limited basis), the rent is not raised.

A plan to remodel the apartments emerged to decrease architectural barriers for an older population. The plan included a "micro-fridge" (combination refrigerator and microwave oven) to replace a small, floor-level refrigerator that was inaccessible, and a stove that had electric burners–a safety concern; a new counter top and sink to replace unsafe burners and an antiquated sink; a step-in shower stall with grab-bars to replace old bathtubs that are inaccessible for a frail person; and a grab-bar near the toilet. Under the plan, each apartment would cost about $30,000 to remodel (*Design for Living*, 2000). At the time of this writing, remodeling for 75 percent of the apartments has been completed.

Childcare Center

Next, the strategic planning team chose a highly visible project which would begin changing the medical-model atmosphere–a childcare center housed within the facility. This project would help meet the childcare needs of staff and the outside community, and bring opportunities for residents to engage with children. With a capital investment provided by the Providence Health System, the strategic planning team launched the Intergenerational Learning Center (ILC). Today, the entire facility is licensed for childcare; children and their teachers move throughout the building and use shared spaces each day. An intergenerational classroom on the third-floor nursing neighborhood serves as a permanent space for one ILC preschool class.

The ILC gives residents the benefit of having more than a hundred "grandchildren" close by and offers opportunities for residents and children to meet anywhere in the building. Residents may interact with children through chance encounters in the halls, lobbies, cafeteria and other shared spaces or scheduled individual or group activities and visits. This project, possibly above all others, increased momentum to build a culture of doing things differently at The Mount.

Nursing Neighborhoods

The nursing home experienced the most radical change, both physically and philosophically. Residents had been assigned to floors based on their level of needed care. As needs changed, residents were moved to other floors, often causing transfer trauma. Resident-directed care brought an end to this arrangement and a new beginning–mixing the acuity levels of residents just as any community would have a population with diverse care needs. A new neighborhood concept was designed programmatically to be flexible in meeting the changing acuity levels of its residents.

The entire building became home to every resident. With movement less restricted, leaders saw decreases in levels of agitation and increases in satisfaction and engagement. For example, a quality indicator comparison of 1995 to 2001 measures indicates that activity-of-daily-living function decline decreased from 82 to three residents (Petitjean, 2002).

The strategic planning team decided to downsize bed capacity from 252 to 215 in order to provide more open space for living. The long corridors were divided into separate, 20- to 23-bed neighborhoods, each with its own décor. At the heart of each neighborhood, a large open area was built featuring a kitchen, dining room, lounge and staffing station called "care team area." In most homes, the kitchen/family room is where people generally gather for meals, entertainment and conversation. The team hoped that the new layout would offer a similarly inviting environment for both residents and staff. (See floor plans 1 and 2.)

Steam tables in the kitchen were installed enabling the staff to discontinue individual tray service and making it possible for residents to choose their food and portion size. Wells in the steam tables allowed The Mount's food and nutrition department to serve a variety of hot, fresh dishes to accommodate special dietary and nutritional needs as well as personal preferences. The flexibility offered by steam tables led to a decrease in special diets from seventeen to six and reduced costly food waste. Additionally, steam tables allowed staff to honor residents' preferred sleep and wake schedules.

Other physical changes in the nursing neighborhoods included the addition of whirlpool baths, a solarium for use as a common space where group meetings or recreational activities take place, and carpeting for halls and resident rooms to reduce noise as well as providing cushioning against falls and injuries. The remodeling for one neighborhood took about three months to complete.

FLOOR PLAN 1

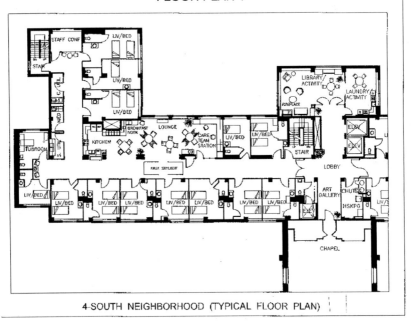

4-SOUTH NEIGHBORHOOD (TYPICAL FLOOR PLAN)

Major Staff Changes

Since the remodel would add common areas while reducing revenue-producing space, major organizational and staff changes were implemented. Thirty-five middle management positions were eliminated to decentralize and add direct-care staffing. This occurred through a process that included natural attrition, terminations with severance packages and retirements. Several department managers were offered and accepted direct-care positions. All floor staff received cross training in every household "chore" including food service, laundry, housekeeping and personal assistance (i.e., resident assistant tasks).

Neighborhood Teams

The neighborhood teams discovered they needed to become flexible, share responsibility and function like a family. Most task-oriented work was incorporated into the daily job functions of all staff. Nurses, for example, might serve food or clean up in the kitchens as well as administer treatments and medications. Resident assistants help in all areas such as serving meals, lead-

FLOOR PLAN 2

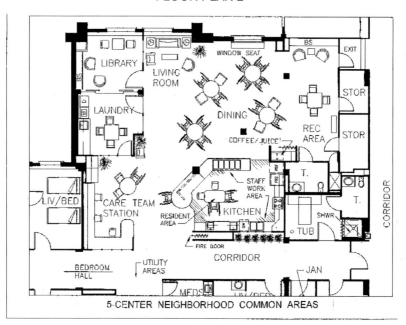

5-CENTER NEIGHBORHOOD COMMON AREAS

ing activities or folding laundry with residents. Recreation therapists helped with rehab as well as other areas. Communication grew much faster and more direct as neighborhood groups replaced a formal hierarchy.

A position called "neighborhood coordinator" was created to serve as a "mini administrator" in every neighborhood. Neighborhood coordinators have full authority over daily activities and are responsible for staffing, supervision, clinical nursing care, budgets, hiring, and firing–*all* aspects of management and operations. As much as possible, decisions are made with input from everyone on a neighborhood team. Careful consideration is given to communication among the staff as well as the residents (Richardson et al., 1997).

During the remodeling, one half of a neighborhood was completed at a time in order to minimize the number of residents who would be displaced. Working in phases allowed for normal attrition among staff to occur and made it possible to avoid moving residents to another facility.

For staff who had worked in a centralized environment doing specific tasks or in a position of medical authority where the "patient" was told what to do, the change process was difficult. Staff were used to having jobs sharply defined by a strict hierarchy. Before culture change, residents adapted their desires to the system.

Most changes were controversial. The Mount lost some managers and direct-care staff who found if difficult to make the transition (Boyd, 1994). During exit interviews, some expressed concern for the safety of residents who were being offered opportunities to make their own decisions regarding health and activities. The most controversial change was the gradual integration of a diverse case mix into each nursing neighborhood. Until 1993, the nursing floors were organized by residents' care needs. Those requiring the least amount of care stayed in rooms on the first floor. Residents requiring the most care stayed on the fifth floor. The fourth floor served as a secured unit for residents with special care needs due to dementia or Alzheimer's disease. People living on the second and third floor especially feared the fourth floor. They worried that if they behaved badly or got too forgetful, they would be "shipped one step closer to heaven." Under the social or community model, residents with dementia are integrated throughout the building. Each neighborhood carries a varied case mix, or residents with a variety of care needs. Neighborhoods function similar to family households. Staff look at strengths and tolerances of each member, realizing that each resident contributes in a different way.

REHABILITATION SERVICES

The Mount's rehabilitation services were increased to offer enhanced services to residents and the community. One nursing floor was divided into two separate programs: a 20-bed subacute, or short-stay, transitional care unit and a rehabilitation center including an adult day health program offering a full schedule of activities for adults needing daytime care and respite to their caregivers.

COSTS

Over the long run, The Mount has found that resident-directed care can be less expensive than the medical model. For the physical remodel, the goal was to keep with minimal capital investment. With the proceeds of a successful capital campaign, The Mount spent approximately $1 million per floor, or $500,000 on each neighborhood. Today, the facility is experiencing improved staff retention rates and employee and resident satisfaction (CORE, 2001), combined with a full census and a wait list for the assisted living apartments, nursing neighborhoods, adult family home and childcare center.

Staffing changes allowed the facility to carry more resident assistants providing direct care to residents and fewer administrative employees. Reducing middle management drastically reduced costs. During the time the remodeling was conducted, the annual consumer price index for the health industry was increasing more than 7 percent each year. When resident charges were raised to a flat rate, The Mount was able to stay in line with the consumer price index increase for general business, which was just 3.5 percent at the time. Generally, the same amount of food is prepared by the central kitchen; but with residents able to choose which foods they want for each meal through fully functioning neighborhood kitchens, far less food is wasted.

Even if the costs of the social or community model had approximately equaled the costs of the medical model, the new model carries a huge advantage: It allows resources to be distributed more directly to the resident. It is customer-service oriented, and provides the option that nearly everyone would choose for his or her own long-term care.

OUTCOMES

According to a 1999 *Christian Science Monitor* article,

> The Mount (after culture change) is the kind of nursing home the U.S. government intended to foster when it passed the 1987 OBRA, which overhauled industry standards. (Kelley, 1999)

In several federal quality-indicator (QI) areas, including pressure ulcers, weight loss and dehydration, The Mount's QI director has seen decreases in negative outcomes (Petitjean, 2002). New systems based on experience with culture change are available for all residents, in a preventive context.

A team of researchers representing a joint effort by the Sisters of Providence and the University of Washington monitored customer satisfaction in the nursing neighborhoods. As a comparison, a typical U.S. nursing home resident spends an average of 25-35 percent of their day engaged in any type of activity. The Mount's measure was 42 percent (see Tables 1 and 2). Additionally, the death curve actually reversed and improved by 83 percent (McNees, 2001).

Neighborhood staff hold quarterly care conferences to discuss the care plan for each resident. Family members are invited to attend these conferences to nurture an environment that encourages communication. Conference participants may include the resident, a primary nurse, resident assistant, spiritual care chaplain, recreation coordinator and the social worker. An annual care

TABLE 1

Providence Mount St. Vincent					
Comparison of Federal Quality Indicators					
Percentages					
1998, 2000 and 2001					
		1st qtr.	1st qtr.	4th qtr.	*Comparison
		1998	2000	2001	Group
Prevalence of falls		21.5	21.3	11.9	16.2
ADL function decline		11.4	10.4	9.6	14.6
(ADL = Activity of Daily Living)					
ROM decline		12.2*	5.1	4.5	9.1
(ROM = Range of Motion)					
Little or no activity		29.8*	29.2	13.8	15.2
Pressure ulcers		7.8*	6.2	4.9	10.1
Incidence of cognitive impairment		3.5	9.4	4.2	12.7
Prevalence of weight loss		18.8	7.3	5	12
		(* denotes 1st qtr. '99)			

*Source for comparison group percentages: 2001 data provided by CMS (the Center for Medicare and Medicaid Services, formerly known as HCFA (Health Care Finance Administration).

conference is scheduled specifically to address any concerns and comments that arise for family members.

Resident council meetings for assisted living apartment residents are coordinated and conducted by the group's elected president and vice president, as written in the by-laws. Each floor elects a representative to serve on the board. A staff member takes minutes. Each nursing neighborhood also conducts resident meetings. The Mount receives some of the most informative feedback through conversations with residents, family, and staff that take place during resident council meetings.

Most successful outcomes with residents are driven by the commitment and satisfaction of staff. The culture change and decentralizing processes have fo-

TABLE 2

Providence Mount St. Vincent Comparison of Selected Quality Indicators (tracked for internal use) 1995 and 2001		Avg. # in 1995	Avg. # in 2001
No toileting plan		52	10
Indwelling catheter		12	1
ADL function decline (ADL = Activity of Daily Living)		82	3
ROM/contractures decline (ROM = Range of Motion)		33	5
Weight loss		20	3
Restraints (body only; does not count side rails)		22	2
Pressure ulcers		11	2

cused administrative leaders on applying the values of a resident-directed model (i.e., dignity, choice, home, privacy and respect) to staff relations as well (Vision, 1994). The Mount works to honor and value workforce diversity and earn the respect of its employees. Decisions are made more locally and, by involving more people in the interview process, more perspectives are taken into consideration for hiring decisions. Real reductions in staff sick leave and turnover have been achieved. In 1992 as the strategic planning process was begun, The Mount's overall turnover rate averaged more than 50 percent. Today, the turnover rate is 22 percent for all positions.

Knowing that every action and attitude of the staff forms the quality of care offered to residents and program participants, The Mount has taken an active role in issues of diversity and the importance of valuing differences among people. The Mount's employees represent 23 different countries of origin. The human resources department has supported the creation of innovative training and development opportunities on-site including a popular Washington state-approved Certified Nursing Assistant program for employees and community members. Materials are translated to languages most common to The

Mount's workforce including Amharic and Tigrigna (East Africa), Tagalog (Filipino) and Spanish. Language courses currently available at The Mount include English as a Second Language and Tagalog.

Staff are involved in committees and workgroups with members representing every position at The Mount to provide input on issues of recruitment and retention as well as cultural diversity. The cultural diversity committee issues a regular newsletter and coordinates special events to celebrate a broad variety of ethnic and religious holidays.

Performance evaluations include input from people who work with and for all staff members so that a full range of perspectives is documented (Ricard, 2001). The HR department conducts an exit interview with each staff member who terminates employment in order to identify and address gaps in employee satisfaction rates. Communications among employees from 23 different countries of origin continues to be a noted gap. Self-directed work teams address issues that former employees have identified as reasons for leaving The Mount. Each year the HR department conducts a salary survey for every position in order to ensure that wages and benefits offered are at or above market. Childcare, wellness and other services available at The Mount are offered at a discounted rate to employees. Scholarships are available for some services including nursing and childcare. An employee assistance program offers free counseling and other crisis services for staff. A tuition reimbursement program helps encourage and provides opportunity for staff to grow professionally.

In a recent Employee Opinion Survey sponsored by the Providence Health System and administered by the System's own Center for Outcomes Research and Education (CORE), The Mount saw significant improvements over 1998 survey results (CORE, 2001). This year, 87 percent of respondents said that they would recommend The Mount as a great place to work. In 1998, that number was just 46 percent. Leaders at The Mount believe that if this survey were administered prior to 1992 and culture change, the results would have been much lower.

The awards noted in Chart 3 summarize the care, environment and innovation of this culture change journey.

RELEVANCE TO SOCIAL WORK PRACTICE, VALUES AND THEORY

Social work as defined by National Association of Social Workers (NASW)

> is the professional activity of helping individuals, groups, or communities to enhance or restore their capacity for social functioning and to create societal conditions favorable to their goals. (NASW, 1973)

CHART 3

PROVIDENCE MOUNT ST. VINCENT

Selected Culture Change Related Awards and Recognition (1996-2001)

- Municipal League of King County, 2001 Civic Awards, "Organization of the Year" for outstanding contributions to the community
- American Association of Homes and Services for the Aging, 1997 Excellence in Practice Award
- Washington Association of Homes for the Aging, 1997 Innovator of the Year Award
- The American Society on Aging and the Brookdale Center on Aging of Hunter College, 1997 Best Practices in Human Resources and Aging
- *Nursing Home Magazine*'s Design '97 Best in Category for Remodeling and/or Renovation Projects
- *Contemporary Long Term Care Magazine*'s 1997 Order of Excellence Awards, Renovation-Architecture Category
- Catholic Health Association, 1996 Achievement Citation, "Innovators in Healing: A Change to Resident-Directed Care"

In effect, The Mount has adopted a model of care very consistent with this social work definition. Culture change at The Mount has made it possible for social workers to work in an environment where the values and theory of their field align with their employer's philosophy and practice of care.

In a medical model, residents are defined by their illness. The focus is on the problem, and the physician is the decision maker. In the traditional nursing home setting, the older adult is deprived of the right to make decisions about even the most rudimentary aspects of daily life. The loss of the ability to affect the outcome has strong potential to produce learned helplessness (Cox and Parsons, 1994).

The Mount's new model of care follows closely the cardinal values of social work–values that are the responsibility of individuals and society: access to resources and opportunities for continued personal and emotional growth; recognition of the needs of the individual person (versus the needs of the group); freedom to enhance independence and self-determination (Hepworth and Larsons, 1993).

The resident-directed model is based on the individual, regardless of his or her needs, with the right to direct his or her care as s/he see fit. The resident is the center (as all clients are in social work practice), his or her needs are assessed and then resources are assessed to meet those needs. The model is based on the principles of choice, dignity, and privacy, with the goal being whatever the resident wishes it to be. "Diagnosis" is not important, and neither are "care needs." What is important is that choices are respected and self-determination is honored. This approach can be taken in such a manner so as not to jeopardize the safety of the resident.

NEXT STEPS

According to the UCLA Center for Policy Research on Aging, Baby Boomers–born between 1946 and 1964–account for a population more than twice the size (75 million) of both previous generations combined and will live until the mid 2030s (Torres-Gil, 2001). This rising tide, and eventual flood, of older Americans during the next 30-plus years is prompting urgent new thinking for leaders beyond the walls of The Mount. Long-term strategies at The Mount are focusing on expanding adult family home services, diversifying the elderly population served by adding an independent living facility and continuing to spread the concepts of culture change through consulting, contracting services and the Pioneer Network.

The Mount has experienced a demand for less costly long-term care options that keep people in their own homes or home-like settings which appears to be much greater than the supply (Boyd, 2001). Another example of The Mount's desire to provide a home-like setting is the development of an adult family home project in 1996. A single family residence, located a few miles from The Mount in a residential neighborhood, was purchased and licensed to provide 24-hour a day care for up to six residents with dementia as an alternative to living in a large institution. Because of the small, secured and supervised living situation, it has proven to be extremely beneficial for individuals who had difficulty with living among a large number of other people. With the help of its Foundation, The Mount has recently purchased additional property to expand its adult family home business. Additionally, The Mount plans to build and run an independent living facility on its existing campus. In the future, residents will include more active, healthy seniors–people in their 70s and 80s who want to live in West Seattle with the security and social benefits of a retirement community.

Through its involvement with the Pioneer Network, The Mount's leaders have been able to spread the word around the country about the success of its culture change process (Williams, 1997). During the past five years, The Mount has served as a resource and learning laboratory for other providers across the country through its Providence Institute, a consulting and training division designed to share the knowledge and lessons learned through the culture change process. Interest and need among consumers, providers and aging-related agencies are swiftly tipping the notion of long-term care culture change onto a scale of social epidemic proportions.

REFERENCES

CORE (Providence Health System Center for Outcomes Research and Education). (2001). Providence Health System Puget Sound Service Area Report, 2001 Employee Opinion Survey. July 19, Contact: Dennis Denfeld, Portland, OR: 503/216-7153.

Contemporary Long Term Care Management Magazine. (1991). 1991 Awards: Mary Conrad Center, Order of Excellence for an innovative approach to urinary continence management and quality control research, December.

Cox, E. and Parsons, R. (1994). *Empowerment-Oriented Social Work Practice with the Elderly.* Pacific Grove, California: Brooks/Cole Publishing Co.

Design for Living. (2000). The Mount's Campaign for Assisted Living Apartment Renovation. Providence Mount St. Vincent Foundation publication.

Fey, David, AIA. (1995). "A Role for Institutional Care? The Nursing Home." *Blueprint for Aging.* Chapter 4: Nursing Facilities. The Center on Aging, Academic Geriatric Resource Program, University of California, Berkeley (proceedings from a two-day conference. June 1-2, 1995. Claremont Resort, Oakland, CA).

Hepworth, D. and Larsons, J. (1993). *Direct Social Work Practice: Theory and Skills.* Pacific Grove, California: Brooks/Cole Publishing Co.

Jennings, Brenda. (2001). Current nurse/neighborhood coordinator at Providence Mount St. Vincent; hired in 1979 as a nursing assistant. Discussion during a meeting of staff who experienced The Mount's culture change. July [unpublished].

Kelley, Tina. (1999). "Pets, kids, and revolution in nursing homes." *The Christian Science Monitor.* May 6. (1999).

King, Marsha. "The pursuit of happiness . . . even in old age." *Seattle Times*, Feb. 21. Local News section, p. 1.

NASW (National Association of Social Workers). (1973). *Standards for social service manpower.* New York: NASW. pp. 4-5.

Ogden, Bob. (2001). Former administrator for Providence Mount St. Vincent and the Mary Conrad Center. Current executive director at Providence Home Care and Hospice of Snohomish County. Discussion during gathering of six members of the Providence Mount St. Vincent 1991 strategic planning team. Onsite at Providence Mount St. Vincent. August [unpublished].

Petitjean, Noel. (2002). Quality Improvement Director at Providence Mount St. Vincent. Member of Providence Mount St. Vincent 1991 strategic planning team. Discussion notes from interview. Onsite at Providence Mount St. Vincent. January [unpublished].

Ricard, Steve. (2001). Providence Mount St. Vince Human Resources Director. Performance evaluation presentation at administrative staff meeting on site at Providence Mount St. Vincent. December [unpublished].

Richardson, Mary PhD. (1997). "Managing for Quality in a Nursing Home: A Resident-Directed Approach." *Health Care Management: State of the Art Reviews.* Philadelphia, Hanley & Belfus, Inc. pp. 31-38. June 1997.

Rimer, Sara. (1998). "Seattle's Elderly Find a Home for Living, Not Dying." *New York Times.* Nov. 22. Late Edition: Final–Section 1, Page 1, Column 1.

Scheer, Kimberly. (2001). Former assistant director and director of nursing services at Providence Mount St. Vincent. Current nursing home administrator at Vashon Community Care Center. Discussion during gathering of six members of the Providence Mount St. Vincent 1991 strategic planning team. Onsite at Providence Mount St. Vincent. August [unpublished].

Torres-Gil, Fernando M. (2001). "The New Aging: Individual and Societal Responses." Opening plenary remarks, Grantmakers in Aging Annual Conference, Denver, CO. Oct. 24, 2001. [unpublished].

Vision, The Mount's. Providence Mount St. Vincent Foundation publication. 1994.

Organizational Culture and Bathing Practice: Ending the Battle in One Facility

Joanne Rader
Joyce Semradek

SUMMARY. This case study describes how, following an experimental study, an Oregon nursing home instituted a new, more effective bathing

Joanne Rader, RN, MN, FAAN, is Associate Professor at Oregon Health and Science University, School of Nursing, and independent consultant and founding member and board member of the Pioneer Network.

Joyce Semradek, RN, MSN, is Professor Emeritus, Oregon Health and Science University.

Address correspondence to: Joanne Rader, RN, MN, FAAN, Oregon Health and Science University, School of Nursing, 514 West Main Street, Silverton, OR 97381 (E-mail: joanne.rader@worldnet.att.net).

The authors would like to thank the following people at Marian Estates whose excellent work is described here: Beth Parker, Brenda Jantz and Laurie Christopherson, CNAs, Donna Bullick, nurse manager, April Diaz, DNS, and Steve Austin, administrator. The authors would also like to acknowledge Beverly Hoeffer and Philip Sloane, the Principal Investigators for the three studies that utilized and tested interventions mentioned in this article, and the members of the interdisciplinary Bathing Project Research Team in Oregon and North Carolina who conducted the studies, including: Ann Louise Barrick, Darlene A. McKenzie and Joyce H. Rasin; Barbara Stewart and Gary Koch; C. Madeline Mitchell, LouAnn M. Rondorf-Klym, and Adele Mattinat Spegman; Charlene Riedel-Leo, Wilaipun Somboontanont, Karen Amann Talerico, Johannah Uriri, and Virapun Wirojratana. Thanks also to the staff, residents and families of the 15 nursing homes who participated in the study.

The specific study referred to in the article, Clinical Trial of Two Bathing Interventions in Dementia, was funded by NINR (RO1 NR 04188).

[Haworth co-indexing entry note]: "Organizational Culture and Bathing Practice: Ending the Battle in One Facility." Rader, Joanne, and Joyce Semradek. Co-published simultaneously in *Journal of Social Work in Long-Term Care* (The Haworth Social Work Practice Press, an imprint of The Haworth Press, Inc.) Vol. 2, No. 3/4, 2003, pp. 269-283; and: *Culture Change in Long-Term Care* (ed: Audrey S. Weiner, and Judah L. Ronch) The Haworth Social Work Practice Press, an imprint of The Haworth Press, Inc., 2003, pp. 269-283. Single or multiple copies of this article are available for a fee from The Haworth Document Delivery Service [1-800-HAWORTH, 9:00 a.m. - 5:00 p.m. (EST). E-mail address: docdelivery@haworthpress.com].

http://www.haworthpress.com/store/product.asp?sku=J181
10.1300/J181v2n03_04

practice for residents with dementia, designed to increase their pleasure and comfort and decrease resistive, self-protective behaviors. Key elements of organizational culture that supported the practice change are examined: creating a shared vision, returning decision-making to residents, empowering caregivers and believing that change is possible. *[Article copies available for a fee from The Haworth Document Delivery Service: 1-800-HAWORTH. E-mail address: <docdelivery@haworthpress.com> Website: <http://www.HaworthPress.com> © 2003 by The Haworth Press, Inc. All rights reserved.]*

KEYWORDS. Bathing, personal care, dementia, aggressive/self-protective behaviors, culture change, Alzheimer's disease, work force issues

INTRODUCTION

In nursing homes throughout the U.S., bathing is often a distressing experience for both residents and caregivers. In most homes it is standard practice to give residents a bath or shower, usually twice a week, even if they verbally protest or physically resist. Most of those protesting residents have dementia (Ryden et al., 1991) and may feel fearful, angry, physically or sexually assaulted by the attempts to provide "good care." As with the use of restraints, which was considered "good care" 15 years ago, more humane approaches to bathing are needed. Such approaches have been evaluated in a series of studies conducted by research teams from North Carolina and Oregon culminating in an experimental study which tested the efficacy of a new approach to reducing resistive, aggressive self-protective behaviors while also maintaining cleanliness (Barrick et al., 2002; Hoeffer et al., 1997; Rader and Barrick, 2000; Rader et al., 1996; Sloane et al., 1995). Despite the enthusiasm of staff who had successfully used the new approaches described in those studies, change in the bathing practices of facility staff not involved in the research was limited. Although the research was not designed to test or demonstrate a change process, it did provide an opportunity to examine the importance of facility culture in the adoption of innovations in practice. This article describes the success of one facility in effectively changing bathing practice beyond the limits of the experimental trials.

TESTING A NEW APPROACH TO BATHING

As background for this case study, it is important to understand certain features of the research. The study was conducted from 1997 to 2001 in 9 facilities in Oregon and 6 in North Carolina. They ranged in size from 81 to 244 beds, and represented a mix of urban, semi-rural and rural facilities as well as proprietary and non-profit auspices. The facilities were randomly assigned to three groups, two experimental and one control. All residents with Alzheimer's disease who had exhibited resistive, self-protective behaviors during bathing were eligible to participate. Two interventions, consisting of an individualized, problem solving approach with either a shower (A) or towel bath (B), were used in each experimental group but were introduced in a different order (AB or BA). The control group received the standard shower experience given in the facilities. Residents' discomfort and disruptive behavior during the bathing procedure, skin condition and bacterial counts were measured during a three-week baseline period and during the last two weeks of each 6-week clinical trial. Agitated, aggressive behaviors and discomfort were coded by blinded raters who viewed digitalized video tapes. Level of discomfort was measured by rating baseline and intervention videotapes using a modification of the Discomfort Scale for Advanced Dementia of the Alzheimer's type (DS-DAT) developed by Hurley et al. (1992). Agitated and aggressive behaviors were evaluated using the Care Recipient Behavior Assessment (CAREBA), a coding system that employs a modification of the definitions found in the Cohen-Mansfield Agitation Inventory (Cohen-Mansfield, 1986). This involves rating baseline and intervention video tapes for the frequency and duration of verbal and physical agitation, as well as for aggression. Skin condition was observed at baseline and at the end of both intervention periods on subjects in the experimental groups using an observational skin assessment form and bacterial counts obtained using skin swabs taken from the axilla and groin areas.

The individualized problem solving approach was introduced to the experimental facilities by the author in the Oregon sites and by a clinical psychologist in North Carolina, each of whom worked with the designated direct caregivers or Certified Nursing Assistants (CNA) in each experimental home. For the first four weeks of each experimental trial they were present in the facilities one or two days a week to assist caregivers in devising ways to reduce resistive, aggressive self-protective behaviors (Talerico and Evans, 2000) and to make the bathing experience as pleasant as possible while keeping each study participant clean. This meant working together, discussing each towel bath or shower, deciding what needed to be changed or adapted and trying out the new individualized plan. Numerous individualized adaptations were tried for each resident in the study within each condition (shower or towel bath), including padding and adapting the shower chairs, keeping people warm and covered, giving a towel bath in bed and offering distractions of food, conversation and objects to hold, depending on the nature and timing of the vocal complaint or resistive behavior. The goal of the new approach was to create a

pleasurable experience for the resident, or at least to decrease distress if pleasure could not be attained. At the conclusion of the study all sites received a facility wide in-service education program on the new approach. (Further details
of the study and interventions can be found in Barrick et al., 2002; Hoeffer et
al., 1997; Rader and Barrick, 2000; Rader et al., 1996; Sloane et al., 1995.)

Following the study, the senior author contacted CNAs at the Oregon sites
who had participated in the research to get an update on practice changes related to bathing. Despite the findings that the new approach successfully decreased resistance, self-protective behaviors and complaints, and increased the
comfort of residents and was practiced enthusiastically by participating caregivers, few of the homes had incorporated the practice changes or had made system-wide improvements. Some facilities continued to use the research-trained
CNAs as bathing experts, referring difficult residents to them, but did not train or
encourage others in use of the new approach. New bathing procedures were not
widely disseminated.

One exception to this tendency was Marian Estates, one of the largest facilities in the study. Though it had staffing ratios and types of residents similar to
those in other facilities, it was able to implement changes in practice to a degree that others did not. Marian Estates, located in rural Oregon, is an independently owned, for-profit, health care campus that includes a 214 bed,
skilled nursing home with three Alzheimer's units. Two of these units took
part in the experimental study. One unit was home to 20 residents with
mid-stage dementia, who were able to identify their own rooms and possessions but required cueing and set up help in order to complete their activities of
daily living (ADLs). The other was home to 30 residents with more advanced
dementia who no longer recognized their rooms or possessions and needed
physical guidance or total assist to complete ADLs. Four residents were included in the study, three from the 30 bed unit and one from the 20 bed unit.
Three CNAs were selected by the facility to participate. One was designated
the primary research CNA; the others were designated for back-up purposes if
the primary CNA was absent or needed additional help and were not consistently part of the study. The primary research CNA was trained to bathe these
residents using the new approach. During the study the new bathing approach
began to be used by other CNAs on the experimental units and following the
completion of the study it became the standard for the remaining units in the
facility. Prior to the study (1999), 100% of the residents on the Alzheimer's
units received at least 1 to 2 showers per week on assigned days as compared
with current reports which indicate that fewer than 25% of the residents still
get in the shower. All residents are currently assessed and consulted to create
individualized bathing care plans. Those who prefer the shower now receive a

shower adapted to their needs. Those who do not like the shower are bathed in a variety of ways in their bed, room or bathroom.

We considered the question of why Marian Estates was uniquely able to adopt the new bathing practice throughout their facility and attempted to identify the facility characteristics that made it relatively easy for the research units to integrate new information into practice and then work to create change in the remaining units. We noted that Marian Estates had key elements needed for successful culture change. Key people held, and were able to create in others:

- a shared vision of how things could be different
- a desire to return locus of control to residents
- a recognition of the importance of empowering the direct caregivers' capacity to be responsive (Lustbader, 2000)
- a belief that change was possible.

Although other Oregon facilities had administrations that generally supported the research interventions, they lacked one or more of these elements, making system-wide change difficult to achieve. The following discussion describes how each of these key elements was critical in creating change at Marian Estates.

A CASE STUDY IN CULTURE CHANGE

A Shared Vision

The research-trained CNA was successful in creating a more pleasant bath or shower experience for the four residents as measured by decreased complaints, fewer resistive, aggressive/self-protective behaviors and more positive comments from residents. Excited by the results, she shared what she learned with other direct care staff and the nurse manager. The enthusiasm grew. Before all phases of the study were completed, the CNAs on the two experimental units, lead by the research CNA and a supportive nurse manager, began revising the bathing care plans on all residents. The CNAs carefully observed residents' reactions and adapted the bathing procedure for each resident. As before, this involved such things as altering the time of day a bath is given, the method used, keeping the person covered and warm during bathing or washing them in bed or while on the toilet. Since CNAs are no longer bound by tradition or experimental protocol to giving a shower, they now bathe most residents with a vegetable oil based, no-rinse soap solution. This might occur in the shower room or the resident's room or bathroom. No problems with skin or odor related to the practice change have been reported to date. In addition, although the general agitation level of the unit was not measured as part of the study, staff described a general lowering of the overall agitation level once they no longer had to "force" residents into the shower.

Culture change, as well as any practice change, requires vision and one or more visionaries to hold steady and lead constant movement toward that vision. These leaders may support, educate and provide consultation to others who are ambivalent about changing, less sure about how to move forward, or feel that they are being "forced" to change. Such leadership existed in Marian Estates at many levels: the administrator, director of nursing, nurse manager/supervisor and direct caregivers (CNAs) all personified the requisite leadership skills.

Although it is crucial for those in administrative and supervisory positions to be visionaries, it was really the direct caregivers' vision of how bathing could be improved that inspired the change at Marian Estates. The CNAs' vision and commitment to change illustrates the existing, often untapped leadership potential of direct caregivers. For example, the research CNA took her success with the four study residents, shared it with other staff and revised how all residents on the two units were assisted with bathing. She also approached the RN who teaches the CNA training class and offered to teach the class on bathing. She has been doing that now for three years.

Returning the Locus of Control to the Resident

One important value in culture change is to keep decision-making very close to the resident (Lustbader, 2000; Misiorski, 2001; Rader and Tornquist, 1995; Williams, 1990, 1999). As Marian Estates implemented the change in practice on the two Alzheimer's units, staff had to shift their perspective from seeing it as "normal" for Mrs. Smith to scream through her shower to recognizing that her resistance meant that they needed to adjust their approach and delay, shorten or stop the bathing. The nurse manager observed that it took from six months to a year for most of the staff, with consistent reinforcement, to be able to make the switch to honoring residents' wishes and creating individualized plans for keeping people clean. Other staff felt that twice weekly showers were necessary, in spite of the residents' protests. The nurse manager and "converted" CNAs had to work with them to show how alternative approaches could meet hygiene needs successfully. Similarly, when facility "float" staff were assigned to the Alzheimer's units, they brought the old standards with them and tried to follow familiar routines. ("It is her shower day so I have to take her into the shower whether she likes it or not.") The regularly assigned unit staff reported this to the nurse manager who assured the "float" staff that a different standard was in place. The nurse manager and the other staff also referred "float" staff to the written bathing care plan or told them to defer the bath until the regular staff person returned.

This resident-directed philosophy was disseminated to other individuals and units when the research CNA (who became the recognized bathing expert in the facility) began teaching bathing techniques in the CNA training class. Thus, new CNAs were oriented to the new culture and clearly understood that the resident had the right to say no and that the staff was expected to be flexible and creative. A telling example of the success of this orientation occurred when a CNA on another unit, with only two months of experience, "reported" a CNA with more than 10 years experience for forcing a person to bathe. The Director of Nursing (DNS) counseled the more experienced caregiver about the changed philosophy and practice and advised her that the former standard was obsolete and unacceptable. The new CNA clearly had embraced the essence of the new culture in which decision-making remained with the resident, and knew that the organizational/administrative structure would uphold caregiver support of resident preferences, the very factors which enabled her to adopt the new bathing approach.

In some study facilities, it was back to business as usual when the study ended as once again residents' wishes and preferences related to bathing generally were ignored. For example, one experimental facility also had the research CNA teach the class on bathing to new CNAs. However, the philosophy that the resident has the right to say "no" has not really taken hold in the facility. The supervising nurses did not perceive forced bathing to be a residents' rights issue. Rather, they felt it was necessary for "good care." Recently at a meeting, a nurse said: "You can't really get people clean with a bed bath." If there is a "problem" person who resists bathing, he or she is referred to the research CNA for care, but the other staff does not believe it necessary to change their approaches. Once new CNAs work with these nurses and unit staff, they fall into the old patterns of showering residents according to an imposed schedule. In contrast, at Marian Estates staff clearly believes that residents retain the right to make decisions about care and that staff have a responsibility to be creative and caring so they can honor residents' wishes and preferences. In this way newly oriented staff find support on the units and the new culture is perpetuated.

EMPOWERING THE DIRECT CAREGIVER

Decision-Making Role of the Direct Caregiver

In the new culture at Marian Estates, direct caregivers have the authority, autonomy and flexibility to decide when and how people are bathed, and in turn are accountable to the resident, family and nurse manager for the quality of care. In practice this means going beyond just accepting the resident's initial refusal to bathe. If a resident says "no," the caregiver is obliged to try a variety of interventions in an attempt to find one with which the resident will agree. If the resident still refuses, the caregiver determines what has to be cleaned for compelling health reasons and does so in the most pleasant, least invasive way. If the decision is made to postpone the bath, the caregiver plans how and when to attempt bathing again and usually implements the plan within 1-2 days. It is never acceptable to simply say, "I asked her and she said no: It's her choice, so there is nothing I can do."

To honor residents' preferences, the caregiver has to adjust how a person is bathed. This requires moment-by-moment decision-making and assessment by caregivers about the best ways to get a person clean. Caregivers may choose from methods which include options such as in-bed and in-room bathing, bathing in the shower using a no-rinse soap, and dividing up the bathing into smaller tasks (Barrick et al., 2002; Rader and Barrick, 2000).

The caregiver also has to be flexible when scheduling baths. The frequency and time of day for baths or showers should be individualized, as it has been on the two Alzheimer's units at Marian Estates. The common, rigid routine of twice-weekly baths or showers is not based on any hard evidence or residents' needs or wishes. Washing the entire body and hair twice a week may be unnecessary. As was mentioned above, many residents at Marian Estates have been kept clean for over two years without getting into a bath or shower. No untoward clinical effects such as skin or odor problems were observed from either reducing the number of baths or eliminating the rinsing and the use of running water.

Caregivers in some of the other study facilities have reported that if they tried to adapt, postpone or shorten bathing, they felt negatively judged by their peers, residents' families and facility supervisors. They reported that their attempts to individualize the bath were sometimes seen as an attempt to get out of work. At Marian Estates, although some of this occurred on the Alzheimer's units during the study and for approximately six months after the study, the majority of the CNAs and families on those units moved beyond this view. Currently, this shift in thinking is in evidence throughout the facility.

Supportive Role of the Supervisor

A direct caregiver in the nursing home cannot continue to be empowered without the consent and active support of a skillful nurse supervisor or manager. This requires a change in the supervisor's role. The old relationship between the nurse and the direct caregivers is reflected in the commonly used title "nursing assistant," which implies that they help the nurse complete her job. This relationship is changing as the licensed nurse moves further away from the bedside because of paperwork and other "hands-off" obligations. More of the decision-making and problem solving is falling to CNAs because they are the ones actually caring for residents.

Despite this shift away from the bedside, many nurses are still supervising CNAs according to a hierarchical model in which they are presumed to know best and which provides them with final decision-making authority, often with little CNA input. In this hierarchical structure, the CNA often feels more responsible to the nurse than to the resident. Too few staff nurses and nurse managers are trained in management skills (Hollinger-Smith et al., 2001) and as they supervise they often resort to what they see or have experienced in the hierarchical management style where communication and decision making flows exclusively from the top down. In addition, too many nurses operate from the perspective of a narrow medical model of care, rather than from a more holistic, biopsychosocial model that recognizes that care is more than medical care (Deutschman, 2001a). Consequently, CNAs often experience nurses as critical, lacking in understanding of residents' needs, and unresponsive to residents' wishes (Deutschman, 2001b).

The model shown in Figure 1 portrays the new culture, and reflects the new relationship between the resident, the nurse and direct care giver. In this model the recipient of care is in the center of the circle. Surrounding that person are the direct caregivers. Those individuals on the outside of the circle, including nurses and social workers, serve those in the middle. Nurses and social workers *assist* the direct care giver in meeting the residents' needs and wishes. They support, rather than simply direct or advise.

This new model was being used as the basis of care giving on the two experimental units at Marian Estates. An enlightened nurse manager, who respected the knowledge and skills of the CNAs, routinely sought direct care giver input and valued their unique contributions and important decision-making role. Because CNAs spent the most time with residents, they sensed when changes were occurring in the residents. The manager listened to and respected their shared information and concerns. She also routinely provided positive feedback and otherwise acted in accordance with the new culture. She encouraged CNAs to decide how best to bathe residents, while also holding them accountable. She supported their requests with administration to assure they could do what they thought was best for the residents. For example, administration initially resisted purchasing a no-rinse soap product and ordered another product. The CNAs tried it, but felt it was inferior. The nurse manager advocated for the new product with administration until the no-rinse product the CNAs initially recommended was ordered. That soap is now a standard product in the facility.

FIGURE 1. At the Center of Good Care

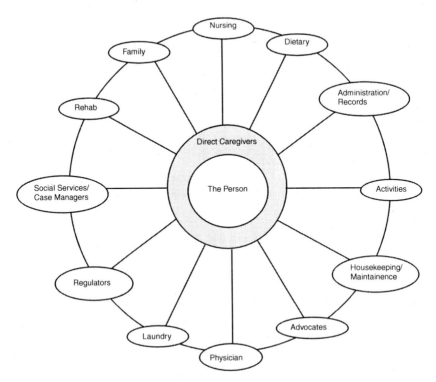

In addition, with this same manager's support and knowledge, the CNA involved in the bathing research began teaching her colleagues what she knew about bathing. At first this occurred informally, in line with the culture of the unit that encouraged team work and sharing useful information about caregiving. With the encouragement of the supervising nurse and DNS, the CNA consulted informally with other units in the facility and spoke to the family support group held at the facility. The nurse manager recognized the special talents and skills of her staff members and supported their professional growth–behavior associated with effective leadership (Hollinger-Smith et al., 2001).

The nurse manager also reinforced the new practice when introducing new families to the facility. When touring prospective families, she explained that the unit had developed alternative ways of maintaining cleanliness. She therefore discussed bathing preferences with prospective residents and families prior to admission and at the first care conference. In addition, she used an open-door style of management that encouraged families as well as staff to seek her help in solving problems.

Supportive Role of Administration

The role of the director of nursing is also crucial. At Marian Estates, the director maintained the vision for new practice standards by working steadily and continually to extend bathing practice changes throughout the facility. Although other nursing units not directly involved with the study had been slower to embrace change related to bathing, facility policies, procedures and forms were rewritten to conform to the new practice. The two units involved in the bath study developed and revised a section on individualized bathing that is being added to all facility care plans to ensure that *how* individuals choose to be bathed becomes part of routine care planning for all residents. The DNS also counseled those who did not change their practice. Recognizing how hard it is for staff to accept that what was previously considered "good care" is now seen in a different light, she remained compassionate but firm. She scheduled opportunities for the research CNA to speak to staff on other units to encourage change. For example, she asked the research CNA to teach an all-staff, mandatory in-service on each shift to describe the new philosophy and techniques related to bathing and also invited her to speak at the nurse managers' monthly meeting to provide information and support.

Although it is no longer acceptable practice in Marian Estates to force someone to bathe, it still happens occasionally, so continual reinforcement and support of the vision are required of administration, nursing supervisors, floor nurses and direct caregivers. Those who have not yet accepted the new bathing practices are generally the nurses and "float" CNAs with many years of experience. They are concerned that alternative methods of bathing are not adequate, and not "the way we have always done it." This attitude also persists in some of the other former study sites, where, without strong administrative commitment to change, the old ways have not been eliminated as has occurred at Marian Estates.

Because the social worker originally assigned to the units involved in the bathing study had left and her position remained vacant for the study period, the social work department at Marian Estates did not have a major role in the practice change. However, as team members they, too, can serve as leaders and visionaries, can influence practice and ask probing questions about resident preferences at care planning conferences, offer suggestions, educate families, share the new philosophy and practice during tours and initial inquiries, and gather information about residents' past and present bathing preferences. In addition, the social workers can help review and revise old policies and procedures that are in conflict with the desired vision. Currently the new social worker at Marian Estates participates in supporting the new practice in her contacts with prospective residents and families, informing them of the innovative and individualized approaches to bathing.

Consistent Assignments vs. Rotation

A common method of staffing used in many nursing homes is to rotate caregivers between groups of residents on a weekly or monthly basis. The underlying rationale is that caregivers need to know all residents. However, rotation does not foster consistency and accountability or promote caring relationships and job satisfaction (Tedros, 1992; Tedros et al., 1993). Many facilities, including Marian Estates, have switched to what is called consistent or permanent assignments in which a CNA on each shift is assigned to care for the same group of people on an open-ended basis (Misiorski, 2001). Although there may be some initial resistance, direct caregivers who have worked under this system generally come to prefer it (Tedros et al., 1993). Marian Estates no longer rotates staff (including activities leaders or housekeepers) between units or groups of residents unless the staff member or resident requests it. The primary CNA provides information by speaking with her colleagues and by writing the bathing care plan so that other caregivers can fill in consistently when needed. The idea is to have as few CNAs as possible providing direct care to each person.

Without consistent or permanent assignments, it is difficult or impossible to build meaningful relationships (Williams, 1999). Having consistent and caring people who know the residents is a part of the culture at Marian Estates that made it possible to institute the new bathing procedures. Consistent assignment is the key to creating individualized care: It enhances the CNA's ability to adjust the time of day, day of week and method of bathing to meet the residents' wishes and changing needs. Being bathed by someone else is a very intimate event, so knowing and trusting that person is a necessary condition for a positive bathing experience. Marian Estates had consistent assignments in place on the two Alzheimer's units prior to the study and now uses this staffing method throughout the facility. Consistent assignments were not used in some of the other study sites whose success in changing bathing practice was more limited.

A BELIEF THAT CHANGE IS POSSIBLE

In order to create change, a change agent must first believe that change is possible. Existing practices are frequently perpetuated by the misperception that they are mandated by federal or state regulations. One such misperception is that the federal nursing home regulations state that residents must bathe or shower twice a week. This is inaccurate. The regulations hold facilities responsible for meeting hygiene needs, but do not specify how it is to be done. Further, using bathing as an example, the State Operations Manual (Health Care Financing Administration, 1999) clearly states the importance of self-determination and accommodation for individual residents' needs. The state surveyors in Oregon had previously been educated about the type of practice changes that were being implemented, and supported the idea of changing the culture to respect residents' rights in general. In fact, some facilities in Oregon had been cited for forcing residents to bathe. Marian Estates, knowing this, felt at ease about the survey process as it related to bathing changes. Having dialogue with regulators prior to implementing systematic change is an essential part of making facility staff feel secure about altering bathing or other practices.

There are many other reasons why facilities and individuals believe change is not possible. Some staff members believe that the corporate culture will not allow it or will not provide necessary resources. Others think that their supervisor or the family might stand in the way of change. Marian Estates took a "can do" attitude towards creating change and worked to overcome obstacles, both perceived and real.

CONCLUSION

Getting research-based best practices into mainstream care is difficult even in facilities that participate in the research process. Following their participation in a study to decrease resistive and self-protective behaviors related to bathing, staff at Marian Estates was able to implement important practice changes, first on the study units and then throughout the facility because they had crucial elements for culture change in place. First, a vision for a new philosophy and practice related to bathing was shared widely by the CNAs, registered nurses, social workers and administration. They all recognized how important it was for decision-making to stay close to the resident, and strove to make that a reality in the daily life of those who lived and worked there. The organizational system on the two study units put the resident-CNA dyad in the center of good care, supported by a nurse manager who respected the decision-making ability of both CNAs and residents. The two units also served as a model for change in the whole facility. Believing that change was needed and possible, administration utilized its expertise to change practice throughout the facility by putting in the policies, providing education, support and equipment needed to create and sustain the desired change. Marian Estates historically had a culture that honored relationships, which allowed the facility staff to operate as a team to create more pleasant bathing experiences for those who live and work there. The state surveyors, having been previously educated about the underlying cultural values and having been informed about this specific practice change, encouraged and supported individualized bathing.

Before practice can be changed and innovative approaches institutionalized, organizational culture must be able to support the changes. To establish individualized care, relationships among staff, residents and family members throughout the facility must reflect a respect for individuals. To ensure that direct caregivers respect residents' rights and listen to their preferences, caregivers must also be respected and their decision making role supported. The actions of all, from direct caregiver to top administrator, must recognize and encourage the contributions that each team member makes in the creation of an environment in which residents can live with dignity and employees work with pleasure. The changed culture also changes the relationship between facility and regulatory agency as both recognize that they are partners striving for the same goal–improved quality of life for those who reside in long-term care settings.

REFERENCES

At the hub of good care. (1999). *Nursing Assistant Monthly*, 5(3), 1.

Barrick, A.L., Rader, J., Hoeffer, B., & Sloane, P. (2002). *Bathing without a battle: Personal care for persons with dementia*. New York: Springer Publishing Company.

Cohen-Mansfield, J. (1986). Agitated behaviors in the elderly ill: Preliminary results in the cognitively deteriorated. *Journal of the American Geriatrics Society*, 34, 722-727.

Deutschman, M. (2001a). Interventions to nurture excellence in the nursing home culture. *Journal of Gerontological Nursing*, 2(8), 37-43.

Deutschman, M. (2001b). Redefining quality and excellence in nursing home culture. *Journal of Gerontological Nursing*, 27(8), 37-43.

Health Care Financing Administration. (1999). State Operations Manual, Interpretive Guidelines, F tag 246.

Hoeffer, B., Rader, J., McKenzie, D., Lavelle, M., & Stewart, B. (1997). Reducing aggressive behavior during bathing cognitively impaired nursing home residents. *Journal of Gerontological Nursing*, 23(5), 16-23.

Hollinger-Smith, L., Ortigara, A., & Lindeman, D. (2001). Developing a comprehensive long-term care workforce initiative. *Alzheimer's Care Quarterly*, 2(3), 33-40.

Hurley, A.C., Volicer, B.J., Hanrahan, P.A., Houde, S. & Volicer, L. (1992). Assessment of discomfort in advanced Alzheimer's patients. *Research in Nursing and Health*, 15, 369-377.

Lustbader, W. (2000). The pioneer challenge: A radical change in the culture of nursing homes. In Noelker, L.S. & Harel, Z. (Eds.), *Qualities of caring: Impact on quality of life*. New York: Springer Publishing Company.

Misiorski, S. (2001). Building a better life: Transforming institutional culture. *Alzheimer's Care Quarterly*, 2(3), 5-9.

Rader, J., & Barrick, A.L. (2000). Ways that work: Redefining the way we meet the needs of persons with dementia during bathing. *Alzheimer's Care Quarterly*, 1(4), 35-49.

Rader, J., Lavelle, M., Hoeffer, B., & McKenzie, D. (1996). Maintaining cleanliness: An individualized approach. *Journal of Gerontological Nursing*, 22(3), 32-38.

Rader, J., & Tornquist, E.J. (1995). *Individualized dementia care: Creative, compassionate, approaches*. New York: Springer Publishing Company.

Ryden, M.B., Bossenmaier, M., & McLachlan, C. (1991). Aggressive behavior in cognitively impaired nursing home residents. *Research in Nursing and Health*, 14(2), 87-95.

Sloane, P., Rader, J., Barrick, A., Hoeffer, B., Dwyer, S., McKenzie, D., Lavelle, M., Buckwalter, K., Arrington, L., & Pruitt, T. (1995). Bathing persons with dementia. *Gerontologist*, 35(5), 672-678.

Talerico, K., & Evans, L. (2000). Making sense of aggressive/protective behaviors in persons with dementia. *Alzheimer 's Care Quarterly*, 1(4), 77-88.

Tedros, N. (1992). Permanent assignment: Key to success. *Long-Term Care Executive Network*, 1(1), 6-7.

Tedros, N., Rice, R., & Krantze, S. (1993). Permanent assignment: Ideal plan for residents and staff. *Brown University Long-Term Care Newsletter*, 5(21), 3-4.

Williams, C. (1999, July). *Relationships: The heart of life and long-term care*. Paper presented at Quality of Care in Nursing Homes: Critical Role of the Nursing Assistant; regional meeting of the American Society on Aging, Philadelphia.

Williams, C. (1990). Long-term care and the human spirit. *Generations*, 14(4), 25-28.

The Power of Circles:
Using a Familiar Technique
to Promote Culture Change

LaVrene Norton

SUMMARY. Social workers can play a pivotal role in bringing about culture change in long-term care, but only if they step out of the narrow confines of case management and client advocacy to use their full spectrum of skills training. By working one-on-one, with groups and with a focus on institutional change, social workers can empower nursing home staff and residents to create a better place in which to live and work. The Learning Circle is a simple and effective methodology social workers can use for achieving these ends. The Learning Circle is a common-sense approach for both conducting meetings and facilitating less formal gatherings in a way that encourages high involvement of all stakeholders in planning and implementing culture change, engenders mutual respect among participants, builds a sense of community and facilitates both personal and organizational transformation. It can be used in all social change

LaVrene Norton, MSW, is the Executive Leader of Action Pact, Inc., a company of consultants specializing in organizational development and committed to culture change in long-term care.

Address correspondence to: LaVrene Norton, 5122 West Washington Boulevard, Milwaukee, WI 53208 (E-mail: lavrene@actionpact.com).

[Haworth co-indexing entry note]: "The Power of Circles: Using a Familiar Technique to Promote Culture Change." Norton, LaVrene. Co-published simultaneously in *Journal of Social Work in Long-Term Care* (The Haworth Social Work Practice Press, an imprint of The Haworth Press, Inc.) Vol. 2, No. 3/4, 2003, pp. 285-292; and: *Culture Change in Long-Term Care* (ed: Audrey S. Weiner, and Judah L. Ronch) The Haworth Social Work Practice Press, an imprint of The Haworth Press, Inc., 2003, pp. 285-292. Single or multiple copies of this article are available for a fee from The Haworth Document Delivery Service [1-800-HAWORTH, 9:00 a.m. - 5:00 p.m. (EST). E-mail address: docdelivery@haworthpress.com].

10.1300/J181v2n03_05

models. This article describes how, where and when to use the Learning Circle. *[Article copies available for a fee from The Haworth Document Delivery Service: 1-800-HAWORTH. E-mail address: <docdelivery@haworthpress.com> Website: <http://www.HaworthPress.com> © 2003 by The Haworth Press, Inc. All rights reserved.]*

KEYWORDS. Learning Circle, culture change, long-term care, social work

INTRODUCTION

Social work pioneer Jane Addams would never have stood for it.

Relegated to finding lost socks when a whole culture needs changing.

Yet such is the dilemma facing many nursing home social workers today. Confined to casework management, resident advocacy and mandatory documentation, they focus on seemingly mundane matters like searching for misplaced clothing and resolving resident and family member complaints. Their advocacy role is itself too limiting, often pits them against other workers, instilling conflict and confusion in the process of serving residents' needs.

Meanwhile, their broader skills, so desperately needed to nurture healthy living environments and meaningful relationships, lie dormant.

Addams undoubtedly would have seen her role in long-term care a little differently than that. Many of the hurdles she helped new immigrants and the urban poor to overcome 100 years ago parallel those for nursing home residents today. That is, the struggle to survive and thrive in strange and often cold, indifferent surroundings.

Addams and her associates established settlement houses to provide social services, educational classes, recreation, workshops, childcare nurseries and theaters in poor neighborhoods where immigrants lived. They not only brought their clientele into the mainstream of society by helping develop the individual skills and abilities of the poor, but also worked to create a sense of community and change in the environment in which they were living (Addams, 1910).

Today's culture change movement has similar objectives in moving the long-term care environment from a medical to a social model of care giving. Barry Barkan's Regenerative Community, Providence Mount St. Vincent's Resident-Directed Care, Lyngblomsten's Swedish-style service house, The Eden Alternative–these and other leading culture change models strive to build community and create a home-like environment, enable greater self-determination and personal growth for residents and create a warm, satisfying workplace for employees (Barkan, 1995, 2001; Kelly, 1999; Thomas, 1998; see also related articles in this volume).

Social workers in long-term care can help achieve these culture change objectives by extending their advocacy role and using their full spectrum of skills and training in working one-on-one, in groups and with a focus on total change within the institution. An effective yet simple methodology they can use toward these ends is the Learning Circle.

LEARNING CIRCLE STIMULATES HIGH INVOLVEMENT IN CULTURE CHANGE

Action Pact, a consulting group that assists long-term care providers in planning and implementing culture change, began experimenting about 15 years ago with what since has evolved into the Learning Circle. The purpose was to devise a technique for involving all nursing home stakeholders–staff, residents, family and community members–in planning, solving problems and creating new relationships during the culture change transition.

High involvement by all is critical to any deep, institutional change endeavor. "Put everybody in the company to work to accomplish the transformation," urges noted industrial quality improvement consultant, Deming (1986). In related fashion the founder of The Eden Alternative stresses that it is imperative that all staff members be involved in creating a vision of how the Eden principles can be implemented (Thomas, 1998).

The Learning Circle is a natural and powerful form in which everyone involved in the nursing home–even residents with severe cognitive losses–can meet, find common ground and take part in the culture change process. When the Learning Circle's techniques are used successfully, mutual respect among the participants is engendered–a vital element in creating a healthy culture.

The Learning Circle has been used to stimulate high involvement and mutual respect in all phases of culture change, from initial planning to final implementation and evaluation, no matter what particular culture change model the nursing home chooses to follow.

Though no data currently exist on its usefulness, anecdotal evidence abounds. At the Meadowlark Hills Retirement Community in Manhattan, KS, for example, residents and staff in each of their five small nursing home households use the Learning Circle daily to connect with each other, address concerns and work through problems.

At White Community Hospital in Aurora, MN, Learning Circles are used between departments to strengthen relationships.

At Meadowood in Worcester, PA, Learning Circles are part of the education and in-servicing the organization uses to develop new skills during their culture change.

Northern Pines Community in Big Fork, MN, uses Learning Circles to give residents more control over their daily activities. Twice daily, residents, including those living with dementia, meet with staff and available family members to determine the day's activities.

THE POWER OF CIRCLES

For millennia, circles have held great spiritual, symbolic and practical significance across diverse cultures and religions, and have been a common means of congregating. The great boulders of Stonehenge silently stand in circles. The legendary King Arthur and his knights sat in a circle to ensure all were equal (Author, 2000). In kindergarten and the United Nations, we sit in circles. Indeed, the world goes around in circles.

As the daughter of a Quaker, Addams would have been familiar with the process typical of Friends worship meetings where participants face each other in a circle, listen and speak from the heart as the Spirit moves them (Addams, 1910; Weening, 1995).

Similarly, the Learning Circle is a leveling technique that encourages quiet people to speak, talkative people to listen and everyone to share in making decisions. Here, everyone is heard as equals.

While on the surface, the Learning Circle is simply a common sense technique for conducting meetings, there are subtle, underlying forces at work that yield results. Sitting face to face in a Learning Circle, especially with people one knows, is itself a powerful learning stimulus.

McCarthy (1998) notes,

> there is something special and fascinating about face perception . . . (which) ties together sensation, recognition, emotion, and memory in different areas of the brain within 200 milliseconds.

Both the verbal and nonverbal sides of the brain are activated when one looks at famous or familiar faces, whereas an unfamiliar face activates only the brain's nonverbal side. One remembers better when there are two (the verbal and nonverbal) ways to get the information into memory (Petersen, 1998).

The Learning Circle also facilitates learning in other ways. Participants observe, interpret and experience not only their own feelings about an issue, but broaden their own perspectives by learning and considering the many other viewpoints around them. Learning Circles encourage and support "inner" shifts in its participants' values, aspirations and behaviors. These inner shifts are as vital as are "outer" shifts in processes, strategies, practices and systems in bringing about profound change in an organization (Senge et al., 1999). As perspectives broaden and inner shifts occur, the individual dynamics of the circle levels out and the group's insight becomes more balanced. A common understanding develops and together everyone can move forward on a plan of action.

THE TECHNIQUE

Participants sit in a circle without tables or other obstructions blocking their view of one another. They may include workers, residents, family and community members or any combination thereof, depending on the purpose of the circle. For example, in trying to build support for undertaking culture change in a nursing home, Learning Circle participants ideally would include all of the above. If the circle's purpose is to resolve conflicts within a particular work team or resident neighborhood, only those involved in that team or neighborhood would participate.

One person is chosen as a facilitator to pose a question to members of the circle, give encouragement and keep the responses moving in an orderly fashion.

The social worker or group leader need not always be the circle facilitator or coordinator. In fact, Learning Circles are most effective when they become a way of life in the nursing home and everyone takes turns facilitating. Social workers can support this by introducing and teaching the usefulness of Learning Circles in a myriad of situations (see below, "When to Use Learning Circles").

The ideal number of circle participants is 10-15. If there are more than 20, the need to limit discussion becomes inevitable.

If the facilitator believes a question will elicit strong feelings of sadness, depression, grief or anger, it is helpful to limit the number of participants to 5-10 and keep them apprised of the time allotted for the circle so they may adjust themselves emotionally. Spontaneous support for respondents such as touch or affirming words is allowed and, indeed, encouraged.

The process begins when the facilitator poses a question or issue. If, for example, the purpose of the Learning Circle is to begin the initial planning phase for culture change, the questions might include: *What is one thing that holds us back? What does "home" mean to you? What would you want for your mother if she were in a nursing home?*

If a universally negative response to a question is predicted, the facilitator might consider shaping the question into two parts. For example: *"Share one thing that worries you and one thing that excites you about culture change."*

A volunteer in the circle responds with his/her thoughts on the chosen topic. The person sitting to the right or left of the first respondent goes next, followed one-by-one around the circle until everyone has spoken on the subject without interruption.

The facilitator prohibits all cross talking during this process. Involuntary laughter and words of empathy are allowed, but others may not add their thoughts or opinions on an issue until it is their turn to speak.

One may choose to pass rather than speak when his/her turn comes. But after everyone else in the circle has had their turn, the facilitator goes back to those who passed and allows each another opportunity to respond. Of course, no one is forced to speak, but there is an expectation that they will. Usually, they do respond with gentle encouragement from the facilitator. Conversely, the facilitator may need to prompt the talkative to be silent and listen while others take their turn.

Only after everyone has a chance to speak is the floor open for general discussion. The main goal of the Learning Circle is merely to ensure everyone's perspective is shared and equally respected. The actual disposition of issues raised in the Learning Circle may be decided by the circle participants, or be resolved through the nursing home's established procedures.

WHEN TO USE THE LEARNING CIRCLE

The Learning Circle is appropriate for practically any gathering–including family nights, open house, inservice trainings, problem-solving and staff meetings–whether or not it is related to an organization's culture change journey. For example, a training session for CNAs about safety issues could begin or end with a Learning Circle in which each CNA is asked to share a concern about safety or "an accident waiting to happen."

Learning Circles may be ongoing, regular meetings of the same participants, or spontaneously organized on an ad hoc basis to deal with a specific issue.

They can be used to strengthen bonds and create a sense of equality between staff and residents so necessary to culture change. Relationships between caregivers and care recipients often are unbalanced, with caregivers playing the dominant role as they hover over the bed or wheelchair bound elders. Everyone who has been injured and had to rely on others to be fed, bathed and dressed knows that helplessness diminishes self-esteem. By meeting daily or weekly in the Learning Circle where everyone is heard and treated with dignity, staff and residents ultimately begin to feel that they all are in this together, working to create an enjoyable world in which to live, work and grow.

Learning Circles at staff meetings can heal minor irritations before they become ulcerating sores. Staff scheduling and the hectic pace of nursing homes often stifle meaningful communication between workers. As a result, many problems never get properly addressed and tensions escalate. Learning Circles help let off steam and promote better understanding before that happens.

Take the case of the outdated sugar packets.

The first shift of dietary workers felt bitter toward workers in the second shift because the latter never bothered to replenish the sugar packet containers in the dining hall. Every morning, the first shift grumbled because they had to refill all the containers due to the second shift's apparent laziness.

It wasn't until the two groups sat together in the staff Learning Circle that the problem was aired and an explanation was forthcoming. As it turns out, the second shift had a good reason for not filling the containers. When they are constantly full, they explained, packets at the bottom never get used and become stale. Thus, a broader understanding and a sweeter disposition between the two shifts evolved.

By introducing the Learning Circle in situations such as these, social workers can help effect culture change at many different levels within the nursing home. Ultimately, workers, residents and family members will begin to listen to each more closely. Respect and sense of community will begin to grow and different possibilities will be discovered for working together to move the environment toward person-centered care.

Helping bring that about is the appropriate occupation for nursing home social workers. Much like Jane Addams and her colleagues enabled the urban poor to take control of their lives in the new, industrialized society around them, social workers today can use Learning Circles to empower staff and residents to create a better life for themselves in long-term care.

It means stepping out of the narrow confines of one-on-one case management and sock searches to reclaim their true purpose in social work. No doubt, Addams would approve.

REFERENCES

Addams, Jane. (1910). *Twenty Years at Hull-House.* New York: Signet Classic.
Barkan, Barry. (1995). The Regenerative Community: The Live Oak Living Center and the Quest for Autonomy, Self-Esteem and Connection in Elder Care. In L. Gamroth, J. Semradek & E.M. Tornquist, *Enhancing Autonomy in Long-Term Care: Concepts and Strategies* (pp. 169-192). Springer.

Barkan, Barry. (2001). Looking for the Candy Store. In *Olam Magazine,* Issue 4, (www.Olam.org/magazine).

Deming, W. Edwards. (1986). Fourteen points for management. In *Out of Crisis* (pp. 23-24); Potomac, MD: The W. Edwards Deming Institute.

Kelly, Tina. (May 6, 1999). Pets, kids and revolution in nursing homes. *Christian Science Monitor.*

King Arthur's Round Table (2000). In Microsoft Encarta Encyclopedia.

McCarthy, Gregory. (1998). Press release, Duke University Medical Center, Feb. 16, 1998.

Petersen, Steven E. (1998). Press release, Washington University School of Medicine, Nov. 10, 1998.

Senge, Peter; Kleiner, Art; Roberts, Charlotte; Ross, Richard; Roth, George & Smith, Bryan. (1999). *The Dance of Change: The Challenges to Sustaining Momentum in Learning Organizations.* New York, NY; Doubleday.

Thomas, William H. (1998). *Open Hearts, Open Minds.* Summerhill, NY: Van Wyk & Burnham Publishers.

Weening, Hans. (1995). *Meeting the Spirit: An introduction to Quaker beliefs and practices.* Religious Society of Friends (www.quaker.org).

SECTION 4
CASE STUDIES:
CULTURE CHANGE BRIEFS

Introduction to Case Studies:
Culture Change Briefs

Judah L. Ronch

This section has been included to share important and illustrative "works in progress." They allow us to include for the reader some of the practical issues that innovators have faced in their culture change projects. In addition, these authors have had a primary focus on changing service models absent a formal research orientation that has precluded them from collecting data of the kind that typically would be included in professional journals. Their stories of culture change are, however, most instructive and should help readers understand how different visions of culture change are being realized in various environments. In some cases, their data sets are in preliminary form or are still too small to yield results that meet standard tests of statistical significance. Nonetheless, their experiences constitute valuable case studies in actual culture change that we believe add helpful insights for the initiatives to come in long-term care settings of the future.

[Haworth co-indexing entry note]: "Introduction to Case Studies: Culture Change Briefs." Ronch, Judah L. Co-published simultaneously in *Journal of Social Work in Long-Term Care* (The Haworth Social Work Practice Press, an imprint of The Haworth Press, Inc.) Vol. 2, No. 3/4, 2003, pp. 293-294; and: *Culture Change in Long-Term Care* (ed: Audrey S. Weiner, and Judah L. Ronch) The Haworth Social Work Practice Press, an imprint of The Haworth Press, Inc., 2003, pp. 293-294. Single or multiple copies of this article are available for a fee from The Haworth Document Delivery Service [1-800-HAWORTH, 9:00 a.m. - 5:00 p.m. (EST). E-mail address: docdelivery@haworthpress.com].

Each Case Study Brief is organized so that readers may gain an overview of the facility/system leading the change, why culture change was initiated, what their vision was, how they went about their process of culture change, lessons they have learned and next steps. Interested readers may contact the authors to gain more detailed information about each project's history and current status. We hope that this section will encourage dialogue between readers wishing to initiate or modify their own culture change programs and the authors represented in this section (and the rest of this volume as well). We also encourage readers to submit Culture Change Briefs for future publications that follow the formatting of the contributions in this section.

Apple Health Care:
Culture Change
in a Privately Owned Nursing Home Chain

Allison Hagy

SUMMARY. The future of long-term care in America is uncertain. As the population ages, it is becoming more apparent that the needs and desires of our elders are changing. Culture Change is an initiative that will provide the individualized care and meaningful interactions that residents, families and staff desire. Apple Health Care, a for-profit provider of skilled nursing services based in Avon, Connecticut, embraced culture change in 1997 and has felt the positive impact of the gradual transition from a medical to a more social model of care in each of its 21 homes. This brief provides a perspective of how to begin the journey from the vantage points of service, care, quality and the for-profit sector. *[Article copies available for a fee from The Haworth Document Delivery Service: 1-800-HAWORTH. E-mail address: <docdelivery@haworthpress.com> Website: <http://www.HaworthPress.com> © 2003 by The Haworth Press, Inc. All rights reserved.]*

KEYWORDS. Nursing home, skilled nursing facility, long-term care, culture change

---

Allison Hagy is the Director of Marketing at Apple Health Care.

Address correspondence to: Allison Hagy, 21 Waterville Road, Avon, CT 06001 (E-mail: ahagy@applehealthcare.com).

[Haworth co-indexing entry note]: "Apple Health Care: Culture Change in a Privately Owned Nursing Home Chain." Hagy, Allison. Co-published simultaneously in *Journal of Social Work in Long-Term Care* (The Haworth Social Work Practice Press, an imprint of The Haworth Press, Inc.) Vol. 2, No. 3/4, 2003, pp. 295-299; and: *Culture Change in Long-Term Care* (ed: Audrey S. Weiner, and Judah L. Ronch) The Haworth Social Work Practice Press, an imprint of The Haworth Press, Inc., 2003, pp. 295-299. Single or multiple copies of this article are available for a fee from The Haworth Document Delivery Service [1-800-HAWORTH, 9:00 a.m. - 5:00 p.m. (EST). E-mail address: docdelivery@haworthpress.com].

http://www.haworthpress.com/store/product.asp?sku=J181
© 2003 by The Haworth Press, Inc. All rights reserved.
10.1300/J181v2n03_07

SYSTEM OVERVIEW

Apple Health Care, Inc. is a privately owned provider of skilled nursing, short-term rehabilitation, respite care, hospice and specialty Alzheimer's and related disorders services comprised of 21 homes in Connecticut, Massachusetts and Rhode Island. Like most providers, quality of care has always been the focus of Apple's mission. In recent years though, the organization's management has become interested in incorporating the progressive approaches known as "culture change" into a mission it could use as its guiding focus. While Apple has been especially interested in adapting the work of the Pioneer Network (see Fagan, this volume) as the basis for these activities, a number of other approaches also served as models for Apple's culture change program, including the Eden Alternative (see Thomas, this volume). To prevent a single, corporate approach from being imposed, an overall corporate philosophy and approach, called "Better Life," was developed and individually expressed in all of Apple's nursing homes.

THE "WHAT" OF CULTURE CHANGE

In order to create nursing homes where people were proud to live and to work, it was decided that Apple's facilities had to move away from the medical model and toward a more social model of care. This direction allowed Apple to work toward its desired outcome–to create a system that honored resident choice. This direction was a continuation of previous Apple initiatives directed toward greater choices and more resident/staff input about aspects of their experiences at Apple that could improve quality of life.

The first step was to identify what was lacking at each of the facilities. It was clear that each home was essentially a traditionally medical model environment that made the public cautious. Although warm and friendly, they were not as "home-like" as possible, and were essentially places in which residents had to give up dignity, choice, privacy, and sense of self in exchange for care. The focus of change was thus identified: how to create a more "home-like" environment and to identify the defining elements that make a place to live a "home." Specifically, the goal was to create environments that Apple's leaders and managers would themselves want to occupy and to identify ways to make choices–about eating, bathing and activities–that they would value as intrinsic parts of the culture.

It was evident from staff meetings, focus groups, and employee satisfaction surveys that the people who worked at Apple facilities wanted more educational opportunities, less use of pool staff, more freedom to spend "down time" with residents and more time to grieve for residents who had passed away. Out of these discussions new priorities emerged, which included educational scholarships, an in-house staffing pool company, and ways to improve relationships between residents and staff. As Apple had also become aware of how frightening it was for children of families and staff to visit a typical nursing home, play areas were built in each of the common rooms in the 21 homes. The level of resident and family involvement in care planning was also enhanced, with special emphasis given to individually monitoring each resident's progress as the "I-Format" care plan was implemented.

The organization's hope when embarking on the culture change journey was that it would center on changing the psychosocial environments, i.e., creating relationships and communities, rather than on changing the physical environments of each home. If relationships were to change, it was assumed that the dollar costs of culture change would be minimized and thus manageable. In the end, the actual financial costs were not prohibitive. Still, there were aspects of the physical environment that were too costly to change, though this might have been preferred. There would still be nursing stations, long hallways, linen closets, medication rooms, and dining rooms in each facility. It therefore became even more important that the culture change program could alter the relationships that existed within the physical environments. If successfully achieved, this change could modulate the undesirable impact of the physical spaces without tearing down walls.

In order to make the culture change program immediate and real for staff, the change leadership at Apple held regional meetings with them to explore the important features that would add to the "home-like" nature of their settings. A slide show was presented that illustrated various aspects of actual environments at Apple facilities. Staff was surveyed about how much they would enjoy living in an environment that featured these desirable and undesirable attributes of an ideal setting, such as lounges filled with wheelchairs and other adaptive equipment, nourishment stations with signs warning about germs, nourishment carts in hallways and cold, sterile bathrooms. Many of those present were shocked that they had walked past those elements on a daily basis for years without a second thought.

The impact of these meetings and the slide show was that staff immediately initiated simple changes to the environment. Staff redecorated dining rooms, placed bird feeders outside of residents' windows, created toy boxes filled with children's toys and games in common rooms and started discussions about having a facility pet. Changes were suggested and facilitated by residents, staff and facility management, marking the first unified work among all three groups in many of the facilities. These changes were possible because the culture change leadership had empowered staff to make changes as they saw fit without having to develop a protocol on paper and waiting for approval. Whatever the change–whether changing the contents of snack carts to items the residents wanted and had enjoyed in the community, initiating a CareerPath program for CNAs, starting community meetings of residents and staff, experimenting with universal worker roles or neighborhood dining–each facility functioned as a self-directed, empowered community.

LESSONS LEARNED

1. *The greatest challenge was to achieve changes in relationships.* If a CNA is seen chatting with a resident, her behavior is recognized as a positive interaction where previously it would have been an occasion for negative feedback and termed "unproductive." Many hands-on staff saw this as a change toward the social model that was rooted in common sense and something they had done everyday when at work. For supervisors and managers buried under the burdens of regulation and paper work, behavior such as this was initially seen as potentially detrimental to good regulatory review. As many of the desired changes in relationships has been modeled by the management of each facility, supervisors and managers are slowly changing the way they view the value of relationships as part of what makes the new culture better.

2. *The financial costs for all the changes were minimal and folded into operating costs.* In the end, all of the changes have had a positive impact on peoples' lives that live and work in Apple's homes and have been worth the minor expense. Increased costs, such as the costs of the expanded choice of foods on the snack carts, the bonuses awarded to the CNAs who completed the CareerPath program and the cost of additional special equipment like gliders, rocking chairs, and raised gardening beds were minimal and strongly supported by leadership.

3. *Successful culture change of this type requires that the organizational structure of the typical nursing home be flattened.* A structure to support culture change in each facility called a "Better Life Committee" has begun to address the central question in operating the home: What can be done to make the home a more enjoyable place in which to live and work? This local control has expedited the process of culture change, and has pointed to an alternate model of facility management for the future.

4. *The positive response to the culture change from residents and families has been the greatest reward of the culture change initiative.* The traditionally high number of positive and enthusiastic letters received at Apple corporate offices has grown significantly. A resounding theme in most of them is the feeling that Apple residents and their families feel that they are staying in an environment that is as close to home as possi-

ble. Traditionally high occupancy rates have improved to even higher levels. Many residents who lived at an Apple facility for short-term rehabilitation have asked, since the culture change initiative was begun, to return to the facility for long-term care. Hospital discharge planners recognize the many benefits of the culture change at Apple homes and are now more likely to refer patients to them.

5. *The survey process remains a challenge.* Since the surveys conducted by State surveillance organizations monitor a medical model of care, Apple involved the State at each step of its culture change process to ensure that there would not be any surprises when they were surveyed. Ultimately, the regulatory organizations and Apple were able to learn and grow together throughout the culture change process. Some surveyors have told Apple that they have started to expect some of Apple's initiatives to begin happening at homes outside the Apple network, which truly indicates the unexpected breadth of Apple's impact on nursing home culture change.

6. *The media have begun to feature positive stories about nursing homes.* Local, regional and national media, which used to cover only labor unrest or poor quality care, have told the story of Apple's culture change.

7. *Culture change is associated with lower turnover rates.* Apple's annual staff turnover rate is between 30 and 40%, as compared with national rates as high as 70%. Employees report higher job satisfaction since the culture change initiative began.

NEXT STEPS

Apple is planning to select one of its facilities that is most deeply entrenched in a medical model of culture and investigate how a neighborhood model of care can best be introduced. Apple also plans to initiate a program of continuing education about what the journey of culture change is and how to begin it at a local level. Though Apple's success with culture change essentially defines the company's competitive edge, corporate leadership believes that this is a resource to be shared in order to change the face of nursing home care on a national level.

Case Study Brief:
The Lyngblomsten Care Center,
St. Paul, MN

Paul Mikelson
Jane Johnson

SUMMARY. Concluding that the medical model nursing home is going to disappear, a Minnesota organization has created a new residential setting for dependent elderly while retaining nursing home licensure and certification. Based on the "service house" system currently used in Sweden, this model has a focus on autonomy and self determination by maintaining the aspects of daily life that are important to every individual. Residents have full apartments and have their own food for breakfast and supper, breaking the age-old facility problem, where mealtimes dic-

---

Paul Mikelson is the President and CEO of Lyngblomsten, a Lutheran related social ministry agency providing housing and services to the elderly in St. Paul, MN. He has a BA in Chemistry from Augsburg College in Minneapolis and an MA in Environmental Health from the University of Minnesota and is a licensed Nursing Home Administrator.

Jane Johnson, LSW, is Admission Social Worker for Lyngblomsten Care Center. She has a BA in Social Welfare from the University of Minnesota, and has worked in various settings as a medical social worker for over 20 years.

Address correspondence to: Paul Mikelson, President and CEO, Lyngblomsten, 1415 Almond Avenue, St. Paul, MN 55108 (E-mail: pmikelson@lyngblomsten.com).

[Haworth co-indexing entry note]: "Case Study Brief: The Lyngblomsten Care Center, St. Paul, MN." Mikelson, Paul, and Jane Johnson. Co-published simultaneously in *Journal of Social Work in Long-Term Care* (The Haworth Social Work Practice Press, an imprint of The Haworth Press, Inc.) Vol. 2, No. 3/4, 2003, pp. 301-306; and: *Culture Change in Long-Term Care* (ed: Audrey S. Weiner, and Judah L. Ronch) The Haworth Social Work Practice Press, an imprint of The Haworth Press, Inc., 2003, pp. 301-306. Single or multiple copies of this article are available for a fee from The Haworth Document Delivery Service [1-800-HAWORTH, 9:00 a.m. - 5:00 p.m. (EST). E-mail address: docdelivery@haworthpress.com].

10.1300/J181v2n03_08

tate your daily routine. Staff act as generalists, which allows greatly improved service with higher staff to client ratios. *[Article copies available for a fee from The Haworth Document Delivery Service: 1-800-HAWORTH. E-mail address: <docdelivery@haworthpress.com> Website: <http://www.HaworthPress.com> © 2003 by The Haworth Press, Inc. All rights reserved.]*

KEYWORDS. Service house, Sweden, autonomy, social model

The Lyngblomsten Care Center was established in 1906 by a group of Norwegian women concerned about the care of the elderly. What began as a 30-bed home was expanded in 1962 and again in 1976 so that it now has 256 skilled nursing beds in two connected buildings. Residents live in private or semi-private rooms with half baths and eat meals in congregate dining rooms.

Contrary to the intent of the acute care medical model that guides procedural and State and Federal regulatory oversight of such settings, short or medium range stays for care and discharge are not the typical experience for 98% of Lyngblomsten's residents. Residents admitted to The Lyngblomsten Care Center come to live out the rest of their lives, not to be "cured" of the infirmities of old age (which of course cannot be done).

WHY CHANGE?

The leadership of The Lyngblomsten Care Center concluded that the medical model nursing home itself had a limited lifespan; that it would succumb to the pressures of poor fiscal performance, workforce shortages, over-regulation and consumer dissatisfaction. The popularity of Assisted Living and other residential options among the elderly and their families adds support to this view. The planning dilemma involved envisioning what would replace the nursing home as we knew it.

The answer began to emerge in 1993 when a group of Swedish colleagues visited Lyngblomsten and described the Swedish Service House model. Their reaction to the medical model setting was: "That's the way we used to do things in Sweden 20 years ago." In response to our shock at this observation, an employee exchange program was established with a Service House in Rottne, Sweden and Lyngblomsten in which two employees from each cooperating facility would spend four weeks at each other's site. Over the course of the next seven years, Lyngblomsten leadership and staff set about to learn about the Service House system to guide their conversion of their American nursing home to a version of the Swedish model.

THE WHAT–
THE SERVICE HOUSE MODEL
AND ITS APPLICATION AT LYNGBLOMSTEN

The Swedish Federal Government requires each municipality to be responsible for housing and services to the aged and handicapped. Services are organized to do everything possible to keep people in their own homes and, when a move to a congregate care setting is needed, to ensure that the setting is as home like as possible. This was a sharp contrast to the service at Lyngblomsten, which was more like a hospital than anyone's home. Each Service House has full apartments, not semi-private rooms, each with a full bath. Unlike the nursing home, there are no nurse's stations or soiled utility rooms.

Care in Sweden is based on a social model, and thus consonant with values that are basic to social workers. The essential focus of care is on increasing autonomy and self-determination by providing options for residents' daily lives. So, for example, residents schedule their daily activity; waking times, eating and bathing are based on resident preferences and may vary from day to day. Activities take place according to resident plans. Residents, who make shopping lists for family members or volunteers, plan morning and evening meals. Residents are encouraged to set the table, help with laundry and perform other daily functions for themselves.

In Sweden, staff are well trained and are expected to function as generalist-direct care providers who perform both home visits and help in residential settings. They are relatively unencumbered by paper work!

Such a model, based as it was on autonomy, privacy, normalcy and dignity of the older person, was attractive in philosophical and practical ways. It was (ideally) a model without layers of bureaucracy and unnecessary regulations and paperwork, one that eliminated departments and the consequent turf issues that arose in medical model care; teamwork and collegiality were core values. The Service House model appeared to function with fewer staff members than the Lyngblomsten nursing home. This was envisioned as a way to support higher wages and ultimately lower turnover at Lyngblomsten.

HOW IT WAS ACHIEVED

In order to develop a demonstration project, pilot version of the Service House at Lyngblomsten and maintain its license as a skilled nursing facility, it was necessary to apply to the Minnesota Department of Health for 69 waivers from state regulations. Fifty-four of these were granted, enough to proceed. An architect from Sweden who was familiar with the type of conversion process was hired and a plan was developed that eliminated 15 private rooms and created nine Service House apartments. Each one was designed for single occupancy and features a small kitchenette, a full bath with shower and a studio type bedroom/living room.

The physical remodeling was done over three months in the Summer of 1997 and cost about $500,000. Nine residents, three from each of the case mix segments (high, medium and low) were selected to occupy the new apartments. Residents who were selected to move to the new Service House were very pleased to shed the regimented daily routine and hectic pace of the nursing home for the freedom and privacy of the Service House. Residents who were not selected to move remained on a waiting list to patiently await their turn to experience the Service House. An independent post occupancy study was performed by a faculty member at the University of Minnesota, supported by funds from a grant from The Retirement Research Foundation (Grant, 2001a; 2001b; 2000). Finally, twelve Licensed Practical Nurses were hired and trained to work in the new House. Following the Swedish generalist model of care, they performed all nursing and support functions that residents needed on a daily basis, including personal care, administering medication and medical treatments, cooking, cleaning, laundry, and social activities, among others. The Lyngblomsten Service House opened on October 1, 1997.

LESSONS LEARNED

1. *Improved resident and family satisfaction were achieved.* Anecdotal results indicate that residents of the Service House had much higher levels of satisfaction than did residents of the traditional medical model nursing home. Resident turnover was lower than in the nursing home, with two residents leaving the pilot program (one died and one developed dementia with a level of severity such that she could no longer participate in the study). Residents and family members indicated that the new setting was much more home like and that they felt more valued as individuals. Residents expressed an increased feeling of responsibility for their own lives; even residents with severe physical limitations enjoyed the increased mental and physical autonomy. Since the model eliminated the hierarchical relationships seen in traditional medical settings, residents, family members and staff were able to act as truly equal partners in care. Staff developed a deeper level of emotional attachment to resi-

dents, prompting residents to say that they felt more as though they were being cared for by members of their own family.

2. *The workload is heavier and staff had responsibilities that are more diverse.* Use of generalist staff makes the workload significantly harder and more physically demanding. Since the Service House is staffed primarily with Care Assistants, most of whom are LPNs, resources can be devoted to direct care staff with an improved resident to client ratio over the nursing home. There are currently 2.5 FTE of LPNs on the day shift, 2.0 FTE on evenings and 1.0 at night. In addition, there is a 10 hour per week Registered Nurse who performs the MDS assessments, coordinates care planning and delegates/trains staff for care related tasks. The Service House Coordinator is employed part time to interview, hire and schedule staff, and supervises the operation of the House. Staff turnover was 50% among the Care Assistants during the two years of the demonstration project, though most of the entire staff complement stayed for the entire two years of the project. The major complaints from the Care Assistants who left were that the work was too physical or that the generalist nature of the position, with no clear delineation of responsibilities, was a problem. Staff now includes Trained Medication Aides, which in Minnesota is a Certified Nursing Assistant with additional education in administering medication, as well as LPNs. Staff retention remains a challenge due to economic difficulties and high turnover rates.

3. *It is not yet less expensive than a nursing home to operate.* For the first two years, expenses exceeded revenues by 25%. While the project was premised on the theory that the simplified, flatter organizational structure would allow the funding of higher staffing ratios using LPNs as caregivers and still be about 90% of comparable costs at the nursing home, major unforeseen cost factors arose. These came about because waivers were not obtained which would have allowed avoidance of the time consuming documentation requirements of the nursing home, using veteran LPNs cost more in salary than the average nursing home staff, and the small size of the project did not afford any savings on the usual complicated, heavily regulated nursing home. Were the entire building devoted to the Service House model, or if it were to be operated as an Assisted Living facility, it is believed that increased cost-effectiveness would be achieved. Of note is that in the four annual licensing and certification surveys since the House has been open, the State Health Department has found only one deficiency and has been generally well received by surveyors.

4. *Regulations are an impediment to realizing the model.* The MDS assessments, case mix documentation, intensive charting responsibilities and

other paper work demanded by regulations are still burdensome. Ideally, with the size of the House and philosophy of the care provided, most of that paper work could be eliminated and staff freed up to promote an even more relaxed environment.

5. *Residents' levels of dependency are high when they enter the House from the Nursing Home.* All the residents of the Service House have come from the medical model nursing home where they have had little or no responsibility for their daily lives. Consequently, the emphasis in the Service House on individual autonomy is foreign to their notion of care, and many choose not to do tasks they are capable of for themselves. It would be interesting to learn how admitting elders exclusively from their own homes would affect the workload on staff and the resulting social aspects of resident-staff relationships.

NEXT STEPS

In 2002, The Lyngblomsten Care Center plans to remodel the entire center into neighborhoods, two of which will be Service Houses. That will bring the number of residents in the new system to 36. Cost prohibitions will not allow the addition of private showers to all rooms and there will be a few semi-private rooms in the new units. Kitchenettes will be added to all units as part of this new phase. Otherwise, the additional Service House units will operate just like the pilot unit. By expanding this program, Lyngblomsten hopes to further its goal of moving the long-term care system in the direction of a truly "normal" setting for nursing home residents. More of the Care Center's units are slated for conversion to Service Houses in the coming years. After all, if we are still providing care according to the medical model and are 20 years behind the times, we still have much to do to catch up!

REFERENCES

Grant, L.A. (2001a). *Putting More Care in Eldercare.* Minneapolis, MN; Carlson School magazine for Alumni and Friends, University of Minnesota, Fall.

Grant, L. (2001b). *Service House Demonstration.* Minneapolis, MN; Center for the Study of Healthcare Management Newsletter, Carlson School of Management, University of Minnesota, Spring.

Grant, L.A. & Anderson, J. (2000). *Lyngblomsten Service House Demonstration: A New Residential Model for Nursing Home Care–Final Report.* Minneapolis, MN; Center for the Study of Healthcare Management Newsletter, Carlson School of Management, University of Minnesota, March 1.

SECTION 5
AN INTERNATIONAL PERSPECTIVE

Using Strengths-Based Practice to Support Culture Change: An Australian Experience

Peta Slocombe

SUMMARY. Workplaces across the globe have experienced an unprecedented pace of change. The effects of a problem focus, de-personalisation

Peta Slocombe, MA, is the Manager of Centrecare Corporate in Western Australia. She regularly presents at conferences and workshops throughout Australia on the application of strengths-based practice to non clinical contexts such as organizational health and employee well-being. She is presently in the process of co-authoring a book describing this approach.

Address correspondence to: Peta Slocombe, MA, Centrecare Corporate, 456 Hay Street, Perth, Western Australia 6000 (E-mail: petas@centrecare.com.au).

The author would like to thank Management and Staff at Centrecare in Western Australia for their collaboration, vision and commitment to supporting the development of this work. Particular appreciation also to Dr. Joseph Eron and Dr. Thomas Lund of Catskill Family Institute in New York for their encouragement and support with the application of the Narrative Solutions model to organizational settings. The increasing success of this work in Australia is a testament to our connection.

[Haworth co-indexing entry note]: "Using Strengths-Based Practice to Support Culture Change: An Australian Experience." Slocombe, Peta. Co-published simultaneously in *Journal of Social Work in Long-Term Care* (The Haworth Social Work Practice Press, an imprint of The Haworth Press, Inc.) Vol. 2, No. 3/4, 2003, pp. 307-323; and: *Culture Change in Long-Term Care* (ed: Audrey S. Weiner, and Judah L. Ronch) The Haworth Social Work Practice Press, an imprint of The Haworth Press, Inc., 2003, pp. 307-323. Single or multiple copies of this article are available for a fee from The Haworth Document Delivery Service [1-800-HAWORTH, 9:00 a.m. - 5:00 p.m. (EST). E-mail address: docdelivery@haworthpress.com].

http://www.haworthpress.com/store/product.asp?sku=J181
10.1300/J181v2n03_09

and over regulation in long-term care settings are experienced similarly by carers, residents, their families and nursing homes as a whole. A pathology focus is no longer appropriate, inviting a paradigm shift to explore how accessing the unique strengths and resources of all parties becomes an imperative role in changing organizational culture. This paper draws comparisons between the experiences and tasks of all those involved in care settings. Adapting the powerful work of Eron and Lund (1996) to organizational settings, this paper describes a clear intervention model and the effects of strengths-based practice on carers, residents, family members and organizational culture when utilized in a nursing home consultation. The model is not only a reactive intervention model, but is a way of re-mobilizing and motivating carers, residents and care settings to be at their best. *[Article copies available for a fee from The Haworth Document Delivery Service: 1-800-HAWORTH. E-mail address: <docdelivery@haworthpress.com> Website: <http://www.HaworthPress.com> © 2003 by The Haworth Press, Inc. All rights reserved.]*

KEYWORDS. Strengths-based, long-term care, organizational culture change, preferred view

INTRODUCTION

In the prologue to *The Alchemist* (1995), Paulo Coelho recites the story of Narcissus, the Greek youth who was so taken with his own beauty that he knelt before the lake each day to admire his reflection. One day he fell into the lake and drowned, and at the spot where he fell a flower bloomed, thereafter named the Narcissus. Coelho writes that sometime afterward, the goddesses of the forest appeared and noticed that the freshwater lake had been transformed into a lake of salty tears. The goddesses asked the lake, "Why do you weep?" The lake answered, "I weep for Narcissus." The goddesses responded, "Ah, it is no wonder you weep for Narcissus, because though we in the forest pursued him for his beauty, you alone witnessed that beauty close at hand." The lake fell silent. "Was Narcissus beautiful?" it asked. "Who better than you to know that?" replied the goddesses, "it was by your banks he knelt each day to admire his own beauty." The lake was still for a long time. "I weep for Narcissus, but I didn't know Narcissus was beautiful. I weep for Narcissus because it was only when he knelt before me that I could see, deep in his eyes, my own beauty reflected."

As helping professionals, Coelho's story has a poignant message about the essence of our role and relationship with our clients. Our culture draws us toward noticing pathology, weakness and dysfunction, particularly with those experiencing the transition of aging. Providing fellow human beings with a reflection of their own *beauty*, or their unique and individual qualities, resources, and strengths and identity, is rarely emphasized in society today. It is a large and never more vital paradigm shift with important implications for carers, residents, their families and organizations. The grief we all feel when we are not reminded of our strengths and unique attributes by those around us is profound and yet rarely acknowledged for the aged, their care givers and care organizations as a whole. Remarkable commonality pervades in a loss of self and identity, and those in care, carers, and care settings themselves are reeling from it–some more silently than others.

Centrecare's Corporate division encompasses an employee assistance program, a large strengths-based training facility, and a range of specialist clinical and consultancy services. It is a revenue generating division of a not for profit organization. In this capacity Centrecare provides counselling, consultancy and training to a large number of care settings regarding staff well being and overall organizational culture, mediation of conflicts and stress debriefing.

The same concerns have been voiced at all levels of organizations. People are increasingly reporting feeling distanced from the reasons they began working in care settings. Professionals who chose care settings because of altruistic or nurturing tendencies report feeling stifled by a language of pathology and illness and a care that focuses more on policy and procedure than connection and "being" with clients. This experience is mirrored in the aged and their families who experience the depersonalization or lack of vitality of even the most well intentioned and professional of institutions.

Gilley (1996) describes that workplaces the world over are experiencing an unprecedented pace of change, often referred to as a silent epidemic or a silent earthquake. Managers and staff alike notice people are lacking in vitality. An increase in stress, workplace conflict, workplace bullying, absenteeism, worker's compensation claims, violence and depression have also permeated to the point where the latter is predicted to become the greatest disease affecting society by 2030. Recent results of a survey of 10,000 employees in the U.K. found that 20% of employees actively switch off in the workplace, with only 17% of employees describing taking an "active role in their work" (*The Australian Newspaper,* 2001). In an attempt to deal with such changes, management and organizational literature has turned its focus to policy, procedure and regulation and a focus on "what we do." Funding limitations and economic rationalism have also exacerbated the difficulties. These trends appear to have asphyxiated the spirit of individuals and organizations even further, promoting problem maintaining cycles of further regulation and greater disconnection and desolation in workplace culture between who people are and what it is they are doing. It would seem that in the continued tinkering of *what we do* in the workplace, we have placed the spotlight entirely in the wrong place.

Of over 9000 documented management theories (Buckingham & Koffman, 1999), barely a handful focus on *who we are* in the workplace. The result of this de-personalization on individual staff, organizational culture and residents is significant and has resulted in work environments that are lifeless and mechanistic in nature (Gilley, 1996; Rankin, 1996; Buckingham & Coffman, 1999). Centrecare consultants report numerous employees who describe a loss of self in their workplace. In an attempt to optimize systems, workplaces have stopped looking for the unique qualities and attributes of their employees in favor of pursuing regulation and "sameness" between employees and residents alike. Given the centrality of work to life for many, employees also appear to have stopped noticing or privileging these attributes in themselves. This increased de-personalization has its origins as far back as the industrial revolution and the introduction of the conveyor belt. Gilley (1996) describes that people were invited to take only a small element of themselves into the workplace and leave that part of them that was not required to complete the task at home.

Perhaps care settings have felt this loss even more profoundly than others since people working in these settings place a strong value on being helpful to the lives of others. The Gallup Organization (Buckingham & Coffman, 1999) conducted an analysis of over 80,000 managers over a 25 year period to determine the factors most indicative of strong and vibrant workplaces. Without exception, the most striking finding of the Gallup study was that great managers don't try to mold or train employees, or treat them all the same. They don't bemoan differences or focus on improving weaknesses. Great managers recognize that the best will come when we bring out the best in each person, so that each person is helped to become "more of who he already is." They summarize, "People don't change that much. Don't waste time trying to put into people what you think is missing. Try to understand and draw out what is left in. That is hard enough."

It is the unique attributes and qualities of the aging, their carers and organizations as a whole that offer the greatest contribution to culture change in care settings. Centrecare staff have noticed that staff in care settings are highly resourceful, well-intentioned people who have chosen a care oriented profession. A deference to "what we do" rather than "who we are" in the workplace has anaesthetized the heart and soul of care settings and caused managers to wonder why they are weak and pale from the effects (Gilley, 1996). Increasing workplace disputes, stress, depression, conflict and general grievances tell us people are not at their best. Indeed the effects of pathology or symptom focussed cultures can be a self-perpetuating phenomenon on the residents themselves, with Kleinman (1988) noting that patients "learn to act as chronic cases, and families and caregivers learn to treat patients in keeping with this view."

Changes to organizational culture need to be integrated on all levels. The answers are not found in a single decision, policy, or training intervention. Change needs to be reflected in individual conversations, within staff and management, *between* staff and clients, and at an organizational decision making level. In this framework, Centrecare bases its interventions on the work of Eron and Lund (1996), co-creators of the Narrative Solutions approach to therapy.

Centrecare has noted profound effects on morale, organizational practices, stress reduction and productivity from reorienting people at all levels of organizations to strengths-based approaches. Reconnecting individuals, staff and residents to their unique qualities and attributes creates passionate and vibrant workplaces. When people are at their best and notice others noticing these qualities and attributes in them, there is a synergy between who people are and their behaviors in the workplace. Chopra (2001) refers to this in the *Law of Least Effort*, stating that when people's action are motivated by harmony and balance, the energy taken to carry out one's tasks is considerably less.

An overview of this model is presented below, including examples demonstrating how the model applies to individual staff, teams, and ultimately how management can utilize the principles of the approach to changing organizational culture. Stories documenting the intervention process appear in italicized form throughout the text to illustrate the various processes undertaken. Mary's story is regrettably familiar.

> *Working as a Nursing Aid at a nursing home for the aged for 15 years, Mary presented for counseling with stress and depression. She described ambivalence toward her work and an increasing lack of energy and motivation toward life in general. Increased absences from work due to stress and ill health, frustration with management, conflict in her team and a loss of connection to the residents were described, somewhat tearfully. Mary spoke of higher patient loads and more of a "production line" approach to care. She became visibly despondent while talking about her experience and began questioning her suitability to the task. Mary disclosed being increasingly frustrated with some of the residents in her care. When I asked Mary how she came to enter this profession, she told a key story about completing volunteer work as a mature age student and formulating a relationship with an older vision impaired resident for whom she used to read. Staff had spoken of the positive effects on her time with the patient with whom few others had been able to connect, and noted her aptitude for working with such residents. Mary*

smiled at her recollection of the resident, and how happy she was to accept a full time position when it was offered.

Eron and Lund (1996) introduce a concept they refer to as *preferred view*, noting that people have strong preferences for how they would like to behave, how they would like to see themselves, and how they would like to be seen by others. These characteristics contribute to defining an identity that offers much in determining when people are at their best.

Preferred view has to do with the *qualities, attributes, preferences, hopes and intentions* people have for their lives and would like to have noticed by others. Organizations, staff, and residents are at their best when they are acting or seen to be acting in line with their preferences, and when they see others viewing them in these ways.

> *For example, Mary saw herself as a caring person who was committed to helping others. When Mary had begun reading to the vision impaired resident, she noticed herself feeling good about her work and looked forward to it all week. When others noticed these qualities and the effect she had on those in her care, Mary was motivated to do more of it, eventually leaving her previous work to pursue work as a nursing aide full time. This was clearly Mary at her best.*

People and organizations are often at their *worst* when *gaps* emerge between how they would like to view themselves, and how they are actually viewing themselves or see others viewing them. At these times, often during transitional or specific events, people may lose sight of the unique strengths and resources they possess. Eron and Lund (1996) describe how people often experience these gaps with intense negative emotion, setting problems into motion which continue.

In an attempt to cope with discrepant views of self, people at their worst may often deny culpability, become angry or defensive, minimize the problem, or even withdraw and accept the negative view of others (Eron & Lund, 1996).

> *In Mary's case, she became angry, stressed, and eventually depressed, missing work and doubting her ability to function in such a setting. Until she was reminded of her reason for entering care settings, Mary had forgotten the attributes that had led to this decision. Mary also began to talk of her distress after a dispute with Linda, a resident's daughter, who felt she was not caring adequately for her mother. Audrey was experiencing dementia and would often remove her clothes after being showered and dressed. She would also report not being given her medication nor being*

*showered even when this had been completed. When her daughter,
Linda, attended repeatedly to find her mother partially unclothed, she
became upset and angry toward staff. Mary reported trying to explain
Audrey's behavior, yet noticed Linda only became more upset and angry
when her mother's degeneration was pointed out. An incident occurred
where Mary lost her temper with Linda, pointing out the challenges of
working with someone with Audrey's behavior and suggesting she was
being unrealistic about her mother's degeneration. Following this, Mary
began avoiding the care of Audrey or ensuring she had a witness with
her when attending to her. Other carers began to avoid Audrey and
Linda also for fear of having to suffer Linda's wrath. Linda complained
to the Aged Care Complaints Board about her mother's care and Mary's
outburst toward her. An inquiry followed, with Mary subjected to extensive interviewing about her care of Audrey by both her organization and
the Board. The Board recommended communication and conflict resolution training of staff and a review of carer's procedures, such as log
sheets regarding patient care being completed indicating time and duties performed. Feeling unsupported by the organization, Mary took
stress leave and the organization appealed her claim. Management, staff
and Audrey's family emerged despondent and relationships deteriorated
significantly.*

*When Linda began making accusations against Mary and stated her view
of her as uncaring and incompetent, Mary became angry, distressed, and
then despondent. She came to believe that both Audrey's daughter and her
employer saw her in ways that didn't fit with the caregiver she wished to
be. Mary noticed that she became frustrated about aspects of her work and
withdrew from contact with other residents, doing the minimum necessary
for their care. The more Mary's behavior departed from her preferred
view, the more stressed she became. Ultimately, Mary's solution to her
predicament was to no longer work at all.*

In this model, the tasks for intervention on individual, team and organizational levels include:

1. Helping people notice and be reminded of their unique qualities and attributes in the workplace.
2. Noticing when gaps emerge between preferred and actual or other's
   views of self.
3. Having the confidence to bridge the gap and encouraging colleagues,
   management and cultures to reflect these qualities as opposed to a problem saturated focus.

As part of my role with the Employee Assistance Program, I asked Mary about her preferences for being as a carer (Step 1). These included questions such as "When were you at your best?" or "What qualities and attributes would you like colleagues and residents alike to recall of you?" and invited Mary to revisit her decision to enter care settings. Mary became visibly animated recalling the vision impaired resident with whom she had connected. With these qualities we completed the left-hand side of the diagram in Figure 1. With sadness Mary noted her own departure from these qualities and the way others had come to see her (Step 2), completing the right side of the diagram. The Gap column reflects the effects of this troublesome gap on Mary and the negative emotions and behaviors that resulted from her attempts to manage it.

The wider the gap between Mary's preferred view, how she saw herself and how she saw others seeing her, the more she became defensive, emotional, angry, and attempted to avoid the situation. As depression and stress increased, she took more time off work. Her Manager came to see her as someone who was not coping and had a problem with communication, and Audrey's daughter saw this as further evidence of Mary's incompetence. When the organization increased reporting requirements and assigned a younger carer to deal with Audrey's daughter, Mary slipped even further into the gap, taking further time off work and reluctantly accepting her doctor's recommendation that she attend counseling. All the qualities Mary had prided herself on during her long carer as a carer appeared forgotten. When Mary talked with others about the events, they were not conversations that reminded her of these strengths and resources. She saw them as seeing her as not coping and deficient, inciting what is often described as a problem maintaining solution.

Exploring how external events had lured her away from her preferred view, Mary was invited to notice whether the behaviors and negative emotions had narrowed or widened the gap. With some distress she noted that her responses had further distanced her from who she knew herself to be. Returning the conversation to Mary's preferences for being, I invited her to contemplate the practices and behaviours that would help to remind herself and others of her at her best (Step 3). Mary recalled a previous experience where she had become frustrated with a resident and had enlisted the help of the resident's family to find solutions. She also reiterated her understanding of the distress Linda must have experienced with her mother's degeneration and spoke of her desire to acknowledge this with Linda at their scheduled review. Refocussed on her unique strengths and positive intentions Mary contacted her employer requesting a return to work plan.

FIGURE 1. Preferred View Diagram of Mary as a Nursing Aide

Preferred View	GAP	Actual View/Others View

Emotions

Preferred View	GAP	Actual View/Others View
Caring	Angry	Uncaring
Dedicated	Frustrated	Disorganised
Patient	Depressed	Avoidant
Gentle	Stressed	Incompetent
		Aggressive
		"Not coping"

Behaviours

Avoidant
Defensive
Tearful

ORGANIZATIONAL LEVEL

Organizations are at their best when they have a synergy between staff identity or preferred view, and that of the organization. The nursing home described above noticed that staff morale declined after the incident with Audrey's daughter. They felt frustrated in their attempts to balance the needs of residents, family, staff and the Aged Care Complaints Board. They worked hard to develop forms and procedures that would enable care plans to be documented and provided increased staff education sessions to inform them of these requirements and improve conflict resolution strategies. Funding reductions had also increased pressure on them to resolve the difficulty to the satisfaction of the Board, as they had been given three months to implement the recommendations offered before facing consequences to their funding classification.

Like Mary, the organization was experiencing a "gap" between its intentions as an organization and the way staff and residents were viewing them. A consultation with Management occurred where management was asked to describe the organization at its best, and to recall how they might like to see themselves or have others (staff, residents and families) view them. These preferences were then plotted against their sense of how others had come to view the organization, and how they had come to view themselves. As with

Mary, the "gap" column of Figure 2 indicates both the effects of this gap on the organization, as well as plotting the way in which the organization attempted to manage this discrepancy.

As the organization attempted to manage the gap and dealt with staff morale issues by increasing regulation and reviewing procedures, staff came to feel more and more despondent and unproductive. They felt that the imposition of these policy changes meant that management saw them as to blame for the complaints or at the very least deficient. They saw increased monitoring as a lack of faith in their ability. A passive work culture began to develop. Staff turnover increased to the point where on selected shifts up to 35% of the staff were temporary staff from a Nursing Agency compared with a usual casual employee base of less than 10%. Several staff refused to attend the development opportunities offered. Some invoked a "work to rule" requirement where they ceased participating in extracurricular duties such as taking residents on outings. Some engaged the union in protest of increased patient loads and work standards. As a result, the organization began utilizing more casual and agency staff to compensate for these losses.

FIGURE 2. Preferred View Diagram of Management/Organization

Preferred View	GAP	Actual View/Others View
	Emotions	
Professional		
Accessible	Frustrated	Rigid
Caring	Embarrassed	Uncaring
Flexible	Angry	Unsupportive
Client centred	Conflicted	Unhelpful
Vigilant		Unprofessional
Supportive of staff		Unsuccessful
Collaborative		
Encouraging	**Behaviours**	
Successful	Defensive	
Dynamic/Innovative team	Increased regulation	
	Increased procedures/paper work	
	Increased staff monitoring	
	Increased staff education	

As with Mary, step one in motivating change was inviting management to revisit their organizational preferred view. I asked management to tell stories of when the organization seemed most to represent itself in accordance with their preferences, or times when they felt they had been at their best.

Many recalled Jack's arrival–a resident who had been placed in the nursing home after a fall and became depressed at being parted from his beloved terrier. Noticing his decline, one of the nurses who lived near Jack's son sought permission from management to collect the dog on her way to work in order that Jack might be able to spend time with him during her morning shift. Jack became motivated to dress and eat breakfast in order to go outside and visit the dog. The dog became a favourite among other residents, who also became motivated to sit in the garden, and was a source of increased interaction between residents. Management recalled Jack's story fondly. This was the organization at its caring, flexible, client-centred best. Management noticed the unique needs of residents, acted in a collaborative manner with carers, and assisted in Jack's recovery. Staff were mobilized by the decision and took turns in returning the dog to its home. Staff also saw the organization as a caring facility in which their suggestions were valued and noted other ways they could cooperate with the preferences of residents. Management also spoke proudly of staff willingness to come up with dynamic, patient-centered solutions. An article had appeared in the local paper and families and other residents were complimentary of the nursing home's actions.

Contemplating how the organization would like to be seen, or how it was behaving at its best, had significant implications. Management noted that at its best, there was synchronicity between the staff's preferences to be caring, flexible, and client-centreed, and the positive intentions and resources of the organization. They also noted that regulation and monitoring widened the gap and further alienated staff from their strengths and attributes. Previous well-intentioned attempts to rectify difficulties had not recognized or mobilized the preferences and intentions of staff. To the contrary, management attempts to ensure the adequate care of Audrey had resulted in disengagement and resentment from staff to the point where staff themselves came to focus on controlling negative behaviors as opposed to bringing out the best in residents. As in step two, they noticed a gap between their preferences and the manner in which staff and residents had come to view them. As with Mary, in step three Management were invited to consider the kinds of practices that would be "gap narrowing," or those practices that would more accurately represent their preferences.

*In the case of Mary, Management stated their preference for client cen-
tred practice and offered their awareness that she had a gentleness
with residents that few of her colleagues possessed. Management
posed a mystery question (Eron & Lund, 1996) to Mary regarding how
it would be that someone who had such a patient and gentle manner
with residents would come to be seen as uncaring and unsympathetic?
They spoke to her as someone who had the compassion and resources
to want to solve the problem and reminded her of the qualities she was
known for. Affirming her resources, Mary was mobilized to contribute
to generating solutions as opposed to the previous problem focus
which had only increased the stress, defensiveness and reduced Mary's
confidence.*

Changing organizational culture in this model requires organizations and
individuals alike to be aware of the unique preferences, intentions, hopes and
attributes they wish to possess. Centrecare consultants often notice that the
majority of discussions, minutes of management meetings, daily procedures
and performance evaluations focus on problematic behavior, and this is translated into problem oriented discussions with staff and residents alike. The effects of this problem focus are de-motivating for all involved, spark a further
spiral of unhelpful behaviors that justify attempts at further regulation, and further the problem.

Once the unique qualities and preferred attributes of staff, teams and the organization as a whole had been identified, the managers were encouraged to
contemplate the practices and procedures that would assist them to act in accordance with these attributes. When gaps emerged, the organization was invited to notice the practices that might best represent their intentions and
preferences, and to focus on a realignment with these preferences. The organization above was also invited to consider the preferences of staff and the
practices that might motivate staff to return to these. They identified that collaborative and resident-respectful practices would invite staff consultation
about problem evolution and problem resolution, as opposed to seeking to
blame or to operate on a deficiency based model. It would also recognize the
inherently positive intentions and preferences of staff, residents and residents' families.

Significant organizational culture changes followed. Management began
stating their preferences and intentions for operation of the nursing home when
communicating with staff and residents so as to reaffirm decision-making processes. For example, when professional development was offered, management noted it as being consistent with their provision of dynamic and
innovative practice, and noted this was also a preference of staff. This was

markedly different from the previously "gap widening" offering of professional development in the context of staff feeling management saw them as skill deficient in some way.

Management also involved staff in a brainstorming session of what they valued about the organization and displayed this preferred view list in the staff and common rooms. These included a list of concrete practices that would represent these preferences. For example, "respectful" would translate into eye contact and use of name with all residents. Some staff suggested it would be as if they were dealing with their own parents, and many other staff resonated with this. In a later team building session, staff were invited to reflect on their reasons for entering the profession and the unique qualities and attributes they noticed and valued in their colleagues. This had a highly motivating effect on staff and resulted in management and staff reinforcing the strengths and attributes of colleagues when they were exhibited. This not only helped staff to remain aware of their unique resources and attributes, it also ensured these were more likely to be exhibited. Accessing preferences and intentions can be done in such settings as this team building and planning process, as well as supervision or performance management contexts. Several organizations with which Centrecare has consulted have built in these preference questions to recruitment and selection processes, where preferred view of candidates may be assessed in relation to organizational preferred view, and this may serve to indicate suitability and hold successful candidates accountable to these preferences following selection. Although in practice for less than 12 months at the time of writing, anecdotal support has been positive. (Sample questions appear in the Appendix.)

As noted, culture change occurs at all levels of an organization. In the nursing home cited, management and staff came to notice that just as they themselves became invited into unhelpful cycles of problem saturation when gaps emerged between preferred and actual views of self, so did residents and their families. For example, Linda clearly viewed herself as a caring, attentive family member who was determined to ensure that her mother received the best of care. When she noticed staff seeing her as difficult and argumentative, she became angry and frustrated. Similarly, Linda had known her mother to be a proud and successful woman who was always impeccably groomed. When Linda came to believe staff viewed her mother as demented and incompetent, the pain of disjunction had significant implications. This knowledge informed how staff might best deal with Linda's concerns when they were presented. If Linda wished to view herself and be viewed by carers as a helpful, caring, involved daughter instead of being viewed as aggressive and overbearing, staff would speak to this in their interactions with her. Instead of becoming frustrated and avoidant, staff in the future may respond to her complaints by saying, "I know it is important to you that your mother get the best of care and be comfortable. We've noticed how committed you are to that. Can we talk with you about some ideas about how this might best happen?" Such a collaborative conversation is likely to reduce Linda's criticism of staff and engage her in more positive outcome searches. It may not alleviate Linda's concern for her mother, but all parties become involved in what Eron and Lund refer to as "the solution team" (1996) based on their statement of preferences and intentions.

Following these consultations, Management and staff noted the increased morale and vitality that resulted from *preference focussed* as opposed to *problem focussed* discussions, with all parties taking responsibility for remaining aligned to their preferences. Presentations to the employee assistance program for work related issues such as bullying, co-worker conflict, management practices and stress all decreased markedly for three consecutive quarterly reporting periods. Staff began to speak of how they could continue the synergy by engaging the positive preferences and unique resources of both residents and also their family members. At a resident and family meeting some months after our initial intervention, they invited families to offer stories of each of the residents at their best. Questions included "Describe an incident or event that would speak of (resident's) qualities and attributes at their best." And "If you were to gather significant people from different stages of (the resident's) life, what qualities and attributes would they most recall about (your parent/resident)?" For those who did not have visiting families, staff recalled their own understanding of resident strengths based on their observations. For example, staff noted the way in which Sarah always greeted staff cheerfully and asked them about their families despite recovering from an uncomfortable hip replacement. Stories of contributions to charity, war service, raising multiple children single-handedly, and even pigeon rearing emerged. Results of these practices were profound. Not only were family members mobilized by recollections of their parents at their best as opposed to problem saturated discussions about illness and degeneration, but they felt encouraged that staff began to understand and be interested in these stories also. Conversations that privileged the strength and identity of the residents had a mobilizing effect on staff, who began to re-engage and recall these stories with residents during their care of them. Conversations were animated, with several staff reporting significant improvements in resident behavior.

CONCLUSION

This paper began with the story of Narcissus and the grief the lake felt when it was no longer able to see its own beauty reflected. Like a pebble thrown into such a lake, we notice a far reaching ripple effect on carers, residents, their families and whole organizations when the culture of organizations, particularly care settings, invites all parties to mobilize their unique attributes and qualities in the workplace. We note that what helps people to be at their best also helps staff and whole organizations to be at their best. These interventions have been used with recruitment and selection, informing empowering performance management interventions, decision making practices, team building, conflict resolution, stress management and strategic planning and organizational culture. It is about consistency of approach and motivating staff to connect with their strengths and resources in the midst of a society that seems often transfixed on pathology and dysfunction, regulation and "sameness."

It is the unique attributes and qualities of the aging, their carers and organizations as a whole that offer the greatest contribution to culture change in care settings. We see people as inherently positive, resourceful, well intentioned and altruistic, even when their behaviors may not always be reflective of these qualities. Not privileging these qualities in our daily conversations does a great injustice to all. The Dalai Lama echoes this in the *Art of Happiness* (1998) when he was asked why, if human nature is essentially gentle, benevolent and kind as he suggests, is so much war, violence, conflict and destruction pervading society. He responded that he believes these behaviors arise when we are frustrated in our inability to have these qualities reflected in those around us and when we are unable to achieve connection. This has significant implications for the care of the aging, who may accept the invitation to become deficiency focussed and who also grieve their loss of self long before they physically cease to function. We are increasingly of the belief that presentations of workplace stress are most often evidence of gaps emerging between preferred and actual view of self, and a symptom of loss of self. This may include psychologists who are bound by paper work and statistics, carers with increased regulation and automated patient care procedures, and teachers doing less talking with children.

Strengths-based or preference focused practice has a great deal to offer care settings. Indeed the effects of not privileging the unique strengths and attributes of staff, residents and organizations have significant implications for emotional, physical, and even financial realms if one considers the often protracted alternatives for problem resolution and positive change.

Just as organizations and those who staff them have much on which to reflect, these tasks are mirrored by society as a whole. Australian Prime Minister

John Howard, in New York on September 11, 2001, was invited upon his return to Australia to reflect on the implications of the attacks. He replied, "I believe we are faced with a task greater than any we have ever faced–the task to see the good in people." As practitioners ourselves, as well as the thousands of people with whom we now work and train each year, we notice profoundly positive effects on those willing to do the same.

REFERENCES

Buckingham, M. & Coffman, C. (1999). *First Break All the Rules–What the World's Great Managers Do Differently.* New York: Simon & Schuster.

Chopra, D. (2001). *The Deeper Wound.* London: Random House.

Coelho, P. (1995). *The Alchemist.* New York: HarperCollins.

Dalai Lama. (1996). *The Art of Happiness: A Handbook for Living.* New York: Penguin.

Eron, J. & Lund, T. (1996). *Narrative Solutions in Brief Therapy.* New York: Guilford Press.

Gilley, K. (1996). *Leading from the Heart. Choosing Courage Over Fear in the Workplace.* Boston: Butterworth-Heinemann.

Kleinman, A. (1988). *The illness narratives: Suffering, healing and the human condition.* New York: Basic Books.

Rankin, M.S. (1996). *The New Bottom Line: Bringing Heart and Soul to Business.* Leaders Press: San Francisco, CA.

The Australian Newspaper. (2001). Oct 21.

APPENDIX

Recruitment and Selection Procedures:
Sample Interview Questions for Accessing Employee Preferred View

- What inspired you to seek a position with this organization?
- What about this organization did you find appealing?
- What do you see as the qualities and attributes you bring to this organization? Why do you see these strengths as fitting with this particular workplace?
- In previous positions when would you say you were at your best? What were you doing? Who noticed? How did they see you?
- How about other times in your life when you were at your best? What were you doing? What effect did you have on people around you? How did they see you?
- Who has been an important influence in your life in shaping who you are? What qualities or attributes do you admire in them? What values have they

instilled that you want to follow? What strengths do they see in you that you would bring to this position?

- What do you enjoy doing? How do you feel when doing these things?
- How would you measure whether you're at your best at work? What indicators would you see as significant?

Implementing the Eden Alternative in Australia

Sarah MacKenzie

SUMMARY. Many Aged Care facilities in Australia are continuing to operate in a traditional medical model, with elders being dependant, living in large institutions and living a life of mere existence. It is Australia's challenge to change the culture of ageing and the perceptions held by the community that elders are powerless and feeble. Australia needs to turn Aged Care facilities into homes, making them attractive for residents, families and staff and to create a life worth living.

In recent times some Aged Care providers have begun to research and implement new practices and philosophies such as the Eden Alternative™ and culture change, believing that they can create an environment filled with animals, plants and children. Australia has seen the positive results and data from the USA, and some homes in Australia are now beginning to gather base data and some comparative data, which in preliminary fashion indicate positive outcomes for staff and residents.

Australia has to continue on the culture change journey, educating and spreading the awareness and positive changes nationally. Other Aged Care operators need to be aware of these new concepts in ageing,

---

Sarah MacKenzie is the Operations Coordinator of *Aged Care Service Group*, Australia.

Address correspondence to: Sarah MacKenzie, 17-21 Ashley Street, Reservoir 3073, Victoria, AUSTRALIA (E-mail: sarahmackenzie@acsg.net.au).

[Haworth co-indexing entry note]: "Implementing the Eden Alternative in Australia." MacKenzie, Sarah. Co-published simultaneously in *Journal of Social Work in Long-Term Care* (The Haworth Social Work Practice Press, an imprint of The Haworth Press, Inc.) Vol. 2, No. 3/4, 2003, pp. 325-338; and: *Culture Change in Long-Term Care* (ed: Audrey S. Weiner, and Judah L. Ronch) The Haworth Social Work Practice Press, an imprint of The Haworth Press, Inc., 2003, pp. 325-338. Single or multiple copies of this article are available for a fee from The Haworth Document Delivery Service [1-800-HAWORTH, 9:00 a.m. - 5:00 p.m. (EST). E-mail address: docdelivery@haworthpress.com].

so that they can begin to practice self-determination; person-centred work and self-directed teams and leadership. Greater knowledge, awareness and Australian proactive data and results will assist and encourage others on the journey to culture change. *[Article copies available for a fee from The Haworth Document Delivery Service: 1-800-HAWORTH. E-mail address: <docdelivery@haworthpress.com> Website: <http://www.HaworthPress.com> © 2003 by The Haworth Press, Inc. All rights reserved.]*

KEYWORDS. Australia, culture change, Eden Alternative™, aged care, person centred care, community model

AGED CARE IN AUSTRALIA

Australia is a large country with a small population which was settled only 213 years ago by the British. Australia's landmass is a similar size to North America, with a population of only 18-19 million people living predominantly around the coastline, leaving the center bare and barren with rugged desert and bush land. Australia's aged population (65 year and over) is about 12.5%. As a relatively young nation and like most countries in the Western world, Australia has an ageing population and with the post World War II baby boomers themselves ageing, the population of elders is expected to hit a peak in the year 2021. It is predicted that by 2050, Australia's population of people 65 years and over will be approximately 25%.

In Australia, Aged Care is organized into three basic areas:

1. Funded Residential Aged Care
2. Un-funded Residential Aged Care
3. Home Care

Funded Residential Care

Funded Residential Care is the sector that has the most financial impact to the government and society in general. All Australians are entitled to federally funded residential care, provided they have official Commonwealth paperwork. This basic funding model revolves around residents contributing 85% of the Aged Care pension (Social Service Payment), which equates to approximately $24 per day with the balance being contributed by the government. This impacts heavily on the Federal Government's budgets, so there is a strict criteria for entering the funded sector of residential aged care. Each person (resident) must be assessed by a community Aged Care Assessment Service (ACAS), which is a team of professionals, including social workers, physiotherapists, nurses, doctors and occupational therapists. The ACAS categorize residents as to whether they are high care (skilled nursing home) or low care (Hostel or assisted living). ACAS paperwork is even required for respite care in the funded sector.

The number of places allocated for both high and low care is linked to a ratio of the population over the age of 70 years. Consequently, in 2001, 5% of people 70 years+ reside in high care places and 4% live in low care places. There are however long waiting lists for residential care in Australia; the wait can be several years for some people, particularly concessional (financially in need) and/or high care beds. As a result of these realities and personal preference a total number of 91% of people over the age of 70 years are still living in their own homes or with family.

Within high and low care there are also sub categories–once a resident is assessed as high or low care, they must have a needs analysis completed [Residential Classification Scale (RCS)] to determine specific level of care needs. Once a resident has been categorized, the government then funds the Aged Care home providers according to that classification. This system is very similar to the Minimum Data Set used in the USA. The funding ranges on a sliding scale from categories 1-8. Category 1 (the residents with highest needs) receives approximately $114 per day (Australian). This equates in April, 2002 to US $61 and Euro $68. A category 7 reimbursement is $25 per day. Category 8 receives nil funding. The resident's needs are continually monitored and assessed at least annually.

A basic social foundation upon which the Residential Aged Care system is based is the concept of the "Concessional Resident." This is a safety net system where an individual with financial hardship is provided with supplementary funding to ensure that they too can enjoy high quality care. All funded residential care homes (except 6% that are extra service homes) must admit a quota of concessional residents as a part of their contract with the Government, thus enabling aged care providers to receive Government funding. An average of 25% of all residents in facilities are concessional. By definition, these residents do not own a home or have assets in excess of $25,000. It should be noted that if one party of a relationship needs residential aged care, then the remaining partner is deemed to retain their home without it impacting on the resident's financial status.

For residents with assets of more than $25,000 (Australian) the aged care provider can request extra funding, i.e., an accommodation bond (refundable when the resident leaves less a small charge) for residents who enter at the low care level. An accommodation fee may be charged for residents who enter at a high care level. The basis of the bond and the charge is to assist the provider to upkeep the standard of the building in which the care is provided. The average accommodation bond is $100,000, although some are as low as $25,000 and as high as $500,000.

Extra service homes are still a part of the funded sector of residential aged care; however, they operate very much on a "user-pays" system. Currently approximately 6% of all homes in the funded sector are "extra service homes." This means a care provider is able to charge an extra fee (over and above the 85% of the aged pension). The purpose of the extra fee is to provide funding for extra hotel services, not care services, as all homes have an obligation to meet the highest standards in the provision of care. The government does, however, reduce the funding provided to extra service homes by a small percentage.

There are a variety of unfunded options for the Australian aged population, which range from assisted care that is totally funded by the resident (this tends to be at the low end of the care needs) through to Retirement Village living. The number of unfunded assisted living residents is relatively small, as the funded option is preferred by most people. The retirement village, on the other hand, is growing in popularity with people aged over 60 years. It is a collection of senior citizens who remain independent, but choose to live in a community environment with people of similar age and ability. Most of these retirement communities have extensive community activities as well as leisure facilities, e.g., pool, community halls, etc.

There are approximately 1% of people over the age of 70 years who receive a Community Aged Care Package (CACPs). These are Government funded packages, provided to assist the aged person to stay in his/her own home whilst still receiving care. These are very popular as they provide an alternative to receiving care in a community setting. Whilst home care is popular and offers a slightly less expensive option to residential aged care, the provision of care is limited due to access to services particularly for 24 hours a day.

Facilities are now called Aged Care homes, rather than the traditional terminology of nursing homes and hostels. Homes are built to offer *ageing in place*, a concept introduced in Australia in 1999. This is a different concept than the conventional separation between nursing homes and hostel facilities. The philosophy of Ageing in Place is that facilities should be structured to provide various levels of care, so that an aged person can remain in the aged care home with familiar friends, family and staff, even when their needs increase.

AGED CARE SERVICE GROUP

Aged Care Service Group was developed in the mid 1980s by private operators in the unfunded sector of residential care. A new 44 bed home was opened in Melbourne, Australia. In the late 1980s, Aged Care Service Group opened another 30 bed facility and in the early 1990s they followed with a 29 bed home. All the residents were low-level care, requiring minimal support with activities of daily living. These unfunded residential care facilities only required the employment of Personal Care Attendants (PCAs or USA–CNAs) and had live-in staff at night who were on call, rather than on duty. All three facilities were typical of the era with most residents in shared rooms with shared bathrooms. These facilities had large communal living areas, with minimal private sitting areas.

In 1995, Aged Care Service Group was granted 45 low care bed licenses, for which Ashley Terrace was opened in 1997. Ashley Terrace has 45 single rooms, all with private bathrooms and private sitting areas in each corridor. This home is currently being extended with the addition of 20 beds, 5 of which are high care, which will enhance the opportunity to offer Ageing in Place.

Since 1997, Aged Care Service Group has grown and developed several homes and has been actively involved in the Australian Aged Care industry. Aged Care Service Group currently own and operate 205 high and low care beds in Queensland and Victoria. It employs more than 150 staff, including registered nurses. Aged Care Service Group has been granted more bed licenses from the Commonwealth Government and was to commence building a retirement village in 2002. This retirement village will offer an integrated high and low care home with an additional 85-90 independent living units. This retirement community will also have a pool, a community centre with a bar, Bowling Green, golf putting green and a children's play ground.

The evolution of Aged Care Service Group over more than 15 years has generated many changes. However, the holistic family approach to staff, residents and the community has remained intact. A philosophy of person-centred care and value of the human spirit has been a part of the group's mission. However, with growing expectations and improved standards, Aged Care Service Group is structurally redesigning its existing homes into a Community Model, creating smaller communities/households for residents to live in a more intimate environment, opposed to the traditional large central lounge and dining areas. All future designs will incorporate this Community Model design.

Aged Care Service Group has sent staff to the USA to work in this model, amongst America's most proactive aged care organisations, including experiences with the Eden Alternative™, Pioneer Network and Action Pact Pty Ltd (see related articles in this volume). Aged Care Service Group has been imple menting the Eden Alternative™ since the year 2000 and has noticed some significant improvements to residents' happiness and independence.

CULTURE CHANGE

Culture change and the Eden Alternative™ are relatively new concepts in Australia and are yet to receive the recognition they are afforded in the USA. Presently only 3 organisations in Melbourne have adopted this model, though recent publicity (such as state radio presentations and several articles written for the Australian *National Health Care Journal*) has resulted in a rapid increase in interest. Aged Care Service Group has been working to implement culture change and the Eden Alternative™ into their Aged Care homes for more than 18 months. Aged Care Service Group began "warming the soil" in early 2000 and after 7 key staff became trained Eden Alternative™ Associates in November 2000, their job was to share the vision, educate others and build a team to implement the Eden Alternative™. As with any new concept introduced, it has come with successes and some failures. Overall, staff, residents, pets, families and the community would agree that the culture change journey is well worth the challenges as it has improved so many lives.

There are many residents who have grown with the environment of love, laughter and companionship.

One case that demonstrates the success of culture change is Harry. Harry is a 76 year-old man with an Eastern European heritage. He speaks fluent English and lives a very Aussie lifestyle. Harry moved into one of Aged Care Service Group's assisted living facilities as a part of a winter bed program in September 2000. The Home provides the local hospital with 3 rooms to place hospital patients, due to the hospitals' chronic bed shortages during winter. Harry was living at one of Aged Care Service Group's homes as a hospital patient for 2 months before a permanent room became available for him. He was admitted with severe leg ulcers, cellulitis, diabetes, depression, CCF (Chronic Cardiac Failure) and could barely walk. Harry had given up control of his finances and had stopped driving. Aged Care Service Group staff were managing his diabetes, wound management and were continually trying to motivate Harry to exercise and become more active, but his depression and physical condition was keeping him predominantly bed bound.

Since introducing the Eden Alternative™ and changing the culture of the home, Harry has gained his independence again. Harry tells staff and families "I've never been so happy in my life." The atmosphere at this home has provided the environment for Harry to have meaningful relationships with staff and other residents. This has helped to alleviate his depression, as well as his physical medical conditions. He no longer requires wound care, as he is actively walking around. He has responded to the lifestyle program, participating in regular activities and outings, and is an important member of the residents' committee. Harry walks the facility Labrador Zeb on a daily basis, he maintains his own vegetable garden, with fruit trees that he picks and shares with other residents. His independence exceeds his own expectation. Harry regularly celebrates his "rebirth" with a nice cold beer, outside in the sunshine with his best friend Zeb. He sits outside, kicks back to admires his vibrant garden. Everyone feels his pride and gain energy from watching.

Harry now helps the maintenance staff by cleaning the fountains in the garden on a weekly basis. Harry is back to driving and has regained full control over his financial affairs. He is able to drive to visit some of his friends in the community. With his content happiness he has more visitors to the home. Harry is just one of the success stories of the change in culture; staff reminisce about Harry and other residents, and staff feel great satisfaction in helping to conquer loneliness, helplessness and boredom and changing the culture of an assisted living home.

Culture change hasn't just reached the residents, but it has also had a substantial effect on the staff at Aged Care Service Group. The staff have embraced the Eden Alternative™ and have become active change agents in the alteration of the culture of ageing. In particular, some of the younger care staff has brought energy, enthusiasm and spontaneity to the homes. Their youth has given inspiration to the team and challenge the traditions of ageing. Their energy and enthusiasm has been carefully nurtured by management, empowering them to speak with doctors and other professionals, deal with conflict resolution and learn report writing skills for government documentation. Many of the staff have developed a strong passion for Aged Care and a sense of self belief from working in a positive team and environment. This has resulted in personal care staff now pursuing further qualifications and academic education in nursing and other health professions. Table 1 details the increase in numbers of staff members pursuing formal training in Ageing and related fields. These data are collected annually from Human Resource personnel files and surveys.

The staff openly informs management of their improved job satisfaction, both verbally and in written surveys. Many staff bring their children to work,

TABLE 1. Ashley Terrace Accumulation of Staff Credentials

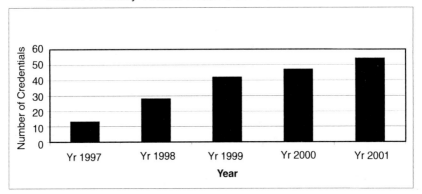

Note: This graph refers to the number of staff as a collective amount per year. It indicates that the staff, as a collective, are gaining in the number of credentials each year through further training and education, a result due in part, we believe to increased respect and job satisfaction.

giving them greater flexibility and availability for shifts and allowing them to have a greater income capacity. The children enhance the environment by building companionship with residents, playing with the animals and participating in activities. The residents have commented on the increased number of grandchildren and great grandchildren who visit. Aged Care Service Group has toy boxes in every sitting room to encourage children to come to the homes. Allowing staff to have their children at work supports staff, enhances the atmosphere and residents' happiness, and invites the community into the home.

The organisation is continually looking to appreciate and value staff, as they view the staff to be the most important component of the organisation. The modest effort it takes to value staff through group and personalized praise and reward has paid dividends with one of the homes having only 2 staff leave in almost 18 months. Table 2 details staff turnover at this facility. These data are collected each year from Human Resource files. Eden Terrace and Albany Gardens, the other homes in the group, have had less documented success in this regard, due to, this author believes, their opening in 2000.

Culture Change has evolved in its first 18 months at Aged Care Services Group, with Ashley Terrace (65 high/low care home) moving into a community model. In February 2002, Ashley Terrace redesigned itself into 4 communities. Ashley Terrace moved away from large style dining and living rooms for residents. Staff no longer cover the whole home. It now has small dining rooms and lounge areas for each community. Communities range in size from 15-21 residents. Resident have been grouped in accordance to their cognitive

TABLE 2. Ashley Terrace Staff Turnover 1997-2001

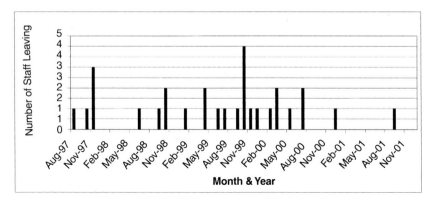

state, with a dementia specific community that caters specifically for their social needs. Staff are now permanently assigned to one community, so they can develop and foster more intimate relationships with residents. Ashley Terrace has also recently promoted several Personal Care Staff to become Community Coordinators, empowering them to be in charge of their team, allowing them to grow their team with the residents, enabling each community to take on its own individual character and operate in a manner that best suits the daily needs of individuals that live in the community. The community with residents who are more independent and cognitively intact are now able to make their own breakfast, without the risk of a person with dementia touching something hot or moving the breakfast equipment. This simple change has allowed the residents of that community to feel more empowered, and consequently they are doing more for themselves and feeling more personal satisfaction.

At the time of writing this article, Ashley Terrace has only been in a community model for 2 months. Yet staff and other residents are capturing success stories. The next step is to introduce this person-centred community model to all of Aged Care Services Group's homes. The Eden Alternative™ and culture change have allowed the organisation to enhance their philosophy of person-centred care; the community of Aged Care Services Group are unanimous in its acclaim. Several comparative resident surveys at Eden Terrace, another of the ACSG's homes, support this view.

Tables 3A/B indicate a substantial increase in self reported happiness and Tables 4A/4B a similar dramatic increase in confidants. Similarly, Table 5 documents increased self reports of emotional well-being. These data were obtained through written resident surveys.

TABLE 3A. Residents' Self Reported Happiness Prior to Admission

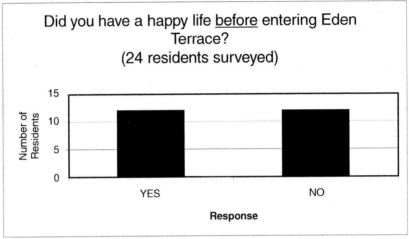

Data were collected through written surveys in 2001.

TABLE 3B. Residents' Self Reported Happiness Post Admission

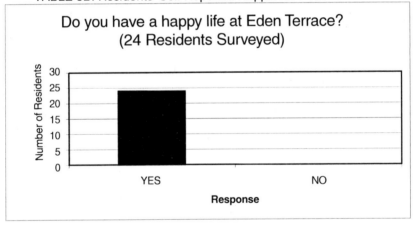

Data were collected through written surveys in 2001.

LIMITATIONS

While Australia faces various limitations when introducing culture change and the Eden Alternative™, several of the challenges are not unique to Australia, but are rather global issues. Australia continues to struggle with drastic

TABLE 4A. Residents' Self Report of Confidants–Pre-Admission

Did you have someone to confide in <u>before</u> coming to Eden Terrace?
(24 residents surveyed)

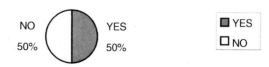

Data were collected through written surveys in 2001.

TABLE 4B. Residents' Self Report of Confidants–Post Admission

Do you always have someone to confide in at Eden Terrace?
(24 residents surveyed)

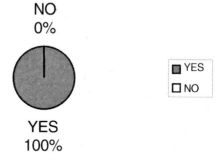

Data were collected through written surveys in 2001.

shortages of Registered Nurses to work in the Aged Care sector. The Aged Care industry has become highly regulated with great documentation, consequently taking careers away from the residents to document in order to receive government funding. This also contributes to the shortages of nurses, as the overload of paperwork makes the industry less desirable.

Aged Care organisations have been urged to increase the size of Aged Care Homes. Family/smaller organisations have been forced to either move out of

TABLE 5. Residents' Self Reported Well Being Pre and Post Admission

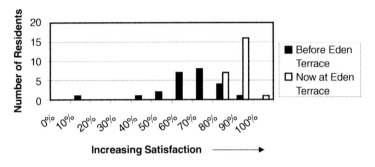

Data were collected through written surveys in 2001.

the Aged Care field or apply for more beds license, for financial viability. In Australia a stand alone low care facility operating with 50 residents or less will struggle to survive economically. This has been the case for Aged Care Service Group, starting as a small business and then forced to expand into 2 states and plan for further growth and development.

In recent years, Australia has introduced the notion of building certification. Certification means that guidelines and standards have been introduced into Commonwealth funded Aged Care homes to ensure that their building meets a satisfactory standard for operation. While theoretically valid, it has meant the closure of many inner metropolitan homes. These bed licenses can be relocated or rebuilt; nonetheless, there is not the land availability in these areas to rebuild or relocate in outer suburbs, subsequently forcing elders to move into areas outside their community.

Homes introducing Culture change and the Eden Alternative™ into Australia still face the challenge of "breaking the norm," "pushing the boundaries" and educating the public and the industry about this social model approach. Most homes still operate in a traditional medical model and view the elderly as receivers, dependent and vulnerable. Organisations such as Aged Care Service Group have already received some backlash from others in the industry related, in this author's view, to the fear of change or the unknown. It is most important to educate the staff and residents about balancing giving with receiving, teaching residents to restore their independence, as well as their social well being. Staff must be trained to re-evaluate their traditional care practises and allow residents to be independent, assist in their own care and have the opportunity to give back. Australia has required people introducing the Eden Alternative™ to promote this concept through journals, radio and other media sources. These Homes must continue to lead the way in changing the culture of aged care in Australia.

RELEVANCE TO SOCIAL WORK PRACTICE, VALUES, THEORY

In Australia, social workers are not commonly found working directly in Aged Care Homes. Social Workers are predominant members of Aged Care Assessment Services, assisting the elderly and their families to find care facilities. Social Workers perform assessments of cognition, psychosocial wellbeing, including depression as a part of an ACAS team.

Awareness and knowledge of culture change and the Eden Alternative™ is vital to social workers working in the Aged Care industry as it provides them with the opportunity to educate clients about positive ageing, maintaining independence and directing people to pro-active Aged Care organisations, such as Eden Alternative™ homes. Philosophies of culture change support social work theories of person-centred care and self-determination. It allows elderly residents to be actively involved in the choice and decision making of their life and their future, empowering them to maintain their "right to risk," and live freely and independently.

Culture change and the Eden Alternative™ build upon formal social work theory such as self-determination, self-directed group work, self-development and person-centered work. It also relies on "informal" social work theory, informal theory being the use of "moral, political, cultural values drawn upon by practitioners for defining 'functions' of social work" (Payne, 1997, p. 39). Formal social work theory such as humanist perspective is important in Aged Care as it supports the culture of self-growth, self-determination and person-centred work. According to Carl Rogers, workers' approach "should be non-directive, non-judgmental and, in later formulations should involve 'active listening,' 'accurate empathy' and 'authentic friendship'" (Payne, 1997, p. 179).

NEXT STEPS

The next step is to spread the awareness across Australia about the Eden Alternative™ and culture change through further national publishing, radio and television. Industry body organizations such as Aged Care Queensland are highly proactive in this regard, offering Eden Alternative™ Associate training and now working to create "Eden in OZ," so that Australian homes can become registered.

People are becoming more readily aware of these concepts; however, Australians still regard it as a USA culture and philosophy with all trend data of positive results also coming from the USA. Australian Aged Care organizations need to develop their own base data and comparative results pre and post culture change, so that Australians can see its relevance and viability here as well. As culture change is still relatively new, time is required before positive results can be disseminated nationally. It is encouraging that strong links have been built between the USA and Australian Aged Care industries. Hopefully in the future our elders can look forward to more independent, happy, healthy ageing in environments they can call home–regardless of the continent on which they live.

REFERENCES

MacKenzie, D. (December 2000, February 2001, May 2001, & August 2001). *National Health Care Journal* NSW, Australia nhj@healthnet.com.au.

MacKenzie, S. (August, 2001). *National Health Care Journal* NSW, Australia nhj@healthnet.com.au.

Payne, M. (1997). *Modern Social Work Theory (2nd Edition)*. MacMillan, Hampshire UK.

Beyond the Medical Model–
The Eden Alternative® in Practice:
A Swiss Experience

Christa Monkhouse

SUMMARY. The medical or institutional model of care has been the standard in most of the 1300 nursing homes in Switzerland. Consequently, staffing problems, increasing costs and poor reputation have become the norm. This case study describes two 60-resident homes in Zollikon, Switzerland, which implemented the Eden Alternative®, beginning in 2000. Based on this model, they are committed to the eradication of resident loneliness, helplessness and boredom. Their tools are companionship, spontaneity and the opportunity to give care to each other, staff, children, animals and plants. The change from a medical model was precipitated by a care and financial crisis. Since then, three

Christa Monkhouse, RN, Clinical Nurse Specialist in Elderly Care, is the Director of Nursing Services and the Deputy Director of APZ Adlergarten, Winterthur, Switzerland. She is a member of the Swiss Association of Expert-Nurses (PES) and the Swiss Association for the Development of Professional Hotel Service in Healthcare Institutions (SIHP).

Address correspondence to: Christa Monkhouse, Speerstrasse 16, 8200 Schaffhausen Switzerland (E-mail: monkhouse@shlink.ch).

Thanks go to Irene Bischofberger, RN, BNS, MSc, Basel, Switzerland, who helped prepare this manuscript and to Gaye Holliday, RN, Regina, Canada, who introduced the author to the Eden Alternative®.

[Haworth co-indexing entry note]: "Beyond the Medical Model–The Eden Alternative® in Practice: A Swiss Experience." Monkhouse, Christa. Co-published simultaneously in *Journal of Social Work in Long-Term Care* (The Haworth Social Work Practice Press, an imprint of The Haworth Press, Inc.) Vol. 2, No. 3/4, 2003, pp. 339-353; and: *Culture Change in Long-Term Care* (ed: Audrey S. Weiner, and Judah L. Ronch) The Haworth Social Work Practice Press, an imprint of The Haworth Press, Inc., 2003, pp. 339-353. Single or multiple copies of this article are available for a fee from The Haworth Document Delivery Service [1-800-HAWORTH, 9:00 a.m. - 5:00 p.m. (EST). E-mail address: docdelivery@haworthpress.com].

steps have been taken. The first, the crisis intervention step, was followed by the implementation of total quality management resulting in significant improvements in clinical outcomes and financial stability. Ultimately, the Eden Alternative was successfully introduced. It was perceived as "the missing link" and appears, at this early stage, to meet the real needs of residents and staff. The change process is described and outcomes are presented and discussed. *[Article copies available for a fee from The Haworth Document Delivery Service: 1-800-HAWORTH. E-mail address: <docdelivery@haworthpress.com> Website: <http://www.HaworthPress.com>*

KEYWORDS. Culture change, paradigm shift, human habitat environment, Switzerland, nursing homes, Eden Alternative®, TQM, elders

INTRODUCTION

Switzerland, a country with 7.2 million inhabitants, is a federal state composed of 26 cantons. The Federal Constitution grants large autonomy to the single cantons in the sectors which are not regulated by the constitution itself, among others the health and social service sector. The decision making autonomy of the cantons in the field of health and social care for the elderly created a strong heterogeneity in the regulations and organization across this country (Crivelli et al., 2001).

In addition to the private, for profit facilities, a majority of the 1300 nursing homes in Switzerland are funded and managed by local political communities. The communities, in turn, are in varying degrees, subsidized by the cantons. The community council, which is elected every four years, determines the annual operating and capital budget, the level and type of staffing, the room rates, building maintenance programs and suppliers for the non profit facilities.

The cantonal health authorities inspect the homes once a year by sending in a local district inspector, who is an elected lay person. There have been no national standards with which homes have to comply, so this inspection is subjective.

Before 1996 care bills had to be largely paid by the resident. In 1996 a new health care law was passed, which entitled nursing home residents to be reimbursed for nursing care by national health insurance. Every facility which provides care for residents is entitled to bill the state funded health-insurance companies and are also subjected to quality assurance programs. Homes are, at present, permitted to slowly implement a system for quality assurance, as standards have not been fully established.

Skyrocketing costs since 1996 and a reputation as a place which is neither desirable for staff or residents frequently stirs negative public discussion about nursing homes.

Solutions put forward suggest better trained staff, regular counseling for staff and better pay. An increasing number of homes have changed their names to "geriatric competence center" or "geriatric rehabilitation center" in recent years. The emphasis on medical terminology is intended to make the facility look more attractive to trained staff by avoiding the stigma attached to the negative image of "nursing home." Other homes now call themselves "center for living for the aged" and introduce pets into their environment. The effect of both approaches is unknown but indicates a search for solutions to the problems mentioned above.

The following case study describes two nursing homes which responded to this crisis in long-term care by implementing the Eden Alternative.

THE CASE STUDY

These two homes are located in Zollikon, a Swiss German town, close to Zurich, the economic and cultural metropolis of Switzerland. Zollikon spreads out on a hillside sloping down to Lake Zurich. It has 12 000 inhabitants, 20% of whom are over 65 years old. There are two elderly care facilities, managed by the community, built in the seventies. Modeled on hospitals, each facility has sixty beds in single and double rooms. There are only a few rooms which have a private bathroom. One home, which is located close to the town's market square, was intended for residents who require very little care, while the other home on the lake front was designed for residents needing more care by incorporating two large bathrooms, wheelchair access and a "medical-equipment" room on each floor. The separation of residents by level of care resulted in married couples being separated from each other. The average age of residents is 87 years. They are 70% women and 30% men; the mean length of stay is 2.5 years. An estimated 20% of the residents have dementia, others have major physical impairments.

In 1999 the author was appointed as crisis manager of one of the homes, on an eight month contract, by the newly elected community town-counselor for health, who was alarmed by the conditions of the homes and was committed to their improvement. Two recent surveys, one conducted by the Alzheimer Society and one by an independent health consulting firm, had indicated a 60% incidence of resident depression, the regular use of physical restraints, 60% staff turnover, high staff absenteeism and extensive use of costly agency staff, thus exceeding the staffing budget by 30%. The reputation in the community was poor and family members appeared to be highly dissatisfied with the home's information policy and billing practice. Beds had to be left empty due to short staffing. This measure resulted in decreased revenue for the homes.

> In late 1998, when I first went to visit the homes, I knew nothing about elderly care at this time, it struck me, how cold and hostile the environment seemed, the place was quiet, residents lined up in wheelchairs in the hall, not moving, many of them tied to their chairs, so they could not get up. My first thought was that there must be a different way to run these homes. (Dr. G. Neukomm, town counselor, 2001)

THE AUTHOR'S ROLE

As noted, the author was hired to "manage the crisis" and then transition the management of both homes to a newly hired administrator. After completion of the mandate, the author remained in contact with the institutions which provided opportunities for an ongoing professional discourse. In October 2000, the philosophy of the Eden Alternative was introduced to the new manager by the author. From September to November 2001 the author was permitted to collect data for the case study (Yin, 1994), in order to describe the change process and to identify outcomes following the introduction of the Eden Alternative. She was permitted to participate in meetings with residents and families, to conduct two hour interviews with the town-counselor, administrator and staff and to record notes. She was allowed to make use of the collected photos, videos, stories, drawings and narrative accounts from members of the nursing, auxiliary, hotel and technical staff.

BEGINNING THE PROCESS OF CHANGE

The framework of Total Quality Management (TQM) (Juran, 1989; Deming, 1986) was initially selected as quality assurance and cost effectiveness were identified as the first priority by the new administrator in 2000.

The TQM model was attractive as it goes far beyond process-reengineering. Rather it recognizes that good leadership can and should result in a culture change and subsequently a new organization (see Figure 1). TQM's focus is on clients' needs and the continuous improvement of services by empowering residents and employees. These measures are intended to also result in cost-effectiveness.

The following preliminary mission statement was put forward by the administrator:

FIGURE 1. TQM–The Transformation

Organization A $\rightarrow$ TQM $\rightarrow$ Organization B
Not Organization A $_{plus\,TQM}$

(Caldwell, 1995)

Elderly care is an exciting field to work in if we consider the residents of our homes as mature decision makers about their care and if we empower staff to follow upon these decisions. (Wapplinger, 2001)

During the first year of this transition, the level of dependency and care needs increased considerably in both facilities. Beds in the homes had been shut down due to staffing shortage, thus new residents, waiting in hospital beds, were given priority for admission. In contrast to prior policy, the administrator decided not to move residents from one home to the other as they became more frail. Therefore more nursing staff positions had to be created and financed by the community. Staff turnover was 60% in the first year as some staff did not accept a new leadership culture and resigned. The turnover in managerial staff was 85%. Room rates had to be raised by 30% to support the increased costs of staffing before a visible difference in the quality of care could be shown to the residents and their families. In the short term this resulted in operational deficits; a financial and a quality audit were therefore conducted by an independent consulting firm. Interestingly, favorable outcomes were attributed to the new administrator. The key outcome of both audits was that budgets were used efficiently and in favor of the residents, resulting in improved quality of care.

Using the TQM model for problem solving, the following results had been accomplished during the first year. More and better qualified staff in nursing, housekeeping and maintenance had been hired. An in-house education system, hosting educational sessions every week, was implemented. Standards for care, meal service and housekeeping were established including flexible mealtimes and more variety of menus from which to choose. Finger-food for demented residents who had forgotten how to use cutlery was introduced, so weight loss of residents could be prevented and feeding time by nursing staff could be reduced.

Most rooms had been renovated. Residents were encouraged to furnish their rooms to their taste and with their own belongings. An interior decorator enriched the hallways and the dining room with new curtains, plants, chairs and tables. Families were invited to participate in decision making by attending family nights at both facilities where an opportunity is provided to share wishes and concerns. A residents' assembly was held every two weeks in order to obtain input from the residents. Residents with dementia were increasingly represented by a spouse or family member at this assembly. The attending physicians were kept abreast and supportive about the changes. Close communication was established and maintained with the staff and the town-counselor of health, as the additional considerable costs had to be paid by the local government (Wapplinger, 2001).

Care had improved and the facilities' finances were stronger when the homes' administrator learned about the Eden Alternative from the author, who had herself encountered this approach to elderly care in a nursing home in Canada through a visit in September, 2000. Following this initial experience, a meeting with the founder, William Thomas, MD, further explained the philosophy and model:

> The medical model had been in the past erroneously generalized as the overall model for facilities which care for frail elderly residents. This approach, which is adequate in hospitals, where "real life" is suspended for a short period of time for treatment, produces life threatening conditions for residents in nursing homes, as they experience loneliness, helplessness and boredom, which are the three plagues and major sources of suffering for the elderly. The necessity for other activities of residents had been recognized, but mostly been fitted into the routines of care and treatment and named "therapy," like activity therapy, pet-therapy. The Eden Alternative provides a paradigm shift, an entirely new way of looking at nursing homes by turning them into human habitats allowing companionship, giving care to animals and plants and where there is spontaneity and decision making by residents and the staff, closest to them. (Thomas, 2000)

The author was convinced that the Eden Alternative had the potential to "replace one conceptual world view–the medical model–by another–the human habitat model" and could therefore foster the necessary paradigm shift (Kuhn, 1970), in elderly care. The homes' administrator grasped that these three plagues, despite the seemingly effective TQM-efforts, still existed in the homes. The Eden Alternative was, at that point, viewed as a potential major enrichment to the culture in both homes.

> The Eden Alternative attached names to the real needs of our residents, which to us no one before Dr. Thomas has accomplished so concisely. I realized, that the plagues were induced by the institutions themselves as

they are based on the medical or treatment model. I became aware of the fact, that despite all quality efforts this model had never been substantially challenged. What we have been trying to do was cushioning the impact of the medical model. We included the residents and staff into decision making and stretched the routines of the institutional model to the limit to fit resident's individuality. A good deal of flexibility had been displayed by all the staff. The key insight, which struck me like a lightning bolt, was that nursing homes could be turned into colorful places for living and growth. The services provided should support living and growth and all staff participate. Residents would not choose to live in a nursing home if they could provide for themselves. (Wapplinger, 2001)

FROM TQM TO THE EDEN ALTERNATIVE

If culture is understood as "shared, learned human behavior, a way of life which is based on accepted rules for living, ideals and values" (Bodley, 1994), the anecdotes and narratives which follow illustrate a change of behavior and attitudes in staff and residents which can be considered valid indicators of cultural change. According to the administrator (Wapplinger, 2001), they represent primarily new behaviors. The insights about the potential of the Eden Alternative as an entirely new way of thinking about nursing homes, can be characterized as a breakthrough, a term defined in the glossary of TQM (Onnias, 1992):

> In the context of quality, the term is applied mainly in relation to obtaining new knowledge that will provide a vision, an understanding at a level never reached before. The new knowledge is so important, so effective, that the problem will have to be re-examined in the light of the new condition reached.

The insights which led from TQM to the Eden approach were conveyed to the staff as a story of enlightenment and inspiration. As put forward by the mission statement of the Eden Alternative (Thomas, 1999), the concept proved to be strikingly simple to communicate and was received with enthusiasm.

> We encountered the Eden Alternative just at the right moment for us, it was, as if we had found the missing link, words for the real needs of our residents. We told the staff that we were committed to re-examining the work we had done so far under the new "compass" of the Eden Alternative. We would do so to further improve the quality of life for residents. (Wapplinger, 2001)

At the weekly scheduled management and staff meetings, staff were familiarized with the concepts of the Eden Alternative. There were lengthy discussions of the three plagues and their remedies. According to Thomas the remedy for loneliness is companionship, for helplessness the opportunity to give care and against boredom, spontaneity. Staff were encouraged to initiate their own remedial experiments. Formal three day training sessions were planned for the spring 2001. Participants completing the sessions would be certified as Eden Associates. For this purpose, the author returned to Canada and participated in training hosted by the Sherbrooke Community Center, Saskatoon. The training was presented by the Region 17 coordinators for Eden. They shared their three year "Edenizing" (Thomas, 2000) experience with the author in great detail and were most helpful in preparing and translating the teaching materials into German. The Eden Associate Training can now be conducted in the German speaking countries of Europe, such as Switzerland, Austria and Germany, starting in Zollikon. By November 2001, 60 of the 120 staff had completed the Eden Associate training.

The staff, residents and families in the Zollikon facilities had been well prepared due to the TQM changes. Thomas (1999), often using gardening metaphors, would have stated that "the soil was warm and ready for new seeds to be planted." Staff in Zollikon were excited by the fact that they were the first nursing home in Europe to transform their facility into a colorful and lively habitat for the residents, families and themselves. Before the training sessions began, the Eden Alternative approach to living for the residents was discussed with family members on three occasions. Family response was enthusiastic. One relative said:

> From my own experience with my mother, helplessness was the worst plague to fear in a nursing home after a long life filled with work and care for a large family, you are doing the right thing. My only question is, all this sounds so simple, why did it not occur to you earlier, to take this route? You could have avoided lots of suffering from residents and families. You know, it makes us feel guilty to place a family member in a facility knowing they will be plagued by helplessness and loneliness.

This statement gave a new insight into the burden of guilt families have to carry. The adoption of the Eden Alternative, it was realized, could alleviate their suffering as well.

After the training and with the support of the administrator and many relatives, results were realized in rapid succession. Stories about fighting the plagues began to take up time at shift handovers. A nurse started to bring her two dogs from home to spend time with the residents who started to care for them.

Residents inquired when the nurse would come back from her days off, as the dogs would be back as well. Residents started sharing stories about their own pets when they were younger. Staff wondered if residents had lost their need to get up in the morning, once their pet had died. This was often followed by mood deterioration and a negative impact on their overall health. Anecdotally staff noted that this was often followed by hospitalization and subsequent admission to the nursing home. As understanding of the helplessness plague increased among staff, and through resident initiation, two guinea pigs, two cats and a few birds and fish were brought into the homes. Careful preparation was carried out with the residents about feeding, care and living with pets.

Residents found planning as exciting as the pets themselves. Plans for more dogs, cats and birds were being discussed in early 2002 by the residents. New residents are encouraged to bring their pets with them. Residents were who don't like animals are encouraged to make their views known. If there is disagreement, a vote is held and the majority prevails. This is an accepted practice in Switzerland, where most of the political decisions are made by democratic processes. No health regulations restrict the housing of pets in nursing homes.

Residents are beginning to assert their own wishes. A shoeshine machine was selected and purchased by residents with the help of the maintenance technician. The same technician, fully committed to the Eden Alternative, took residents in a van to select a new barber chair for the hair salon. Residents immediately took ownership of their new purchase and suggested that there should be a beauty salon as well. It opened in October 2001; it is successful, as business hours had to be extended by 20%.

Male residents, who are in the minority, have been encouraged to take part in light repair of the home. They change lightbulbs, one man painted the newspaper stand, others repotted plants with the maintenance crew. A maintenance staff member, a passionate hobby gardener himself, suggested planting lettuce and herbs in window boxes so that residents who are chair- or bedbound can garden on their balconies. This initiative was received as a remarkable step forward to fight helplessness, because it came from a man who had worked quietly in one of the homes for over twenty years. When he was recognized for his initiative he was very happy.

> In early November when we had the first snowfall, I saw a nursing assistant sneaking out the back door to gather up some snow in a bucket and bring it back in for a bedbound resident to feel it and play with it. The resident had memories of winter as the most pleasurable season of the year. He was so happy he had the assistant take a picture to show his visitors. Staff started photo albums about "Eden-moments," recording incidents on video and writing down vignettes of such moments which then could

be shared with colleagues, residents and visitors. The activities going on in this regard are most exciting. (clinical nurse specialist, 2001, personal communication)

Earlier in my career I did everything to help people sleep. I quietly walked the aisles and distributed sleeping pills wherever required. Residents who get their day and night rhythm mixed up were gently coaxed back into their beds to sleep. With Eden in mind I act differently. Residents who wake up and don't want to go back to sleep are given coffee or even breakfast if they want. They can talk about how they feel and later they often offer to wash the dishes they had used. We got to know each other better and loneliness has no chance as I turned from a "warden of peace and quiet" into the nighttime companion of waking residents. Often they go back to bed in the early morning hours and are now allowed to sleep in. I think there will be evidence that the use of sleeping pills has decreased considerably. There are times when a few residents are awake and we have started a nighttime coffee-shop. Eden does not stop when the night falls, I am so proud of my work and find it very rewarding. (night-nurse, 2001, personal communication)

The author herself noticed that every time she visited the homes, the lobby and the cafeteria seemed busier, noisier, with more visitors during weekdays, many of them bringing their dogs. More children are seen visiting the homes. Staff bring their children along on Sundays or have them visit after school. A nurse invited her neighbor, a mother of three, to come for coffee to her workplace as they never seem to have time to meet privately. The children and the mother found the residents such good company that they decided to come back.

I can now do such things, knowing that I can counter loneliness and boredom. This is fun and rewarding and it makes so much sense to me. We have the resources, there is no extra work involved. My instincts had often told me that there is more to caring than doing a good hands-on nursing job, sometimes I followed my instincts. Secretly, on Sundays, I brought my godchild in, and the residents liked her, but I never knew, if this was allowed. Now I know and this knowledge is very liberating. (unit manager, 2001, personal communication)

There are many more stories to be found in the "Eden Albums" which have been created by staff. In addition to the narrative outcomes, data has been tracked for quantifiable results. The administrator states:

We have been collecting baseline data like falls, infections, use of physical restraints, these will be evaluated by the end of the year. Sick leave times have decreased by 15%, occupancy rate is up from 85 to 97%. We have evidence that staff turnover is on the decline (from 45% to 30%). If all this is due to Edenizing, the future will tell, given the short period, we treat the data with caution. From five open posts last year we have advanced to a small waiting list of three qualified nurses, while other homes are still terribly understaffed. Staff seem to be the best advocates for the Eden Alternative outside the homes when they talk to family and friends about it. Increasingly we get applications through word of mouth. We observe a decrease of medication supply orders by an estimated 20%. We have at least three phone calls of prospective residents, saying they want a place as they had heard good things about us from the press. We kept the local newspaper informed on the changes in our homes. (Wapplinger, 2001)

We would have had increasing costs anyhow, with or without the Eden Alternative, there is no way to run a nursing home cheaply. The Eden Alternative does not cost more money, I am convinced of that. We seem to save money as staff stays longer. If I had opened a heart-transplant center, money would have been given to this supposedly prestigious project with no questions asked. Spending money on nursing homes is different, there is no prestige attached to that. So I work hard to attain consent on every cent spent on the homes from my counsel colleagues, I talk a lot with them and assure their support. I am sure that one day the inert attitude towards nursing homes will change and it will be of advantage to political parties, to show concern for the elderly population. I personally support the Eden Alternative as I remember too clearly the first impression I had when I was newly elected and inspected the homes. I then had wished for an alternative, today we have one. (Dr. G. Neukomm, 2001)

LIMITATIONS

This case study represents twelve months experience of an Edenizing process of two nursing homes in Switzerland. The results appear very promising. It can be assumed that many homes in the US "doing Eden " would be able to give similar accounts of their experience. Numerous anecdotes about a change in behavior of staff and residents indicate an irreversible and successful culture change towards "a life worth living" (Thomas, 2000). Anecdotal evidence of culture change is therefore treated as valid as statistical evidence. Quantitative data, due to the short time frame, cannot serve as a basis to draw final conclusions. It is critical to note that staff turnover rate might have decreased without the Eden Alternative, as the TQM culture is also an empowering one, thus having the capacity to retain staff.

DISCUSSION

The impact of the Eden Alternative has been demonstrated by Ransom (2000), in her measures of clinical outcomes in Texas nursing homes. She found a 60% reduction in behavioral incidents, 57% decrease in pressure sores and 18% reduction in use of restraints. Increase in census (11%) and decrease of staff absenteeism (48%), were also attributed to Eden. Drawing from social support literature, the concept of companionship (Wills, 1991) can be seen as a strong agent to buffer daily stressors and therefore being conducive to health. Residents in nursing homes suffer from the stress of the institutional environment in addition to their chronic illnesses. More stress is often created by having to accept help and assistance. Caring companionship appears to be a powerful tool alleviating the feeling of indebtedness, resulting from having to receive help. It makes it easier for people to receive help when they have the opportunity to reciprocate (Nadler, 1991). Social support can enhance self esteem and an overall feeling of mastery. Being able to give support is found to enhance one's sense of self efficacy and self image (Spacaban & Oskamp, 1992). Thus depression triggered by the experience of helplessness can be prevented (Jones, 1991). There is an abundance of evidence to be found in the literature (Veiel & Baumann, 1992) on meaning, measurement and practical applications of caring support, which is a key concept of the Eden Alternative. However, further discussion would be beyond the scope of this case study.

From the perspective of employees, who are close to the residents and thus add to the variety of social contacts available to them, and who appear to stay longer in an Eden Alternative environment, the theory of Salutogenesis, developed by Antonovsky (1997) holds a promising explanation. He explored factors which keep human beings healthy, despite severe physical or emotional stress factors, which are known to be a major cause of immunological, cardiovascular and psychosomatic diseases. He identified as the core concept of salutogenesis the "sense of coherence" which means:

> one has an enduring though dynamic feeling of confidence, that the world one lives in is structured, predictable and explicable. That the resources to meet the demands of this world are available and that these demands are challenges worthy of investment and engagement.

The work environment within an Edenizing home appears to be "comprehensible, manageable and meaningful" (Antonovsky, 1997). As employees stated and the above anecdotes attest, the plagues of loneliness, helplessness and boredom are comprehensible for staff as they can intuitively relate to them. Staff efforts to remedy the plagues draw from their own needs and inner resources to provide companionship, meaningful activities and spontaneity. This is not perceived as extra effort but unleashing tremendous untapped resources within the staff. These are, in fact, resources which have unknowingly been there but not utilized by the medical model approach to elderly care. Staff agree that the Eden Alternative has added a new meaning to their work. A sense of coherence has been shown to be a powerful predictor of coping with stress and thus staying healthy (Schüffel & Brucks, 1998). It can be concluded that an environment implementing the Eden Alternative promotes the health and wellbeing of staff who in turn can provide a nurturing climate for the residents.

NEXT STEPS

The focus of further development will be on the full transformation of both nursing homes into a "human habitat" (Thomas, 2000). The process can be visualized by using Figure 2, as it is clear, that after the TQM transformation (from A to B) there will be a new transformation from "a very good institution" (from B to C) to a human habitat.

The course of action will not differ from what has been described in this case study, other than there will be training for every existing and new staff member. There will be a combination of organic changes initiated by staff and residents and planned changes. Planned changes are specified in the managerial goals for the year 2002, for example, the establishment of an effective complaint management system. There are also plans to reach out into the community by having school classes or daycare in the homes.

Both buildings need major reconstruction in the next years and it was decided to use the Eden Alternative as a guideline to this process.

FIGURE 2

Organization B→ Eden Alternative® →
Organization C
Not Organization B plus Eden Alternative®

(Adapted from Caldwell, 1995)

"We are not modernizing a hospital by putting in private bathrooms and modern appliances. We will create a big household where there is professional support available to the residents," the town-counselor says. "This is the way we approach our architects, as we are their clients who try to make the world a better place for our elderly population." (Dr. G. Neukomm, 2001)

A conference on the Eden Alternative© featuring Dr. Thomas and the Zollikon staff was held in November 2001 for other interested home-managers, politicians and press. Funding for research will be pursued. It is felt that there should be quality of life measurements available which support the view of residents, staff and management that the Eden Alternative is the "right thing to do as it fulfills the needs of residents and staff" (Thomas, 1999) and that it is indeed a solution for the pressing problems institutional elderly care faces today.

The administrator summarizes her experience:

The true added value of the implementation of the Eden Alternative is that every employee, beside doing a very good job in his or her field, contributes to remedying loneliness, helplessness and boredom. This is achieved by being a companion, explore what is meaningful in the life of the residents and provide opportunities to give care. Being spontaneous means laughing, joking and the power to alter routines. Staff are familiar with the TQM-tools and use them if there is systematic improvement to be achieved. At the same time the Eden Alternative provides the overarching philosophy to everything we do. All this is tremendously fulfilling, for me and my staff. (Wapplinger, 2001)

REFERENCES

Antonovsky, A. (1997). Salutogenese. Zur Entmystifizierung der Gesundheit. Tübingen: dgvt.

Bodley, J.H. (1994). *An Anthropological Perspective.* http://www.wsu.edu:8001/vchsu/commons/topics/culture/culture-index.html.

Caldwell, C. (1995). *Mentoring Strategic Change in Health Care.* Milwaukee, Wisconsin: ASQC Quality Press.

Crivelli, L., Filippini, M. & Lunati, D. (2001). Effizienz der Pflegeheime in der Schweiz. Lugano, Svizzera: Quaderno N. 01-06 Decanato della Facoltà di Scienze economiche.

Deming, W.E. (1986). *Out of the Crisis.* Cambridge, Massachusetts: MIT-Press.

Jones, S. (1991). Education and life in a long stay ward. In Denham, M. J. (editor), *Care of the Long-Stay Elderly Patient* (p. 161-182). London, New York, Tokyo, Melbourne, Madras: Chapman and Hall.

Juran, J.M. (1989). *Juran on Leadership for Quality.* New York: Free Press.

Kuhn, T. (1970). *The Structure of Scientific Revolutions.* Chicago: The University of Chicago Press.

Nadler, A. (1991). Help-Seeking Behavior. In Clark, M. S. (editor), *Prosocial Behavior* (p. 290-311). Newbury Park, London, New Delhi: Sage Publications.

Neukomm, G. (2001). Interview minutes November 7th.

Onnias, A. (1992). *The Language of Total Quality.* Castellamone, Italy: TPOK® Publications on Quality.

Ransom, S. (2000). *Eden Alternative: The Texas Project.* Texas: Texas Long Term Care Institute, College of Health Professions, Southwest Texas State University.

Schüffel, W. & Brucks, U. (1998). Handbuch der Salutogenese. Wiesbaden: Ullstein Medical.

Spacaban, S. & Oskamp, S. (1992). An Introduction to Naturalistic Studies of Helping. In Spacaban, S. & Oskamp, S. (editors), *Helping and Being Helped* (p. 1-15). Newbury Park, London, New Delhi: Sage Publications.

Thomas, W.H. (1999). *The Eden Alternative Handbook.* Sherburne, New York: Summer Hill Company Inc.

Thomas, W.H. (2000). Life worth living. Acton, Massachusetts: VanderWyk & Burnham.

Veiel, H. & Baumann, U. (1992). *The Meaning and Measurement of Social Support.* New York, Washington, Philadelphia, London: Hemisphere Publishing Corporation.

Wapplinger, R. (2001). Interview minutes November 15th.

Wills, T.A. (1991). Social Support and Interpersonal Relationships. In Clark, M.S. (editor), *Prosocial Behavior* (p. 265-289). Newbury Park, London, New Delhi: Sage Publications.

Yin, R.K. (1994). *Case Study Research.* Thousand Oaks, London, New Delhi: Sage Publications.

Changes in Long-Term Care
for Elderly People with Dementia:
A Report from the Front Lines
in British Columbia, Canada

Nancy Gnaedinger

SUMMARY. Recent changes in dementia care in Canada, based primarily on successes in Sweden and Australia, include clustering small numbers of residents together, delivering care in a flexible and individualized manner, and permanent scheduling of front line multi-skilled staff. This model, generically referred to as "resident-centred" care, has

Nancy Gnaedinger, MA, is Research Affiliate of Simon Fraser University in Vancouver, and Independent Consultant in Gerontology based in Victoria, British Columbia, Canada. The Hospital Employees' Union of British Columbia, a provincial union with over 13,000 members providing long-term care, contracted the author to design and conduct the exploratory study summarized in this article.

Requests for copies of the full research report should be sent to: Marcy Cohen, Research and Policy Planner, Hospital Employees' Union of British Columbia, 5000 North Fraser Way, Burnaby BC Canada V5J 5M3 (E-mail: mcohen@heu.org).

Other correspondence should be directed to: Nancy Gnaedinger, MA, Consultant in Gerontology, 2705 Arbutus Road, Victoria BC Canada V8N 1W8 (E-mail: ngnaed@islandnet.com).

The author acknowledges the wisdom, passion and true caring of the front line workers who participated in the study.

[Haworth co-indexing entry note]: "Changes in Long-Term Care for Elderly People with Dementia: A Report from the Front Lines in British Columbia, Canada." Gnaedinger, Nancy. Co-published simultaneously in *Journal of Social Work in Long-Term Care* (The Haworth Social Work Practice Press, an imprint of The Haworth Press, Inc.) Vol. 2, No. 3/4, 2003, pp. 355-371; and: *Culture Change in Long-Term Care* (ed: Audrey S. Weiner, and Judah L. Ronch) The Haworth Social Work Practice Press, an imprint of The Haworth Press, Inc., 2003, pp. 355-371. Single or multiple copies of this article are available for a fee from The Haworth Document Delivery Service [1-800-HAWORTH, 9:00 a.m. - 5:00 p.m. (EST). E-mail address: docdelivery@haworthpress.com].

10.1300/J181v2n03_12

been embraced by practice leaders across Canada, and yet there remain challenges to its implementation in the front lines. An exploratory, qualitative study focussing on front line workers' experience in British Columbia was conducted in 2000. Results revealed five key barriers to full implementation of resident-centred dementia care: workload, resistance to change at all levels, operational realities, resident characteristics, and the design and scale of the built environment. Keys to successfully implementing this approach were identified as: higher staff-to-resident ratios, effective leadership, formal involvement of front line staff in decision making, on-going education and training for all providers, and some rotation of staff scheduling. *[Article copies available for a fee from The Haworth Document Delivery Service: 1-800-HAWORTH. E-mail address: <docdelivery@haworthpress.com> Website: <http://www.HaworthPress.com> © 2003 by The Haworth Press, Inc. All rights reserved.]*

KEYWORDS. Dementia care, resident-centred care, front line workers

INTRODUCTION

Across Canada, the approach to long-term care is changing to accommodate the increasing number of residents who have dementia. Based primarily on successful Swedish and Australian models, architectural design, programming and staffing patterns are changing (Beck-Friis, 1988; Tooth, 1994; Dow & Gnaedinger, 2000). Some facilities are being built or adapted, based on what is variously called a "cottage," "neighbourhood" or "cluster" model,[1,2] where no more than 12 residents with dementia (and as few as eight) live in one dwelling unit, which is residential in character. Typically, several of these units are attached to a central administrative core. The approach to the provision of care has moved from a highly scheduled and task-oriented approach to a flexible, resident-centred approach based on the activities of daily living. Staffing patterns are also changing from task-specific with considerable rotation, to multi-skilled with deliberate continuity of staff and teams in each dwelling unit.[3]

Many practice leaders and health managers in Canada[4] regard these changes as appropriate and desirable in meeting the needs of elderly long-term care residents who are more frail, and more likely to have a dementia, than any previous cohort. As a consequence, various health authorities across Canada are embracing these ideas and attempting to implement changes in dementia care.[5] They are doing so, however, with very few Canadian references: In 1999, when this study was designed, there was a dearth of published reports based on Canadian dementia care practice,[6] and more specifically, there was a lack of research that *focussed on front line workers' experience and assessments of these new approaches to dementia care in long-term care.*[7]

Within this context, a study was commissioned by the Hospital Employees' Union of British Columbia (HEU),[8] and carried out in 2000. Its purpose was three-fold: (1) to learn about the changing approaches in long-term care for elderly people with dementia, specifically in the province of British Columbia; (2) to understand HEU front line workers' experiences and assessments of this model of care, more specifically, how it "plays out in practice"; and (3) to make a positive contribution to policies and practices that will result in supportive environments for both residents and staff in dementia care in British Columbia.

STUDY DESIGN AND METHODS

The nature of the study was exploratory and practical,[9] its scale was modest, and its scope was provincial, in keeping with the provincial mandate of the union. There were four phases and five different research methods used. First, recent literature on resident-centred care and other changes in dementia care was briefly scanned, to help prepare questions for interviews with key informants (Jones, 1996; Barnes, 1996, 1997, 1999; Johnson, n.d.). Second, in-depth telephone or face-to-face interviews were conducted with eight key informants, people considered "practice leaders" in the field of dementia care in British Columbia, all of them with a nursing background as well as administrative and/or educational experience.[10] They were asked about the philosophical roots, evolution, key components, challenges and benefits of changing approaches in dementia care. Third, a written survey was sent to HEU representatives to determine which long-term care facilities in British Columbia served by the union had the key characteristics of the new approach to dementia care: (1) small clusters of residents, (2) resident-centred programming based on the activities of daily living, and (3) multi-skilled staff with no or minimal rotation in assignments. From this list and in discussions with a number of HEU servicing representatives, sites which had at least two of the three characteristics were chosen as potential sites for focus groups with front line staff. Fourth, focus groups were conducted with front line staff in four long-term care facilities in different regions of British Columbia.[11] Thirty front line workers, including Care Aides, Licensed Practical Nurses, Housekeepers, Food Service and Maintenance staff, and Activation Assistants[12] participated in focus groups. Together, they represented 429 years' experience working with residents with dementia. They were asked about their experiences and assessments of the new approaches in dementia care. Participants' responses were recorded on a flip chart, then reviewed for confirmation with each group at the end of each session. The researcher also made diary notes immediately following each focus group session. Fifth, on-site, ad-hoc interviews were conducted with Administrators before or after the focus groups.

RESULTS

Tenets of Resident-Centred Dementia Care

The most fundamental change in long-term care for residents with dementia is a move from a medical and hierarchical model, which stresses residents' incapacities and staff's obligation to follow rigid schedules, to a social model, which emphasizes each resident's individuality and abilities, and empowers staff to flexibly provide support and care. This social model of care, known generically as "resident-centred care," is based on several sources, including Swedish and Australian experiences. In British Columbia, this model was initially introduced as the Gentle Care® philosophy[13] (Jones, 1996), which in turn was adopted, adapted and disseminated by the British Columbia Ministry of Health in the early 1990s, and has been implemented, unevenly, across the province since that time.

The key elements of a resident-centred model of dementia care are: a work culture that values the residents first; flexibility of residents' schedule and care; multi-skilled or multi-tasked workers; permanent assignments for front line staff (little or no rotation); front line workers' involvement in care planning; a respectful management philosophy; and small clusters of residents. Following is a description and discussion of each of these components, based on the findings from this study.

A Work Culture That Values the Residents First

The resident-centred model, as implied by its name, focuses on and values the residents first, before all else. It is apparent that this philosophy has been embraced by the front line workers who participated in this study. When asked to identify the best things that happen during their work day, their responses were almost exclusively resident-focussed.

> Getting a smile, a hug.
> Reaching a resident–finding the key.

Similarly, the worst things that happen during their work day are almost entirely resident-focussed.

> When a resident dies, it is hard, it is like loss in the family, in your life.
> Not having enough time to meet the emotional needs of the residents.

Flexibility of Residents' Schedule and Care

In resident-centred care, the goal is to create a natural "daily rhythm." The agenda for the day is not task-oriented and rigid, as in a hospital for instance, but instead is intended to be more like the predictable daily routine in a family, where each individual's abilities, preferences and personal history are taken into account. For example, if a resident had been a farmer, accustomed to getting up very early in the morning during the summer, this familiar habit would be accommodated.

Flexibility in the work day is generally regarded, by practice leaders and front line staff alike, as a positive feature of this model of care. Practice leaders observed,

> This approach to care taps into their creativity.
> Workers become empowered to make decisions about their work day.

Front line workers remarked,

> You organize your own time.
> You are more relaxed about scheduling residents' days.

There are challenges, however, to "creating the resident's day"–one of the credos of the resident-centred approach. According to key informants, many of the residents in long-term care these days are both "heavy physical care *and* severely cognitively impaired," unable to participate in activities of daily living. They require significant effort and time to toilet, bathe, dress, groom, and help with meals. This heavy personal care, coupled with the time required to manage residents' uncomprehending or agitated behaviour, results in a situation that is frustrating for front line staff who cannot spend the "social time" with residents that they would like to.

Multi-Skilling or Multi-Tasking

Another characteristic of the new approach to long-term care for residents with dementia is "multi-skilling" or "multi-tasking," which means that front line staff are required to do more than one category of work, just as a homemaker looking after a family does many different categories of work. Multi-skilled work may involve tasks that were formerly done by four different workers in long-term care facilities: Care Aides, Housekeepers, Food Service staff and Activation staff. There is no standard "multi-skilled worker" in dementia care in British Columbia, although it is fairly standard that Care Aides have become multi-skilled, whereas other service providers, in Dietary, Laundry and Housekeeping, are still single-tasked. Multi-skilling is in the early stages of evolution in this province.

One benefit of multi-skilled work is that it allows flexibility in routine and allows front line staff to become more familiar with each resident. On the other hand, multi-skilling can be frustrating for some front line workers.

> The housework tasks take away time from care time and one-to-one time!

Another limitation is that multi-skilling works best in a small scale environment, such as a large house, with small groupings or "families" of residents–for example, six residents for each worker. It does not work well in large facilities with long distances to travel and large numbers of residents in each wing.

Permanent Assignments for Front Line Staff

For front line staff to be able to create flexible and meaningful days for their residents, they must be very familiar with the individual residents. Giving front line staff long term or permanent assignments (working the same shift with the same group of residents for long or indefinite periods) facilitates this familiarity. It also makes it easier for family members to get to know staff members, and to share details of the residents' lives–information which is extremely helpful to staff. Another benefit of permanent assignments, according to both practice leaders and front line workers, is that continuity of staffing has been seen to reduce residents' agitation.

There are both advantages and disadvantages to permanent assignments. On one hand, being on permanent shifts and therefore familiar with individual residents, makes it easier for staff to anticipate residents' needs, which in turn makes staff more efficient in their work. On the other hand, non-rotation of staff, although important for residents' sense of continuity, is not always good for staff or for staff morale. Front line workers warned,

> Some staff members burn out.
> [It] is a mistake; it breeds impatience. . . . It also results in stagnation and higher expectations of staff among residents and families.

Front line workers recommended rotation every four to six months. This would allow them enough time to become familiar with residents, so that they could provide individualized care, but would also allow them to look forward to a refreshing change. It was indicated that front line staff also need flexibility in certain situations; for example, if they find it extremely stressful to work with a particular resident, they want to be able to change their shift or assignment.

Front Line Staff Involvement in Care Planning

An essential component of the resident-centred approach to dementia care is formal involvement by front line staff, especially Care Aides and Licensed Practical Nurses, in care planning. This involvement requires communication with other team members and with family members, careful documentation of the workers' activities and observations, and specialized knowledge in dementia care, provided through education and in-services. Involvement in care planning is considered meaningful and desirable by front line workers, who maintained,

> It makes you a valued member of the team.
> It is based on our familiarity with residents.

It appears that front line workers' involvement in care planning in long-term care in British Columbia varies by both workplace and supervisor, however. Front line workers noted,

> [The amount of involvement] depends on the RN. Some listen, some won't. It's hit and miss. Sometimes we are consulted on the spot.

Respectful Management Philosophy and Practice

Ideally, a resident-centred care environment can be developed and will thrive if management is respectful of staff, involving them in decision-making and the change process. Strong leadership and respectful management practice are critical. Practice leaders advised,

> You must treat your staff the way you want them to treat the residents—with respect and nurturing.
> Management must support, involve and consult, and be seen to support, involve and consult front line staff.

It is not easy to change from a traditional, hierarchical approach to a resident-centred approach. Change must be made in small increments, with each small change tested ("trialed") and assessed by all the people involved, including front line staff. Practice leaders cautioned,

> It is necessary to spend time and allow time for change to be implemented.

Involving front line staff in the change process requires leadership skills that many Administrators and Registered Nurses do not possess. A number of the practice leaders commented that this lack of leadership limits the implementation of the resident-centred approach.

Small Clusters of Residents

An important component of resident-centred dementia care is small groups or clusters of residents. Clustering residents in small groups in a home-like environment that is residential in scale can increase social interaction among residents, reduce noise and other aggravating stimuli that agitate residents, and ultimately, facilitate the implementation of flexible care. A practice leader asserted,

> When it looks like a house, you act like a house.

A front line worker warned, however,

> When you have to walk long distances to meet the needs of large numbers of residents, and use, and wait for, elevators, you cannot provide multi-skilled and flexible service to residents, nor do you have time for one-to-one contact.

In this study, the most frustrated and discontent front line workers were those who worked in the largest facilities, where they were being asked to "act like a house" in a large institution.

Barriers to Implementing Resident-Centred Dementia Care

Practice leaders and front line workers identified several barriers to implementing a resident-centred care model of dementia care. These are: workload, resistance to change, operational realities, resident characteristics, and the design and scale of the built environment.

Workload

It is apparent that one of the main barriers to implementing a resident-centred model of care is workload. The workload for all health care providers has increased steadily in recent decades, because residents' average age at placement, level of acuity and complexity of care needs have all increased significantly. At the same time, budgets are tighter for both service delivery and continuing education, there are higher expectations among residents and family members, and, added to this, there is a push to deliver individualized, resident-centred care. One practice leader and administrator professed,

> Administrators are between a rock and a hard place!

Similarly, front line workers are under pressure. As the weight of care becomes heavier, it is more and more difficult to provide individualized, flexible care and one-to-one attention to residents. This is a source of frustration and stress for front line staff, who declared,

> I work harder now than I ever have in my life.
> Some days you don't have time to go to the washroom!

Practice leaders say input from front line staff is essential in measuring workload; so is consistent use of a workload measure or tool. Workload measures should include residents' behaviour and cognitive status, and should be based on the "weight" of work involved, rather than on the number of residents per staff person, since one resident may entail three times the work of another. Two problems related to workload measures were identified by practice leaders:

> There is no valid workload measurement tool yet for multi-skilled staff.
> Managers are in a difficult spot . . . bureaucrats do not want to see the results. . . because the evidence points to the need for more staff.

Resistance to Change at All Levels

A fundamental problem identified by both practice leaders and front line staff is that some people at all levels of the organization are unwilling or unable to change the way they do their work. Some Directors of Care find it difficult to involve front line staff in the change process, and some Ward Registered Nurses resist the flattening of the hierarchy, the sharing of decision-making and on-going communication that are hallmarks of the resident-centred model. Some front line workers resist the change because they think it is unreasonable to expect them to do more with residents whose care needs are heavier and heavier, while staff-to-resident ratios do not increase.

Operational Realities

At least four operational realities create barriers to implementing a resident-centred model. First, many Administrators are now covering several facilities, which may be many kilometres apart. They are "grasshoppers, moving from one to another!" This lack of continuity means they are less able to participate in and receive feedback during the small, incremental changes that are part of the multi-faceted transition to a resident-centred approach. Another consequence of their "grasshopper" existence is that they are not able to become as familiar with their staff and residents as is expected in this model of care.

A second operational fact is the extensive use of "casual" front line workers. Casuals may be sent anywhere there is a need. They do not have the opportunity to become familiar with residents–a basic tenet of resident-centred care–yet they are expected to provide individualized care to residents with dementia.

A third operational challenge, according to some of the practice leaders, is that the "benchmarks" currently in use do not adequately take into account the skills and attitudes required to work effectively with people with dementia. (A benchmark is a generic job description that states the key skills and training required for a particular job classification. It is negotiated between employers and unions.)

Another operational factor, according to some practice leaders, is that unions allocate jobs based on seniority, not suitability. Others say that this is not a problem, because front line staff eventually "self-select" to work where they feel most comfortable and competent.

Resident Characteristics

The fourth barrier to implementing individualized, flexible care to long-term care residents with dementia is that they have much more complex diagnoses and heavier care needs than they did 10-20 years ago, when the first models of resident-centred care were developed and exported from Sweden. Both practice leaders and front line workers point out that "generalist" or multi-skilled workers may not be suitable in an environment where residents have "complex psychiatric problems and cognitive deficits." More specialized skills may be required.

Design and Scale of the Built Environment

The fifth barrier to implementing care with flexible work routines and multi-skilled staff is the large scale and hospital-like design of the typical long-term care facility in Canada. The larger the facility, the less likely it is that this model can be delivered successfully. For example, in a large building or complex, staff have to spend so much time simply getting from one point to another that they do not have time for one-to-one social interaction with residents. Similarly, multi-tasking does not work well in a large building or complex, where a staff member may have to travel a hundred metres, or wait for elevators, to retrieve meals or do a resident's laundry.

Keys to Successfully Implementing a Resident-Centred Model of Dementia Care

Six keys to success emerged during this exploratory study. These are: higher staff-to-resident ratios and/or a mix of residents, leadership, formal involvement of front line staff in decision-making, team work, education, and, some rotation in staff scheduling.

Higher Staff-to-Resident Ratios and/or a Mix of Residents

It is apparent that if all the residents in a unit have dementia and require heavy physical care as well, it is very difficult for front line workers to "create the day" with each resident, since so much time and energy is spent doing basic personal care. Practice leaders and front line workers agree that there need to be higher staff-to-resident ratios than currently available. (These ratios vary across the province. In this study, they ranged from 1:6 to 1:8 in dementia care units. The ideal expressed by front line workers is 1:4 to 1:6.) In addition, a mix of residents–in terms of the weight of their care needs–for each front line worker would lighten the load.

Leadership

Leadership skills among Directors of Care and Ward Registered Nurses is key. It is clear that leadership training is needed. Practice leaders warned,

> Without good leadership and role models, this change will not happen. The Ward RN is key. If the Ward RN doesn't buy it, forget it!

Good leadership, among both managers and front line workers, could make a significant difference to the change process and could help overcome resistance to change.

Formal Involvement of Front Line Staff in Decision-Making

Formal and effectual involvement of front line staff in decision-making is considered a key to success. Ideally, front line workers are involved on two levels. On a macro level, they participate in decision-making about changes in the practice of care delivery, and in decisions about who is hired to work with residents with dementia. On a micro level, they participate in developing and modifying individual residents' care plans and making personal decisions about the rhythm of the residents' days.

Team Work

Front line workers appear to miss the teamwork that was part of the "old school," although they do not miss other aspects of a traditional, task-oriented, hierarchical approach to care. They desire more collective and less isolated decision-making, and more information transfer with on-coming front line shifts. If they worked in smaller facilities, and had adequate time for direct communication between workers (including casuals) on different shifts, they would feel that they were less isolated, more of a team.

On-Going Education and Training

Education and training for Registered Nurses, Licensed Practical Nurses and Care Aides is critical to the success of a resident-centred model of care, because, first and foremost, a worker cannot implement a "model" without first understanding what that model is addressing; in this case, dementia. Practice leaders advocated,

> Education is critical–education of both Care Aides and RNs!
> Administrators must be willing to pay for education, training [and up-grading].

Education and training are required for both managers and front line workers, so that they can become more knowledgeable about the various types of dementia and more skilled in providing dementia care. In addition, union leaders need to become more knowledgeable about the new approaches to dementia care, and Directors of Care need to become more aware of front line workers' everyday reality. Increased knowledge, skills and awareness, for all parties, would reduce stress and conflict on the job.

Some Rotation in Staff Scheduling

Although permanent assignments for staff, in terms of both their shift and their unit, is a basic building block of the resident-centred model of dementia care, it is not considered ideal by some front line workers and practice leaders. Instead, it is considered more desirable to give staff the option of rotating their shift, or unit, or both, every four to six months. This length of time in one unit allows staff to become familiar with their residents. A change of shift allows them to see their residents at different times of day, helping them become familiar with the whole person. A change of unit gives them a break from residents and other staff whom they may find noxious; as the workers say, they have got to know them "too well." Some rotation of staff scheduling is considered necessary in long-term care where residents are physically frail and cognitively impaired.

Benefits of Resident-Centred Care

Despite difficulties in implementing a resident-centred model of care in today's financially strapped health care system and with today's heavy-care resident population, the philosophy and values of this model are generally embraced, and the benefits of the model are recognized by practice leaders and front line workers alike.

Benefits to Front Line Workers

In the two facilities where the new approach to dementia care has been most successfully implemented, front line workers "get a lot of pride in their work and internal satisfaction" from being empowered to make decisions about their workday, and from being involved as a team member in care planning, according to their managers. This was endorsed by a front line worker, who observed,

> Your day is your own. It is a good feeling.

Another important aspect of this model of care is that front line workers are able to develop relationships, "to bond," with their residents and their residents' families, relationships which they value highly. In addition, front line staff claim that familiarity with the residents and information that they glean from family members can make them more effective and efficient in their work.

Benefits to Residents

Residents benefit from a resident-centred model of care in ways that directly relate to their interaction with front line staff. For example, both practice leaders and front line staff claimed that continuity of staffing can reduce residents' frustration, confusion and agitation. The fact that staff members get to know them well increases the chances of their receiving appropriate and individualized care. Furthermore, the relationships that develop with staff members can enrich their lives. In some cases, the front line workers are the residents' most devoted advocates and friends. For example,

> . . . we may be their only social relationship.
> They have to be protected; we are their angels!

A Vision: The Ideal Long-Term Care Setting for Elderly People with Dementia

Front line workers were asked to describe an ideal long-term care facility for elderly people with dementia, a place to which they would be comfortable moving one of their parents. Their responses underscore the importance of creating home-like, rather than institutional, environments.

According to front line staff, the ideal facility would be a clean, bright, safe, comfortable, residential-scale environment that "looks like a house," all on one level, with plenty of natural light and access to gardens. Each resident would have a personalized, private bedroom and private bathroom. No more than 10 residents would live in one unit, or eat together in one dining room. Activity areas would be separate from the dining room, and there would be some sports and recreation opportunities suitable for men. The ambience would be "home-like," with soft window dressings, "homey furniture," "pretty china" and music playing on the stereo. In or near this facility there would be a suite for visiting family members.

In this ideal setting, there would be a staff-to-resident ratio of 1:4 or 1:5. Front line staff would be "fun, motivated, team workers, caring, compassionate and part of a family." They would "love what they do," have "the right nature" and appropriate training, and would "work as a team." Registered Nurses would be "involved." Workers would be multi-trained and multi-skilled *only if* the home were a small-scale facility. In this context, there would be "no rushing staff"; the atmosphere would be "laid back."

Residents' days would be flexible, providing a choice of meaningful activities and chores. Food would be very good and culturally appropriate: "It's an important part of their day!" Wherever possible, residents would be able to converse in their mother tongue with staff.

DISCUSSION

Results from this exploratory study suggest that there is a great deal to be learned from front line workers in dementia care: They are a gold mine of knowledge and experience. The long-term care providers in this study embrace the philosophy of resident-centred dementia care, and their values and vision largely agree with the professional wisdom in the field. The *implementation* of the ideal resident-centred model of dementia care, however, is very challenging.

Several key steps required to successfully implement resident-centred dementia care in long-term care environments were identified. First, to increase the understanding and acceptance of this model of care, Registered Nurse Team Leaders and front line workers alike should receive leadership training, as well as on-going, paid education in dementia and training in dementia care. It is also essential to involve front line workers (including casuals, when possible) in all aspects of change: decision-making in approaches to care; hiring decisions; and care planning. This involvement requires good leadership skills, an incremental approach to change, and considerable invested and elapsed time. To reduce staff stress and burden of care, a staff-to-resident ratio of 1:4 or 1:5 is considered ideal in units where residents are both cognitively impaired and physically frail. Other solutions for reducing staff stress are to: mix residents (in terms of weight of physical care) to make it easier for front line staff to spend one-to-one time with them; and allow for rotation of shift or unit every four to six months and/or some flexibility in assignments. Finally, it is clear that this resident-centred model of care is difficult to implement in large scale, institutional long-term care facilities. These environments need to be modified to create small clusters of six to 12 residents, with all the amenities of a home attached to each cluster.

NOTES

1. The "Swedish model" is the result of serendipity. Approximately 20 years ago, a long term care facility for elderly people was being renovated in Sweden. A small cluster of dementia residents and a small group of their care providers were moved to a house, while the renovation took place. During the time spent in the house, staff observed and reported marked improvement in residents' functioning and mood (Beck-Friis, 1998). The "Australian model," refined, applied and disseminated by Dr. John Tooth of Tasmania, is based on the elements of the Swedish model, with a practical bent: Several small houses, or cottages, are clustered around (and typically attached to) a central administrative core. This averts administrative redundancy and increases emergency response capacity. A national study, *Home-Like Environments for Elderly People with Dementia*, conducted for Health Canada in 1999-2000 by Dr. Elizabeth Dow and Nancy Gnaedinger, as yet unpublished, includes case studies of 10 dementia care facilities in Canada that were either designed or retrofitted according to evolving versions of this model.

2. The terms "cottage," "neighbourhood," "cluster," and more recently, "household," are used synonymously by different practice leaders in dementia care.

3. At the time of research, the main source of information on multi-skilling was gathered by word of mouth from colleagues and from dementia care experts in several provinces.

4. Before gathering information and opinions for this study from practice leaders in British Columbia, the author was already familiar with the topic through: (a) attendance at numerous conferences, workshops and meetings in gerontology and Alzheimer's disease, at various venues in Canada over the previous 12 years; and (b) conducting in-depth telephone interviews with, and receiving documentation from dementia care directors, managers or experts in Alberta, Saskatchewan, Manitoba, Ontario and New Brunswick, while carrying out six case studies during 1999, as part of the Canadian national study quoted in 1 above.

5. This statement is based on: (a) information gathered during the national study quoted above; and (b) conversations with colleagues and attendance at numerous conferences.

6. In 1999, the author could not find any published studies on the Canadian experience of this new model of dementia care. (One evaluation study had been conducted in Alberta, but results had not been published.)

7. The sponsor of this study (see below) requested an exploratory, qualitative study limited to their members' experience and assessments of this model of dementia care.

8. The sponsor of this study, the Hospital Employees' Union of British Columbia (HEU) has approximately 46,000 members, of whom approximately 13,000 work in long term care in varying roles: Licensed Practical Nurse, Care Aide, Activation Assistant, Housekeeper, Maintenance staff, Food Service staff and Laundry staff.

9. The study was not intended to be academic, nor was it intended to compare different models of care: It was designed to inform the HEU union executive and membership about the principles and key elements of resident-centred dementia care and about HEU workers' experience and assessment of its application.

10. The practice leaders chosen as key informants for this study were, and are, recognized as people who have broken new ground and made a significant contribution to dementia care in British Columbia. Their "credentials" typically include graduate degrees, experience in direct care, research, change management, and travel abroad to observe dementia care in other countries.

11. Focus group #1 was held in an attractive, modern two-storey 100-bed multi-level facility built in 1992, designed on a "village" model, with a "shop" and "bank" opening onto a sunny, open communal area on the main floor, and plenty of natural light everywhere in the facility. The staff-to-resident ratio for mixed Intermediate and Extended Care wards and for the Dementia Care ward is 1:6 for the day shift. The second focus group was conducted in an older 157-bed facility with three wings. The building which has been added to over the years, is a maze with a number of twisting hallways. Communal rooms include a chapel, several activity and lounge areas, and seven dining rooms, four of which are in a new Dementia Care unit, where the staff-to-resident ratio is 1:8 for the day shift. The third focus group was held in a new, 194 bed multi-level care facility near Vancouver, which opened in 1998 to replace two older facilities in the area. The facility is very large in scale, with wide hallways and plenty of natural light. An effort has been made to provide a residential ambience, with the use of wood detailing, fireplaces, homelike furniture and a small dining room in each unit. Residents are clustered into units according to their needs/characteristics: extended care with dementia; extended care and cognitively intact; mobile with de-

mentia; frail with dementia (but not to the degree that they require special care); and dementia care. Most units have 27-44 residents, split into groups of 12-22. Approximately 70 percent of the residents have dementia. (Staff-to-resident ratios were not available.) The site of the fourth focus group was a multi-level care facility with 196 beds. The three storey facility has the look and ambience of a nursing home of the 1960s, although it is clear that a great deal of effort has been spent to reduce the institutional look of the facility, by adding wallpaper and curtains, photos of residents, plants and other homelike furnishings. The hallmarks of "institution" remain, however: nursing stations, long corridors, shiny floors, flourescent lighting. Residents are divided into different programs of care: cognitively well but physically frail, those with mild to moderate dementia, and those with moderate to severe dementia. The staff-to-resident ratio is 1:7 for residents who have moderate to severe dementia. Approximately 70 percent of the residents have dementia, and most have multiple diagnoses.

12. Activation Assistants are people trained at community college to assist professionals, such as Recreation Therapists and Occupational Therapists, who direct the activation and recreation programs in long-term care facilities.

13. GentleCare® is the registered trademark of Moyra Jones Resources, of Burnaby, B.C.

REFERENCES

Barnes, I. (1996). "The Hidden Joys on a Dementia Unit," *Canadian Nursing Home*, Nov./Dec.

_____. (1997). "Toward a Caring Dementia Unit," *Canadian Nursing Home*, Feb./Mar.

_____. (1999). "Making a Difference in Dementia Care," *Canadian Nursing Home*, Feb./Mar.

Beck-Friis, B. (1988). *At Home at Baltzargarden: Caring for the geriatric senile in a small scale group environment*. Uddevalla (Sweden): Bohuslans Grafiska AB.

Dow, E. & Gnaedinger, N. (2000). *Home-Like Environments for Elderly People with Dementia*. Unpublished report funded by Health Canada, Division of Aging and Seniors, for the Housing Sub-Committee of the Canada Co-ordinating Committee for the International Year of Older Persons, March.

Johnson, L. (no date). *Creating Caring Environments for the Person with Dementia–A Guide*. Contact the author Louise Johnson at Louise_Johnson@telus.net.

Jones, M. (1996). *Gentle Care®–Changing the Experience of Alzheimer's Disease in a Positive Way*. Moyra Jones Resources, 8264 Burnlake Drive, Burnaby, BC, Canada V5A 3K9. Email: jonesb@direct.ca.

Tooth, J. (1994). A presentation on Home-like Dementia Care, sponsored by and presented at the Oak Bay Kiwanis Pavilion (long-term care residence for people with dementia in Victoria, British Columbia, Canada).

SECTION 6
IS CHANGE REALISTIC?

Quality Oversight and Culture Change in Long-Term Care

Deborah Wilkerson
Christine MacDonell

SUMMARY. The culture of long-term care is changing as the Baby Boomer generation ages, needing long-term care but finding that the quality of care is such that many would rather die than enter a long-term care facility. While quality oversight mechanisms are looked to for protection of consumers, in fact regulations have been seen by the industry as restrictive in this changing culture. This article explores the ways in

Deborah Wilkerson, MA, is Chief Research and Education Officer for CARF, The Rehabilitation Accreditation Commission; her academic training is in cultural and medical anthropology.

Christine MacDonell is Managing Director, Medical Rehabilitation, Adult Day Services and Assisted Living programs for CARF; her academic and clinical training is in occupational therapy.

Address correspondence to: Deborah Wilkerson, MA, Chief Research and Education Officer, CARF, 4891 East Grant Road, Tucson, AZ 85712 (E-mail: dwilkerson@carf.org).

[Haworth co-indexing entry note]: "Quality Oversight and Culture Change in Long-Term Care." Wilkerson, Deborah, and Christine MacDonell. Co-published simultaneously in *Journal of Social Work in Long-Term Care* (The Haworth Social Work Practice Press, an imprint of The Haworth Press, Inc.) Vol. 2, No. 3/4, 2003, pp. 373-395; and: *Culture Change in Long-Term Care* (ed: Audrey S. Weiner, and Judah L. Ronch) The Haworth Social Work Practice Press, an imprint of The Haworth Press, Inc., 2003, pp. 373-395. Single or multiple copies of this article are available for a fee from The Haworth Document Delivery Service [1-800-HAWORTH, 9:00 a.m. - 5:00 p.m. (EST). E-mail address: docdelivery@haworthpress.com].

which quality oversight organizations attempt to address quality and proposes a model for conceptualizing quality oversight alternatives that may help mediate the conflict between the quality oversight and changing long-term care cultures. Finally, challenges are summarized regarding what the various stakeholders in long-term care might do to form partnerships in meeting the needs and desires of the long-term care consumer population. *[Article copies available for a fee from The Haworth Document Delivery Service: 1-800-HAWORTH. E-mail address: <docdelivery@haworthpress.com> Website: <http://www.HaworthPress.com> © 2003 by The Haworth Press, Inc. All rights reserved.]*

KEYWORDS. Quality oversight, long-term care, accreditation, regulation, licensure, certification

INTRODUCTION: CULTURE OF QUALITY

This special volume focuses on culture and culture change–the changing culture of the long-term care service environment, changes in consumers' expectations of long-term care, and changes in the population needing (or soon to be needing) long-term care. When invited to make a contribution to the issue on the topic of the regulatory environment, we were presented with the challenge of exploring how "regulation" could support–and not impede–the positive culture change under way in the long-term care service world.

The literature is replete with critiques of long-term care quality and with challenges to government and other authorities to take action (Schnelle et al., 1997; Walshe, 2001; Kane & Kane, 2001). The Institute of Medicine's 1986 report on quality of long-term care and the subsequent new regulations contained in the OBRA 1987 were major events in the evolution of attention to improving the quality of long-term care. Outside the regulatory environment, guidelines for how to address many of the more difficult problems in long-term care (Schnelle et al., 1997) also exist.

For those concerned about the quality of care delivered in and quality of life experienced by recipients of long-term care, there is abundant responsibility and even blame to go around. Providers are faulted for poor quality of service (Kane & Kane, 2001); the government is faulted for lack of attention (Kane & Kane, 2001); insurers are faulted for not covering long-term care (Burgess & Riley, 2000); the regulatory process itself is faulted for being misdirected and burdensome (Schnelle et al., 1997; Walshe, 2001), and people looking for long-term care are observed to be "naïve shoppers" (Kane & Kane, 2001, 118).

Who Cares? "It's the Demographics, Stupid"

One could paraphrase James Carville in answer to the question: "Where can we look to learn how the need for long-term care will be changing over the next couple of decades?" The facts before us should wake the industry up to the coming changes in the culture of long-term care, and the corresponding challenges the industry and its regulatory enablers must address. These facts include (U.S. Census Bureau, 2001):

- The 2000 Census data show nearly 40 million people (or 12.4% of the population) in the US are aged 65 and older, and over 4 million of those are 85 and older;
- Of those, 10.6% live below the poverty level;
- The 2000 Census data show almost 10 million single-person households are of people aged 65 and older;
- But, there are nearly 70 million people now 45-64 years old waiting in the wings (the pool of new 65 and older people for the next 20 years);
- In 1999, the older population (persons 65 and older) represented 34.5 million people or 12.7% of the US population. By the year 2030, there will be 70 million older persons or 20% of the US population (Administration on Aging, 2000).

The long-term care continuum in the year 2000 included: 17,799 licensed nursing facilities, 43,102 Board and Care facilities and 33,000 licensed assisted living facilities (Older Americans Report, 2001; Osborn, 2002). These numbers illustrate the sheer magnitude of the challenge in reviewing health and safety, the outcomes of services, rights of individuals, performance improvement, care planning, training and competence of staff, and many other facets of the long-term care service system.

The implications of these facts for the need for long-term care and the magnitude of the "system of care" are enormous. Baby boomers who are now shopping for care for their parents will in the next 20 years begin to need care themselves. To the extent that beliefs and values among baby boomers now are reflected in their shopping habits for parents, those beliefs and values will be brought to bear on their demands for their own care. In other words, the culture of long-term care will be influenced in the near term by a large influx of a new population relevant to long-term care.

WHAT DO WE MEAN BY "CULTURE?"

Anthropologists study culture as a way of understanding the way human beings live in their environments and with each other, and in the course of studying culture, touch on every aspect of human physical, social, and cognitive being. Many fields of inquiry emphasize different aspects of human beings–psychology the cognitive, sociology the social, medicine the biological, and so forth, and these fields naturally overlap. It is an elusive concept, but understanding what culture is, is nonetheless central to trying to understand how to change it.

In his work on *Organizational Culture and Leadership*, the organizational psychologist Edgar Schein tackled the definition of culture for practical use in understanding organizations, drawing from the "deeper, more complex anthropological models" (Schein, 1992, 3). Schein's (1992, 8-10) composite definition is useful herein and includes the following:

1. Observed behavioral regularities when people interact: language they use, customs and traditions that evolve, and rituals they employ
2. Group norms for expected behavior
3. Espoused values
4. Formal philosophy
5. Rules of the game ("the way we do things around here")
6. Climate (look and feel of the place and people's interactions)
7. Embedded skills and competencies (passed on to others)
8. Habits of thinking, mental models, and/or linguistic paradigms
9. Shared meanings (how people understand each other)
10. "Root metaphors" or integrating symbols

Culture involves shared meaning, beliefs and activities regarded as normative for the group. A classic anthropological reference describes: "A society's culture consists of whatever it is one has to know or believe in order to operate in a manner acceptable to its members" (Ward Goodenough quoted in Geertz, 1973, 11).

Let us assume here that Schein's package of traits can be examined at different levels of analysis. As we consider culture, culture change, and the role of quality oversight organizations, we might consider contrast between the culture of long-term care versus that of some other enterprise (such as trauma care). Consider also the cultures of one kind of facility (e.g., a skilled nursing facility) versus some other kind of long-term care organization (e.g., a home care agency or group residential facility).

With that distinction in mind, let us return to the central question for this article: What is the role of quality oversight in the changing culture of long-term care?

1. If culture involves shared meaning, and norms of behavior, do and should quality oversight organizations (QOOs) reflect (i.e., derive from) or enforce (i.e., produce) those behaviors, or both?
2. Since culture involves underlying beliefs and values, do quality oversight organizations and their requirements allow or counteract those beliefs and values?
3. Since culture includes explicit rules and rituals, how do the requirements and review events of QOOs fit in the cultural environment they intend to monitor?
4. If there are conflicting interests that emerge (e.g., between long-term care provider staff and the consumers, or between policymakers and payors) in whose interest does quality oversight operate?

In order to approach these questions, let us first define the scope of quality oversight and the kinds of organizations that perform it.

THE FIELD OF QUALITY OVERSIGHT

President Clinton's Advisory Commission on Consumer Protection and Quality in the Health Care Industry (1998), a treatise that introduces the Health Care Bill of Rights, used the term "Quality Oversight Organization" (QOO) to refer to a collection of efforts that are somewhat different in their tactics and locus of control, but can generally come under a "regulatory" umbrella. We here use the term "quality oversight organizations" in referring to the various systems of reviewing the quality of a provider organization and awarding a license, certificate, or accreditation designation. Each system serves a somewhat different purpose and each is typically offered by different entities: federal, state, or local governments; professional boards and associations; and private not-for-profit bodies. Each may draw upon and/or seek to enforce regulations that appear in the law or public administration's regulations. In addition, each may augment formal regulations as a basis for quality oversight with requirements or guidelines that are generated elsewhere.

Dictionary definitions of the relevant terms can help guide us (*Webster's Encyclopedia Unabridged Dictionary of the English Language*, 1990) clarify the differences. Definitions below are augmented with brief descriptions of how the oversight is usually carried out.

Regulation: A rule or order prescribed by authority, as to regulate conduct; a governing direction or law. To regulate: To control or direct by a rule, principle, method, etc.; to adjust so as to ensure accuracy of operation. Regulations appear in the form of rules established and published by federal, state, or local agencies to detail the implementation of laws. They can be found in publications such as the *Federal Register* and comparable state legislative and policy documents.

Licensing: Formal permission from a constituted authority to do something, as to carry on some business or profession. Thus, licensing is often the most basic and necessary form of quality oversight, and required in order to conduct business. Most licensing is conducted by state or local government agencies responsible for regulating the quantity and/or acceptable level of quality of a service provided by an organization or an activity performed by individuals requiring a certain level skill to ensure public safety.

Certification: Act of assurance, endorse reliably, inform with certainty. Certifying bodies review individual practitioners to assure competence to provide certain services. This distinction is important because of the focus on individuals rather than organizations or programs, which are the focus for licensing and accreditation.

Accreditation: Accredit: to ensure an organization, program, or service has met all formal, official requirements. Generally a review is performed by a private not-for-profit entity, and if standards for quality services are met an accreditation award is made, often with different levels or categories.

In addition to the formal quality oversight mechanisms defined above there is also provider industry self-evaluation and monitoring that may be required or stimulated by a QOO, or may be instigated by the quality-seeking organization. The difference is that self-evaluation lacks the external review and an indication to the public that an unbiased assessment of the organization has been conducted.

Each form of quality oversight fulfills a different role in the effort to ensure that services are delivered in a safe and effective manner, but they can (or should) work together in a complementary fashion. It is where overlaps, inconsistencies, or worse, conflicts between requirements of the different QOOs appear that the greatest "hassle factor" exists for providers.

Moreover, when rules or standards require that the provider act in ways counter to what is perceived as quality care or a positive culture change, there is great conflict for the provider. Anecdotally, providers report such situations, and complain that it is the quality oversight environment that deters change of the type being highlighted in long-term care today. Examples of such dilemmas include:

- A surveyor finds that a therapeutic recreation department begins and ends activities at times other than those specified on the provider's activity schedule. If spontaneity and availability of activities on a 24-hour basis are "hallmarks" of resident-centered care, shouldn't the organization have the latitude to make alterations to a schedule or calendar on the seeming "spur of the moment"?

• A standard might state that the evening meal and breakfast should be offered no more than 14 hours apart. If, in a resident-centered environment a resident is "allowed to be awakened" at a time of their preference (or not awakened by staff at all), then breakfast may be more than 14 hours after dinner. How is the organization to accommodate both the QOO and the resident-centered philosophy?

Let us examine key concepts in both quality oversight and long-term care before we consider how such dilemmas might be resolved–and by whom.

Key Concepts Relating to Quality Oversight in Long Term Care

Two conceptual frameworks are mentioned here because they offer an opportunity to understand the domains of concern for quality oversight, the domains for attention to the needs of the persons served in long-term care, and a common language to enhance the development of shared meaning among the stakeholders in long-term care.

First is the now-classic work of Donabedian (1966, 1983, 1988), which defines key dimensions for the assessment of quality. (See also Fratalli, 1997, pp. 3-4, for an excellent discussion of Donabedian's framework.)

Structure–refers to the relatively stable tools and resources available to providers of care; the physical and organizational setting; the human, physical, and financial resources needed to provide care.

Process–refers to activities that take place within the setting of care, including both technical (diagnostic and treatment) and interpersonal (social interaction) aspects of care.

Outcome–refers to change in the health or status of the person served attributable to the care provided, including physical, social, psychological and attitudinal changes for the person.

Added to the Donabedian framework in recent years is the notion of access as a fourth domain of quality. Potentially thought of as a part of structure, but crossing the border into process, access has been incorporated by several systems of performance indicators and measurement systems from professional groups and accrediting bodies (ACMHA, 2001; CARF, 1998; NCQA, 1997). Therefore, let us add:

Access–refers to the availability of care and the degree to which those who need it get it.

Any of the four domains of quality presented–access, structure, process, outcome–can and are addressed in varying degrees by QOOs, and requirements for quality oversight may fall into any or all of these domains. We will refer to these domains later in the discussion of different oversight types and the changing focus away from structure and toward access, process, and mostly on outcome.

Regulation and licensing often contain requirements for structure in physical facilities and organizational arrangement to ensure that safe and appropriate resources are in place. Licensing and certification also focus to a large extent on process issues, and less on access and outcomes. It is in the arena of accreditation where the domains of access and outcomes are more likely to appear, though much of this attention is to the process-requirements for organizations to examine and try to improve access and outcomes, as opposed to specific benchmarks or targets for access and outcome levels. It is in the focus on these two domains that we believe lies the opportunity for quality oversight to address the culture changes underway in the long-term care field. We will address this point later.

The second conceptual framework to keep in mind is the World Health Organization's (WHO) *International Classification of Functioning, Disability and Health (ICF)* (WHO, 2001). First developed in draft form in 1980 by the WHO as the *International Classification of Impairments, Disabilities and Handicaps (ICIDH)*, the framework has been much debated around the world, but especially in North America where reference to the term "handicap" inflamed the disability rights and independent living communities and prompted a changed for the better. The WHO framework and its key terms have now been revised and reflect a positive outlook on the notion of functioning at the levels of the body, the whole person, and the person operating in society. Moreover, the new ICF adds domains of environment and the personal factors that influence a person's choice and ability to participate in life. The concepts of the ICF, we believe, are particularly germane to the culture change underway in long-term care. Key terms are defined in Chart 1 (WHO, 2001).

The third and final concept related to the changing long-term care environment is the notion of "independence" as conceptualized by the disability rights and independent living social and civil rights movement of the 1970s and 1980s. One impetus for passage of the Americans with Disabilities Act, the independent living (IL) model, features the ideas that people with impairments/disabilities should be able to live and choose as the rest of society; that accepting assistance does not constitute dependence, and disability does not equal sickness (Heumann, 1977; Frieden,1978; DeJong, 1979). People should not be devalued just because they have impairments or need assistance with activities, and the social and physical environments should be the primary focus of change needed so that people can participate in the life situations they choose.

CHART 1. Definitions from the ICF

- *Impairment*–Problems in body function or structure such as significant deviation or loss. (Examples: schizophrenia, loss of limb, Alzheimer's disease)

- *Activity*–The execution of a task or action by an individual. (Examples: Taking care of oneself, activities of daily living)

- *Participation*–Involvement in a life situation. (Examples: taking part in community activities, being a qualified voter)

Originally discussed primarily within the context of young people with disabilities receiving and providing services in community-based independent living centers (ILCs), the notion of independence is making its way explicitly into the literature on aging where the very same values are being espoused (e.g., Kane, 2001). Moreover, the change in the language of the WHO's ICF to emphasize activity and participation (relevant to all people) assists in deflecting attention from the socially charged concepts of disability and "handicap," and becomes more relevant to a normally aging population now experiencing limitations in activity and restrictions on participation and choice. The combined political strength of young people and elders who share a desire for and a determination to obtain quality services leading to positive outcomes in terms of choice and participation will be powerful in enacting policy and regulatory change. It is our belief that the "culture change" under way in long-term care is, in fact, a feature of the growing visibility and voice of the large demographic of people whose parents, and who themselves are aging and facing the evident needs for long-term care. The massive population of aging baby boomers will change the system to reflect their preferences–whatever they are–and these preferences are now beginning to focus on long-term care.

CHANGING NOTIONS OF QUALITY IN LONG-TERM CARE

At the heart of the issue is the fact that virtually no one chooses "long-term care" as a way of life. People mostly do not seek to enter nursing homes; in fact, many would rather die than enter one (Kane & Kane, 2001). But, people do get old, they often need care, and unless they die traumatically and accidentally, quickly from an illness, they may need care for a long time–hence, long-term care. Thus, on the one hand long-term care is almost inevitable as an alternative to early death, and on the other hand, it is considered worse than death itself (Kane, 2001).

What do people want? There is a growing and compelling literature documenting what older people want. They want the same things younger people (with or without disabilities or who need assistance) want: as much activity to one's taste as possible; freedom to do what they choose where and when they choose it; comfort and companionship with one's family and friends; and a safe environment.

But the institutional notions of safety at any cost, quantity over quality of life, and the convenience of uniformity in an institution have taken precedence over these features of personal preference (Kane, 2001). What is new may be more the *recognition* of older people's preferences by the many aging baby boomers rather than the preferences of older people themselves.

Kane (2001, 295) places at least part of the fault at the feet of the larger culture:

> Blatantly put, long-term care policies and practices in the United States are flawed, particularly for those long-term care consumers who are old. Moreover, the quality of life for long-term care consumers is compromised by a societal reluctance to come to grips with these flaws.

Yet, the answer is not necessarily to simply legislate or regulate the specifics of quality care. If it is part of the "U.S. culture" to devalue the quality of life for our old people, changing this value is striking at real culture change–a major task and one not easily or quickly achieved. Kane acknowledges, "Real change in the way most Americans can expect to receive long-term care is strikingly difficult to achieve" (Kane, 2001, 295).

But Kane's own arguments illustrate the conflicts inherent in this discussion. She argues on the same page (2001, 295):

- "Regulators and policymakers often expect too much of nursing homes and other LTC providers"
- " 'Just not living' and 'rather be dead' are such dismal outcomes for life in nursing homes that the various quality-of-life indicators should be rendered almost irrelevant against such indictments."

In other words, the quality of (and quality of life in) long-term care is completely unacceptable AND requirements attempting to improve the quality of long-term care are 'expecting too much' of providers. There is something wrong with this picture.

What is wrong centers on the mismatch between domains of focus, using Donabedian's structure-process-outcome domains. The quality of life goals articulated by and for consumers are *outcomes* focusing on the person, and they speak largely to participation and choice, including but not limited to physical and environmental safety. Yet, quality oversight requirements are most often attempts to specify the *structural* and *process* parameters that are (a) easier to observe, (b) clearer for QOOs to require and (c) more palatable to providers who rightly argue they can not control or provide every element of a person's quality of life. What, then, can or must QOOs do to accommodate–or even promote–the shifting culture in long-term care toward real and meaningful outcomes?

Where quality oversight does look at outcomes, they are often stated negatively, i.e., as sentinel events such as unwanted weight loss or the occurrence of pressure ulcers. While these events can be important outcomes to monitor, doesn't a resident-centered environment argue for a focus on positive outcomes? What about the process of caring, or the satisfaction of residents that they are safe and able to participate as they wish in life? How can quality oversight and provider organizations mutually acknowledge and address both avoiding untoward outcomes and promoting the positive ones?

CHANGING QUALITY OVERSIGHT IN LONG-TERM CARE

We must change the way we view quality oversight; that is, it should be viewed less with dread for the burden it creates, and more with an eye toward its potential to mend a "dismal" system. Changing this view will require adjustments of both the provider and the quality oversight organization communities.

Walshe (2001, 129) traces the history of nursing home regulations and concludes that

> fundamental regulatory reform is needed but that greater attention should be paid to the lessons of regulation in other settings, and more use should be made of research and formative evaluation to improve the effectiveness of nursing home regulation.

Walshe (2001) also acknowledges that the regulations of CMS (HCFA) are "administratively complex but conceptually straightforward" (Walshe, 2001, 130), essentially aimed at seeing that providers paid by Medicare or Medicaid funds comply with regulations. State licensing entities may add requirements, and often check to see that providers meet regulations regardless of payment source (Walshe, 2001, 131). While researching the impact of regulation is challenging for several methodological reasons–no clear control group, data collection inconsistencies, and questions about validity and reliability of data–it is acknowledged that some, but not enough, progress has been made since OBRA 1987 reforms (Walshe, 2001; Kane, 2001). Inappropriate use of restraints and hospitalization have declined, but pressure sore rates, malnutrition, dehydration and bowel incontinence have not. As a result of regulation, large, multi-site providers have been favored over small single-site owner operated providers, perhaps because of being able to spread the cost of compliance (Walshe, 2001). Moreover, the spending on quality oversight (e.g., state licensing and certification) by long-term care providers and publicly-funded agencies is significant, but also in direct (survey) and indirect (preparation and compliance) costs (Walshe, 2001).

Regulation and quality oversight are one mechanism for changing behavior, even if the values of the majority have not changed. It is this feature of QO that is both offers the potential for quality improvement–regulatory requirements can force or stimulate structural and process changes that match the outcome and quality of life goals of consumers and others. But they can also get in the way of real improvement where the structural and process requirements of QO miss the mark, are irrelevant–or worse, counter to–good outcomes. Thus a challenge is presented for the role of QO to promote the structural, process and outcome features matching the desired goal of high quality of life for consumers of long-term care without constraining solutions to reach the stated goal. Others have suggested that QO might be used as an indirect incentive to insurers to attend to quality and to increase access to good long-term care (Burgess & Riley, 2000).

Why is the enterprise of QO in long-term care such a challenge? First, we don't know enough–exactly which requirements work to, in fact, promote quality of life? Second, the long-term care industry might prefer to limit regulation, preferring its own freedom from constraint and pressures. In turn, pressures are directed toward QOOs to limit rules. Yet, if the larger culture–not to mention the individual long-term care provider–does not embody the beliefs, values, norms, shared meaning of how long-term care should be delivered, freedom from QO will not result in the desired goals of independence, support, and participation for consumers.

Kane (2001) presents a well-thought-out proposal for consideration of all who would improve the effectiveness of regulation in long-term care. Her recommendations include:

- "Assisted living and the unbundling of housing and services" (Kane, 2001, 300). Kane argues that the housing provider should not be held responsible for care outcomes. "Assisted living offers the opportunity for home-like environment, choice, participation . . . and a normal lifestyle" but with assistance close by. Yet, quality varies widely, and there is a need in the industry for some kind of QO.

- "Culture change in nursing homes" (Kane, 2001, 300).
- Attention to ways the environment and assistive technology play into quality of life (Kane, 2001, 300). This is a relationship long attended to (if not well paid for) in disability issues for younger PWD.
- Information is needed for consumers to choose a provider (Kane, 2001, 300).
- Moreover, information on quality and QI is needed for providers, though measurement and political issues surrounding the definition, collection, cost, reporting and interpretation of uniform data abound (Kane, 2001, 302).
- Service providers should focus on building supportive environments.
- Yet providers must learn how to allow residents to accept a level of risk in life consistent with having and making choices (Kane, 2001, 302).
- While this poses an issue of balancing liability and responsive services for providers, solutions must be discussed in order to make these settings livable for older people.

Several prominent themes emerge in this recent literature on regulation and changing notions of quality in long-term care (Kane, 2001; Kane & Kane, 2001; Walshe, 2001; Schnelle, Ouslander & Cruise, 1997).

- Increased attention to measuring, communicating and improving performance, while allowing latitude for providers in how to improve performance;
- An emphasis on person-focused services; a strong emphasis on participation (and the activities supporting participation) of the resident/client;
- The need to build structure and process around the central goal of participation of persons served (rather than the other way around; participation as the dependent variable and structure/process as independent variables). In other words, we need to *begin* by focusing attention on outcomes and then on structures and processes that support or produce them.
- The need for balance at the person, organization, and systems levels. At the person level, recognizing the validity of balancing risk and independence and choice; at the organization level, balancing accountability with independence and creativity; at the systems level, balancing cost of regulation with the diversity and array of good providers.
- The need to re-think the incentive structure such that good performance and responsive care are rewarded; this will challenge the quality oversight organizations and put the burden on the QOOs to develop "responsive" regulation that both protects consumers and allows providers enough flexibility to respond to consumers' needs and choices.
- The need to identify needed information for consumers, develop strategies and methods to validly and reliably gather data, and use the clout/imprimatur of the QOOs to make information available for consumer choice if providers are not willing to do it themselves.

We believe the underlying current here is a shift in whose interest quality is defined, that is, the balance is shifting in favor of choice and participation of the consumer in broader terms and away from narrower prescriptive structural and process requirements. This shift will require providers to be responsive to consumers, holding them to indicators of consumer outcome and satisfaction, and forcing them to compete on value (outcome for relative cost) and not cost alone. The shift will also require quality oversight organizations (regulators, certification boards, licensing agencies, and accrediting bodies) to incorporate these new notions of quality into their requirements, standards, and review procedures.

A MODEL FOR UNDERSTANDING QUALITY OVERSIGHT

It has been suggested that there is a need less for changing regulations than for "reforming the regulators themselves and changing the culture of the regulatory process" (Walshe, 2001, 142). We suggest here that both are essential in order to ensure that the interests of people seeking service are to be served over those of the providers, payers, or QOOs.

Following we summarize the array of quality oversight options by laying out a conceptual framework for the classification of purposes and types of quality review. The organizing principle of this framework is the degree of prescriptiveness involved. Four degrees of prescriptiveness are described: non-negotiable prescription (most prescriptive); general prescription; flexible parameters; and topical guidelines (least prescriptive). Across this continuum, one can map where the various forms of quality oversight tend to focus, as well as dimensions, such as the use of evidence versus consensus in developing guidelines. The model is depicted in Chart 2; definitions and examples are summarized as follows.

Non-Negotiable Prescription

What–provide in the highest level of specificity what should be done (structure or process)

When–safety and health at issue requiring absolute level; known documented evidence of relationship between level achieved and safe operation or outcome

How–regulation, licensure, grading

Examples–minimum temperature of food; maximum temperature of hot water tap; architectural design specifications; square footage; time between meals.

General Prescription

What–provide specific type of structure or process that should exist (moderate specificity); broad outer limits of operation

When–safety and health at issue but allowing moderate flexibility in level to be reached; known relationship between structure or process and

How–licensure, certification, accreditation

Examples–type of degree required for certification; staffing ratios; space designations; uniform outcome measures and data elements; times for completion of assessment and reports; training hours and types for staff.

Flexible Parameters

What–provide outline or range within which structure, process or outcome should fit

When–effectiveness and/or efficiency at issue, but allow moderate to substantial flexibility in level to be reached or manner of operating with the parameters

How–accreditation, some certification

Examples–involvement of persons served; domains of outcome measurement; safety drills required; documentation topics to be covered.

Topical Guidelines

What–provide the most broad, flexible direction, options, or suggestions as to process or outcome

When–access, effectiveness, efficiency, satisfaction, or style at issue; providers and their consumers can benefit from "best practice" knowledge but they are not necessarily required; a substantial amount of flexibility is allowed the organization

How–accreditation, consultation

Examples–education on designing outcome management systems; options for organizing records of persons served; approaches to planning and financial stability.

Our intention in proposing this model is to offer a framework for not only reflecting the concepts and alternatives in quality oversight, but to suggest that progress can be made in solving some of the dilemmas in the culture change/quality oversight intersection. As consideration is given to accommodating a resident-centered environment, the future of QOO may move more toward the flexible end of this spectrum. Although a level of prescriptiveness may be needed to ensure that consumers of the long-term care service process are pro-

CHART 2. A Model for the Understanding of Quality Oversight Mechanisms

F R A M E W O R K	Non-negotiable Prescription	General Prescription	Flexible Parameters	Topical Guidelines
	Restrictive ◄─────────────────────────────► Flexible			

Q U A L I T Y O V E R S I G H T	Licensure ├───────────────┤ Certification ├──────────────────────────┤ Accreditation ├───┤ Practice Guidelines / Clinical Pathways ├───┤

O R I G I N	Research / Evidence-based ├──────────────────┤ Consensus-based ├───┤

tected (e.g., do not incur pressure ulcers), quality oversight must allow for–and ultimately demand–positive outcomes on behalf of the persons served. Providers must have the flexibility to provide a resident-centered environment.

Returning to our anecdotal examples of how QOO are seen to impede culture change in long-term care, let us consider how changes could accommodate the new culture.

- The therapeutic recreation service could craft its activity schedules in such a way that choice and flexibility are stated values and options. The QOO could look not for specific time frames for activity, but for evidence that the provider is attending to alternatives and posting an accurate reflection of options for residents.

- The scheduling of meal times and availability of food could offer a range of alternatives to residents such that no one is *forced* into long periods of time between meals (the consumer protection factor), but that food is available for those who choose an alternative schedule (e.g., to sleep in). Quality oversight organizations could focus providers on monitoring weight, health, and nutrition outcomes rather than become overly prescriptive regarding the process (e.g., time frames for meals).

Reaching a balance between needed prescriptiveness and allowable flexibility in quality oversight requires more knowledge than we currently have. Research into process-outcome relationships and the effects of organizational structure on process and outcome is needed to guide evidence-based practice and quality oversight.

Partnerships: Potential for Collaboration Among QOO

Several approaches could help facilitate a culture of collaboration between regulators, accreditors, consumers and providers.

1. *A concerted effort to move from adversaries to partners.*

Accreditation and certification complement the roles of regulators. Assuming there is a range of prescriptiveness needed to ensure the simultaneous health, safety, choice and participation of consumers in long-term care, and considering the QO model just presented, there remains a need for more than one type of QOO. There is a need for the concrete foundation that regulations offer. There is a need, however, for regulators, consumers and providers to have more information about actual performance and improvement activities. Accreditation standards address full disclosure of performance (what happens for consumers), admission and discharge criteria, fees, rates, responsibilities of all parties, etc. This type of information would only add to a relationship, not distract from it. Joint surveys between regulators and third party accreditors could improve the process, reduce duplication, enhance information, and spend fewer dollars on survey site visits.

2. *Deliberate movement toward performance indicators that could be used across the long-term care continuum.*

Indicators of provider performance offer information for consumer choice and provider accountability. Performance indicator systems require the continued development of tools that would answer the questions that consumers, regulators and providers have. By measuring the direct results of services (outcome) and the indicators of the efficiency of achieving the outcome and the satisfaction of the consumers and other stakeholders, the industry could increase its capacity for providing services that make a difference–caring but cost effective services. The value of long-term care would be clearly defined. People would know actual quality and its cost. When dealing with real data decisions around locating and paying for good care can become more informed rather than emotional.

3. *A shift in philosophy from cost to value.*

Throughout the debate of the impact of regulations on the long-term care industry there has been the continual discussion around the fact that the payment structures created providers who were in a "business" mode and that they "did not care" about consumers, but attended to their bottom lines instead. If we could discuss value (defined as "value = quality/cost") then some of the distrust of providers might dissipate. Either cost or quality considered in a vacuum has little merit in humanitarian or financial terms.

4. *A move toward consumer focused care and consumer involvement.*

When consumers consistently have the ability to influence policy in the long-term care continuum, assist with standard development and revision, take a place on state task forces and accrediting bodies' governance boards, then both regulations and standards can be used to help differentiate and assist consumers wanting value for the services that they purchase and receive.

Each of the stakeholders in this discussion has a set of incentives that motivate them to perform. It is necessary to develop, through ongoing dialogue, some common incentives across the stakeholders to better facilitate solid communication and collaboration. Examples of common incentives might be:

- All providers and regulators want each consumer to receive quality and appropriate care, no matter the setting.
- Maintenance–and in some cases, improvement–of function and participation is critical for consumers. Performance in this area should be disclosed to consumers.
- Adequate resources to achieve quality for each consumer should be utilized but done while controlling costs. This means making sound business decisions. As noted earlier, accreditation standards tend to complement regulations in the business side of care delivery.

- All stakeholders must believe that the care continuum has value. Stakeholders should be able to identify their contribution to value. Stakeholders need to be accountable to embrace the cultural shift and their unique role in it.

RESOLVING CONFLICT:
HOW QO CAN SUPPORT CULTURE CHANGE IN LONG-TERM CARE

As with other culture change and conflict situations the way out of conflict is not necessarily to choose one side or the other, but may lie in finding the common ground between two belief systems. In the case of long-term care, there is tension between the desire for clarity and simplicity in oversight (facilitated by higher prescriptiveness in the model), and flexibility and choice in the structure and process of services (facilitated by lower prescriptiveness).

The challenge for all stakeholders in this situation is to maintain the safety, protections and feasibility features of the regulatory/oversight process while allowing for the new quality culture with its emphasis on consumer choice and provider responsiveness in the service setting.

The Challenge for Quality Oversight Organizations

Given that QOOs, consumers of long-term care, and providers all share these common goals, there are certain steps quality oversight organizations themselves can undertake to address the need for and take a positive role in culture change for long-term care:

- Re-examine the true goal and scope of quality review: In whose interest is the QO enterprise?
- Review QO requirements to ensure that they are meaningful, clear, non-conflicting to the degree possible
  - Where multiple types of oversight must be obtained, e.g., licensure and accreditation, the two types should not be at odds with each other. This is difficult when one QOO is national or international (e.g., accreditation) and another is state- or locally-based (e.g., licensure), but efforts should be made to avoid blatant conflicts and where possible to streamline duplicative requirements.
- Be clear about the level at which requirements are applied, i.e., for the individual practitioner (e.g., certification), for the physical facility (e.g., licensure) or for the organization and its processes and outcomes (e.g., accreditation);

- Identify where prescription is necessary and warranted to ensure a desirable level of safety *and* a desirable level of independence and participation on behalf of persons served;
- Where it is not, work to train surveyors/reviewers about a valid range of options for operating a safe, effective, *and* choice-accommodating environment;
- Inform providers and consumers about quality oversight rationale, benefits and options;
- Develop requirements that are meaningful but not unnecessarily burdensome.

The Challenge for Providers

Providers too must examine their role in the quality oversight enterprise. While provider organizations and QOOs may seem like natural enemies, this need not be the case, especially considering the common goals. Quality oversight can provide not only assurance for consumers, but an advantage for providers. Providers can:

- Recognize consumer-protection rationale for quality oversight;
- Work with QOOs to develop appropriate rules/standards/monitors/reviews to ensure quality services and consumer protection;
- Inform consumers about quality oversight rationale, benefits, options, and their own status;
- Provide consumers and their sponsors/advocates with information about providers' quality oversight activities and status;
- Focus on needs and preferences of persons served first, and secondly on the convenience of the provider staff; staff members are human too, and their satisfaction may derive as much or more from providing excellent service than from pure convenience of routine.

The Challenge for Consumers

Finally, QOOs, providers, and payor/sponsors as well as consumer advocacy organizations can capitalize on the theme of consumerism to educate people on how to choose long-term care, including how to:

- Look for and ask for information about quality of providers
- Be concerned about and ask about quality oversight: licensure, certification, accreditation of provider organizations and its employees.

CONCLUSION

Culture change entails the building of new beliefs, values, and meanings on the platform of old ones. It also involves the change of behaviors, habits, language, and rituals. The enterprise of quality oversight should both reflect the ambient culture and accepted quality standards, and also nudge (or even push) the field toward new ones in the interest of the persons served. We have tried to show that to accommodate consumer interests in participation and quality of life, all stakeholders in quality services may have to adapt to the culture change underway in long-term care. If–or rather, when–there are conflicts along the way, *it is the person served in whose interest the system should operate.* This will take time.

We have also proposed a model for the assessment of quality oversight that ranges from prescriptiveness to flexibility, and suggested that there is work to be done to sort out the proper mix of quality oversight standards and requirements along this continuum. The changing culture of long-term care could benefit from, and be accommodated by, refinements in the mix of prescriptiveness for consumer protection and flexibility to allow for choice.

If one believes that in the long-term care continuum through collaborative partnerships there could be roles for regulators, accreditors, consumers, and providers, there are concerns that need to be addressed:

1. Quality oversight organizations should form public/private partnerships. It should be recognized that there are roles for each of the stakeholders in producing quality care that has value for consumers, and that is effective and efficiently delivered.
2. We need a clear definition of value and quality. There has to be acceptance that in the care continuum there most likely will be limitations. These need to be disclosed to all parties. There are also opportunities to open up quality oversight so that it can accommodate the flexibility and creativity required to promote the values of independence, support, and participation as defined in this paper.
3. We need to determine what has value for each stakeholder. The term quality alone has little use when discussing a new culture of accountability. Stakeholders should include consumers, regulators, licensing agencies, accreditors, and providers. If there are other identified stakeholders the circle should be inclusive versus exclusive.
4. Recognize long-term care as a continuum. No one setting should take precedence or a more prominent position over others; rather services should be appropriate to the needs of the consumers. To have value there should be opportunities for people to enter and to move throughout a continuum of care if possible. With this in mind, regulators and

accreditors need to partner to create meaningful surveys and consultation for improvement in all areas of the continuum.

5. The relationship between reimbursement and quality needs to be examined. If outcomes are not produced should there be payment in this new culture?

6. To facilitate this shift in culture there has to be unbiased education and communication among all stakeholders.

7. We need strategies to share and manage risk among all stakeholders. There is a shared risk among all stakeholders if this culture is to be embraced, but the question is no longer how to eliminate the risk, but how to ensure choice and quality of life while providing safe, quality services.

A transparent continuum of care for long-term care needs would certainly better address the future needs of consumers. Many of these individuals are people like the authors and many readers of this article–baby boomers caring for aging parents and anticipating their own retirement. We ask ourselves about the current state of quality and our ability to assess value in long-term care. Is this the service and quality culture we want, or is it time for change?

REFERENCES

Administration on Aging. (2000). *A Profile of Older Americans: 2000*. Washington: U.S. Department of Health and Human Services.

American College of Mental Health Administration [ACMHA]. (2001). *Proposed Consensus Set of Indicators for Behavioral Health*. Report of the Accreditation Organization Work Group. Pittsburgh, PA: Author.

Burgess, K. L. & Riley, P. (2000). Can accreditation solve the insurance crisis? *Provider, 26*(10):71-74.

Commission on Accreditation of Rehabilitation Facilities [CARF]. (1998). *Performance Indicators for Rehabilitation Programs, Version 1.1: Working Draft for Comment*. Tucson: CARF.

DeJong, G. (1979). *The movement for independent living: Origins, ideology, and implications for disability research*. East Lansing: University Centers for International Rehabilitation.

Donabedian, A. (1966). Evaluating the quality of medical care. *Milbank Quarterly, 44*:166-203.

Donabedian, A. (1983). Quality, cost and clinical decisions. *Annnals of the American Academy of Political and Social Science, 468*:196-204.

Donabedian, A. (1988). The quality of care: How can it be assessed? *JAMA, 260*(12):1743-1748.

Frieden, Lex. (1978). IL: Movement and programs. *American Rehabilitation, 3*(6):6-9.

Fratalli, C. (Ed.). (1997). *Outcomes Measurement in Speech-Language Pathology*. New York: Thieme Medical Publishers, Inc.

Geertz, C. (1973). *The Interpretation of Cultures*. New York: Basic Books, Inc.

Heumann, J. (1977). Independent living programs. In: Susan Stoddard Pflueger (ed.), *Independent Living: Emerging Issues in Rehabilitation*. Washington, DC: Institute for Research Utilization.

Institute of Medicine [IOM]. (1986). Improving the Quality of Care in Nursing Homes. Washington, D.C.: National Academy of Sciences Press.

Kane, R. A. (2001). Long-term care and a good quality of life: Bringing them closer together. *The Gerontologist, 41*(3):293-304.

Kane, R. L. & Kane, R. A. (2001). What older people want from long-term care, and how they can get it. *Health Affairs, 20*(6):114-127.

National Committee for Quality Assurance [NCQA]. (1997). *HEDIS 3.0: Volume 1 Understanding and Enhancing Performance Measurement* and *Volume 2 Measurement Specifications*. Washington, D.C.: National Committee for Quality Assurance.

Older Americans Report. (2001). Business Publishers Inc., December 14:403.

Osborn, E. (2002). Who Should Regulate? *Assisted Living Success*, January, 2002:32.

President's Advisory Commission on Consumer Protection and Quality in the Health Care Industry. (1998). *Quality first: Better health care for all Americans*. Final Report to the President of the United States from the President's Advisory Commission on Consumer Protection and Quality in the Health Care Industry. (Consumers' Bill of Rights). Washington: President's Advisory Commission.

Schein, E. (1992). *Organizational Culture and Leadership, Second Edition*. San Francisco: Jossey-Bass Publishers.

Schnelle, J. F., Ouslander, J. G. & Cruise, P. A. (1997). Policy without technology: A barrier to improving nursing home care. *The Gerontologist, 37*(4):527-532.

U.S. Census Bureau. (2001). *Profile of general demographic characteristics, 2000. DP-1*. Census 2000 Summary File 1 (SF 1), 100 percent data. Available from U.S. Census Bureau web site, *http://factfinder.census.gov*.

Walshe, K. (2001). Regulating U.S. nursing homes: Are we learning from experience? *Health Affairs, 20*(6):128-144.

*Webster's Encyclopedia Unabridged Dictionary of the English Langua*ge (1990).

World Health Organization [WHO]. (1980). *International Classification of Impairments, Disabilities, and Handicaps*. Geneva: Author.

World Health Organization [WHO]. (2001). International Classification of Functioning, Disability and Health (ICF). Geneva: Author.

Policy Values and Culture Change in Long-Term Care– The Role of State Government in Catalyzing Change

William E. Reynolds

SUMMARY. Despite some improvements that can be attributed to the provisions of OBRA '87, the quality of care in nursing homes remains far from optimal. Excessive reliance on a medical model of care fails to address residents' desire to be treated with kindness, courtesy and consideration. In addition, the issue of improving quality of care is linked to addressing growing concerns about nursing home staffing. One solution

---

Willliam E. Reynolds, DDS, MPH, is Public Service Professor, University at Albany, School of Social Welfare, and Clinical Associate Professor, University at Albany, School of Public Health, Department of Health Policy and Management. Until his retirement from the New York State Department of Health in October 2001, Dr. Reynolds served in a variety of positions including Director of the Bureau of Standards Development and Project Director in the Office of Continuing Care.

Address correspondence to: William E. Reynolds, DDS, MPH, 1515 Keyes Avenue, Niskayuna, NY 12309 (E-mail: wreynol1@nycap.rr.com).

The author is grateful to Elizabeth Pohlman and Rose Marie Fagan for their helpful comments on an earlier draft of this article. In addition the author wants to acknowledge Beth Dichter for her substantial contribution to the development of the RFA for the NY State Dementia Grant Program which was cited in this article. David Levine's assistance in the literature review is greatly appreciated.

[Haworth co-indexing entry note]: "Policy Values and Culture Change in Long-Term Care–The Role of State Government in Catalyzing Change." Reynolds, William E. Co-published simultaneously in *Journal of Social Work in Long-Term Care* (The Haworth Social Work Practice Press, an imprint of The Haworth Press, Inc.) Vol. 2, No. 3/4, 2003, pp. 397-410; and: *Culture Change in Long-Term Care* (ed: Audrey S. Weiner, and Judah L. Ronch) The Haworth Social Work Practice Press, an imprint of The Haworth Press, Inc., 2003, pp. 397-410. Single or multiple copies of this article are available for a fee from The Haworth Document Delivery Service [1-800-HAWORTH, 9:00 a.m. - 5:00 p.m. (EST). E-mail address: docdelivery@haworthpress.com].

10.1300/J181v2n03_14

is for government to play a role in catalyzing a change in the organizational culture of nursing homes to address the concerns that both residents and staff have with the existing culture. A number of states are providing grants to nursing homes to implement culture change. This has included New York State which has emphasized culture change in its Dementia Grant Program. *[Article copies available for a fee from The Haworth Document Delivery Service: 1-800-HAWORTH. E-mail address: <docdelivery@haworthpress.com> Website: <http://www.HaworthPress.com> © 2003 by The Haworth Press, Inc. All rights reserved.]*

KEYWORDS. Nursing homes, quality improvement, regulation, workforce, culture change, public policy

WHAT IS GOVERNMENT'S ROLE IN IMPROVING QUALITY IN NURSING HOMES?

The Institute of Medicine (1986) in its landmark report on nursing home quality articulated a widely held view of government's role in assuring quality in nursing homes:

> State and federal nursing home regulators have a mandate to protect the public's health and safety in nursing homes. There are three components: establishing explicit criteria to govern nursing home behavior and operations; establishing and carrying out standard methods for monitoring nursing home performance; and taking enforcement action where unsatisfactory performance is substantiated.

A similar view of government's role was recently expressed by an Assistant United States Attorney who represented the United States in a case that applied the False Claims Act as an enforcement mechanism to ensure proper care:

> The protection of our older adults residing in nursing homes is one of the most important functions of government, whether federal, state or local. While recognizing that the nursing home industry is one of the most regulated, enforcement of those regulations, by whatever means, is paramount to ensuring appropriate care. (Hoffman, 1997)

However, some authorities advocate that government must also provide leadership that goes beyond enforcement actions to improve quality. Nearly 15 years after it issued its 1986 report on nursing homes, the Institute of Medicine

(2000) called for such leadership when it issued a report on quality in health care.

While the Institute of Medicine's Committee on the Quality of Health Care in America's report did not specifically address quality of care in nursing homes, the findings and recommendations apply and provide a useful background for this discussion. Government is in a unique position to provide leadership that is beyond the capacity of nursing home providers or advocates. The report is a call to action to improve the entire American health care delivery system in all of its quality dimensions. The approaches described below provide a potential agenda for addressing the inadequacies in nursing home operations as well.

The Institute report (2000) begins by noting that the American health care system is in need of fundamental change.

> Quality problems are everywhere, affecting many patients. Between the health care we have and the care we could have lies not just a gap, but a chasm (p. 1). The need for leadership in health care has never been greater. Transforming the health care system will not be an easy process. But the potential benefits are large as well. (p. 5)

The Committee proposed an ambitious agenda for redesigning care processes, which includes calling upon purchasers, regulators, health professions, educational institutions, and the Department of Health and Human Services to create an environment that fosters and rewards improvement.

The Committee stressed that health care should be patient-centered, which means providing care that is respectful of and responsive to individual patient preferences, needs, and values and ensuring that patient values guide all clinical decisions. The report recommends that health care processes should be redesigned in accordance with a new set of rules, which notably includes "The patient as the source of control" (p. 8).

This paper will briefly describe the failure of the current federal and state regulatory approaches to improve quality of care in nursing homes. While a detailed review and evaluation of the effectiveness of each of those efforts is beyond the scope of this paper, there is substantial evidence that efforts to date have fallen short (U.S. General Accounting Office, 1998; U.S. General Accounting Office, 1999; U.S. General Accounting Office, 2000; Harrington, 2001). More fundamental changes are needed that are consistent with the recent recommendations of the quality committee of the Institute of Medicine and the principles of culture change as described throughout this publication. As will be described, New York State's recent initial effort to encourage the wide scale adoption of culture change strategies is one example of the kind of governmental leadership that could produce fundamental change in long-term care consistent with the Institute of Medicine (2000) recommendations.

THE SHORTCOMINGS OF THE CURRENT REGULATORY MODEL

Other authors (see, for example Thomas, Kehoe, Fagan, Gilbert, Rader, Brecanier and Boyd in this volume) have proposed strategies to improve quality at the facility level. Once these are accepted as promising practices, the next step is to determine how society can achieve wide scale implementation of the kind of changes necessary to improve quality in all facilities and identify the ways that government may provide the necessary leadership for this to occur.

While many agree that a regulatory approach that includes setting minimum standards and conducting surveillance and enforcement activities in some manner is essential to ensuring quality (Harrington, 2001), opinions on how this regulatory role might best be carried out depends upon how the industry and its motivations and behaviors are viewed. Day and Klein (1987) have characterized the overall model of regulation used in the United States as legalistic and adversarial, in contrast to European models, which are informal and consensual. They (Day & Klein, 1987) point out that these two models rely on significantly "contrasting systems, styles or strategies" (p. 307) of regulation.

Europeans generally rely upon a *compliance model.* This model focuses on preventing problems and on encouraging investment of time and money to improve the situation. The inspector's role is to cajole, negotiate and bargain. Legal prosecution is seen as the last resort. The relationship between the regulator and the regulated party is part of the process of improving quality.

The other model, the one favored by the United States, is the *deterrence model* (Day & Klein, 1987). This model emphasizes punishing wrongdoing. The style is accusatory and adversarial. Recourse to formal legal proceedings is typical. The underlying assumption is that effective punishment of rule breaking will lead to improved behavior in the future. Most regulatory systems tend to be a blend of the two styles but there is usually a bias toward one style or the other in any given system (Day & Klein, 1987). Day and Klein's (1987) analysis of the body of literature on regulatory approaches leads them to conclude that while the deterrence model is ineffective in stimulating health care providers to "do good," it may be effective in preventing providers from doing the "bad" things they might otherwise do.

Shortly after Day and Klein's (1987) research was completed, the Omnibus Budget Reconciliation Act of 1987 (OBRA '87) raised standards for nursing homes and strengthened federal and state oversight. A limited number of studies have found evidence of improvement in the care processes studied, such as accuracy of information in residents' medical records and comprehensiveness of care plans. Use of restraints and indwelling catheters also declined. There were also increases in good practices, such as the presence of advanced directives and participation in activities (Hawes et al., 1997). Yet these and other researchers point out that quality of care still is far from optimal (Reinhardt & Stone, 2001; Harrington, 2001; U.S. Department of Health and Human Services, Health Care Financing Administration n.d.; Eaton, 1997). While more effective implementation of the OBRA '87 legislation may be warranted (Harrington, 2001), there is limited research to demonstrate that OBRA '87 has been effective in enhancing quality of life, which is a key goal for quality improvement efforts (Hawes et al., 1997).

CULTURE CHANGE: THE INTERSECTION OF ADVOCACY FOR IMPROVING QUALITY IN NURSING HOMES AND ADVOCACY FOR ADDRESSING THE WORKFORCE SHORTAGE

Improving quality of care in nursing homes is a persistent public policy issue that has perplexed government regulators. At the same time, nursing home operators are faced with serious problems as they attempt to improve the quality of services in nursing homes. One significant barrier to improving quality is the high rate of staff turnover at all levels. A most desirable goal would be to create nursing homes where residents want to live and workers want to work.

The issue of improving the quality of care of residents has been linked with addressing nursing home staffing concerns (Eaton, 1997; 2000; Harrington, 2001). Nursing home administrators, state and federal regulators, and consumer advocates share a growing recognition that poor quality of care can be traced, in part, to at least one root cause, namely staffing shortages and inadequate training (Reinhardt & Stone, 2001). While each individual facility must play a key role in solving this problem through improving its own human resources management, collective action involving government leadership will be required as well (Faculty Workgroup on Peopling Long-Term Care, 2001; Willging, n.d.). Nursing home operators are unable to implement strategies available to employers in less regulated industries. Substantially increasing pay for workers in nursing homes probably would attract more workers, but this solution would require that government, the primary source of funding of long-term care, raise payments to providers. Despite numerous studies and proposed solutions to the workforce problem, government response has been limited in part because of its unwillingness to spend the additional money (Faculty Workgroup on Peopling Long-Term Care, 2001; Harrington, 2001).

While more money is part of the answer, a more fundamental change is needed at the policy level to guide the actions of regulators so that they match the changes that need to take place at the facility level. In other words, all stakeholders in the system must participate in formulating and executing the changes needed in the system as a whole to enable improvements in quality at the individual facility level. A "systems thinking" approach is needed by government, providers and advocates who typically have pursued limited solutions based upon their simple explanations of complex problems (Senge, 1990).

GOVERNMENT'S INITIATIVES

Government can, and should, address the workforce shortage in a way that goes beyond merely putting more money into the system by catalyzing the change of the organizational culture of nursing homes (Faculty Workgroup on Peopling Long-Term Care, 2001). Culture change is at the intersection of the concerns of the workers, the administrators, the residents and the advocates for better resident care. The current perception of nursing homes is such that the elderly dread entering them and few workers are attracted to enter or remain in employment in the industry. Even under the best of circumstances, caring for the typical elderly nursing home resident who inevitably declines and dies can be seen as an unrewarding task (Day & Klein, 1987; Eaton, 1997). The rate of pay, lack of benefits, poor quality of supervision, and other human resource management factors compound the inherently unattractive nature of the work (Faculty Workgroup on Peopling Long-Term Care, 2001; Eaton, 1997; 2000).

Day and Klein's (1987) evaluation of New York's system of regulating nursing homes concluded that the entire conceptualization of nursing home care was too skewed toward the medical model given that a large number of the residents will eventually die while living in the nursing home. Most residents did not come to the nursing home with the expectation of being cured of an acute illness. These and other researchers (Eaton, 1997; 2000) concluded that the way in which residents are treated–hopefully with kindness, courtesy and consideration–would always be more important than intermediate measures of quality based upon the medical model. Eaton's (1997) study of nursing homes in Pennsylvania and California also identified the problems associated with application of the medical model to long-term care. She found that many discrete medical problems are treated without adequate consideration of how the treatments affect quality of life. She pointed out that the potential for developing a new concept for the long-term care of the elderly to focus on supporting their functional independence and quality of life remains largely unexplored.

Acting by themselves, providers have had limited effect in obtaining the necessary response from government to address the workforce issues. However, coalitions that include all stakeholders are beginning to demonstrate success in addressing workforce issues and the culture of care simultaneously. Advocates who worked together in the political process that led to OBRA '87 have joined forces with those progressive nursing home providers and other professionals who created the Pioneer Network (see Fagan, this volume) to collaborate in overcoming the barriers faced by nursing homes which seek to provide high quality care. The National Citizens' Coalition for Nursing Home Reform, for example, participated in the original meeting of the Pioneers in 1997 and continues to be closely associated with the Pioneer Network. A number of Long Term Care Ombudsman Programs at the state level have played a major role in the promotion of culture change in their states (Frank, 2000). As a result of such advocacy, a number of state governments have taken actions to address the workforce shortage in combination with efforts to encourage the change of nursing home culture.

Notable among regional coalitions is the Southwestern Pennsylvania Partnership for Aging (SWPPA). SWPPA is a 10-county, 403 member coalition of providers, business and community organizations, and governmental entities which is leading a 5-year culture change project to change the way aging services are provided, organized and staffed in the region. Statewide coalitions have been formed or are forming in Ohio, Florida, New Hampshire and Illinois (Pioneer Network, 2002). The goals of these coalitions typically include improved funding and demonstration grants from states to address workforce issues and culture change.

Statewide coalitions have been formed with the assistance of the Eden Alternative (see Thomas, this volume) organization in Michigan, North Carolina and South Carolina. The results of this advocacy have included grants to nursing homes to implement "Eden" projects in these three states. The Michigan program, Bringing The Eden Alternative to Michigan (BEAM) was established in 1998 with support from the Michigan Office of Services to the Aging. Since its inception it has assisted 48 nursing homes to pursue implementation of the Eden Alternative (Culture Change Now, n.d.).

North Carolina and South Carolina have awarded funds garnered from nursing homes fined for being out of compliance with Medicare and Medicaid standards to support facilities engaging in culture change (Warner, 1998). The South Carolina program has provided grants to 25 nursing homes for projects which began in 1999 and concluded in 2002. The state provided another series of awards in 2002 (State of South Carolina, n.d, State of South Carolina, 2002).

The state of New Jersey awarded two-year grants of $20,000 each to ten nursing homes in December 1999 to implement the Eden Alternative. The New Jersey Department of Health and Senior Services worked with the Rutgers Center for State Health Policy to develop measurement tools to assess the results at both the resident and nursing home industry levels. Meetings of grantees to share experiences were also supported and state inspectors visited the homes to collect documentation. New Jersey built its program on results obtained from evaluations conducted by South Carolina and Texas (State of New Jersey, 1999).

Texas has used $100,000 in funds recovered from overpayments made to nursing homes to conduct what is called the Rider 26 Project. This project studied the performance of 101 nursing facilities that used one or more quality improvement interventions. Some facilities used the Wellspring Innovation Solutions model (see Kehoe, this volume), while others used the Eden Alternative model. A third group used the Facilitator Program, a quality improvement model proposed by the Texas Health Care Association based upon a data-driven approach that gives resident feedback to providers, while a fourth group serves as a control (State of Texas, n.d.a; State of Texas, n.d.b).

Along with their interest in supporting culture change, most advocates have not abandoned their zeal for higher standards, increased surveillance and more enforcement. But they, as well as policymakers, researchers and the public, see a place for these new approaches in the mix of strategies needed to improve quality since they have seen the limited progress made over the past 25 years by continuing the same old strategies.

NEW YORK STATE'S DEMENTIA GRANT PROGRAM AND ITS ROLE IN CATALYZING CULTURE CHANGE

Background

The New York State Department of Health (The Department) created the Dementia Grant Program in response to the concerns providers and advocates expressed about the implementation of New York's Medicaid case mix reimbursement for nursing homes in the late 1980s. In that system, many ambulatory residents with dementia who presented with difficult to manage behaviors (like wandering) were classified into Resource Utilization Groups (RUGs) which were tied to low levels of reimbursement. As a result, hospitals found it difficult to discharge persons with dementia to nursing homes that did not want to admit them because their low reimbursement rates were unattractive in view of their many service needs. Advocates for persons with dementia saw the new reimbursement system as one that perpetuated inadequate and inappropriate services for residents with dementia whose low RUGs scores were based not upon a realistic comprehensive assessment of their overall care needs but rather upon needs as assessed in a medical model of care and services. These residents would have scored high on need for socialization, structured opportunities to behave competently, and other psychosocial needs in a different classification system. The Department responded by providing slightly higher additional Medicaid reimbursement to facilities for each resident with dementia and by developing the Dementia Grant Program in 1988. Under this program nursing homes were competitively selected to conduct research projects designed to develop and evaluate innovations in dementia diagnosis, care and program development.

The projects funded by the program have the potential of having a broader impact than the title of the program might imply because a large portion of nursing home residents can benefit since so many have dementia. Many promising practices which have been developed under the program have implications for the care of persons without dementia, and they have been replicated in ways that benefit all residents regardless of diagnosis.

A notable example of such a benefit is the Eden Alternative, an early and probably the best-known example of culture change which was one of the first projects funded by the program. The positive evaluation of the project conducted under the Dementia Grant Program contributed to the widespread interest in its underlying concepts.

LINKS BETWEEN THE DEMENTIA GRANT PROGRAM AND THE PIONEER NETWORK

More recent projects supported by the grant program have included work with facilities in implementing culture change in Rochester, New York. The work of Fagan and her colleagues at the Nursing Home Culture Change Project has produced evidence of change in the entire community of long-term care providers in the Rochester region as many facilities pursue culture change (Frank, 2000).

The Nursing Home Culture Change Project in Rochester originated in the Monroe County Ombudsman Program and grew out of the Lifespan Long Term Care Community Forum (The Forum). The Forum was started in 1991 by the Ombudsman Program to bring together providers, regulators, advocates, family members and residents to explore the intention of OBRA '87 and to understand the meaning of restraint-free care. The Forum sought to remove obstacles that providers felt stood in the way of removing restraints by seeking the advice of experts such as lawyers, nurses and others who could address providers' concerns (Frank, 2000).

In 1994 the Forum established a steering committee comprised of practitioners who were ready to consider implementing facility-wide evolution toward individualized care. By 1996 two nursing homes in Rochester had committed to begin the process of transforming their culture. They volunteered to be the site for a grant funded demonstration project to adopt approaches that had been successful in a few facilities elsewhere. In 1997 the Nursing Home Culture Change Project received funding to bring together innovative practitioners from around the country to identify what their approaches had in common and how to measure the outcomes of their efforts (Frank, 2000).

In 1998, the Nursing Home Culture Change Project received funding through the Dementia Grant Program as well as from a foundation for a three year study of the culture change process and its outcomes in these two Rochester nursing homes. The funding enabled the project to bring consultants to the two homes and make them available to all the homes in the community through public education programs. Through the Community Forum, these nursing homes engaged in local sharing and exchange to create a network of mutual support. By 1999, 10 of the 36 nursing homes in the county were engaged in culture change to varying degrees (Frank, 2000).

The Nursing Home Culture Change Project subsequently implemented culture change strategies to shift nursing homes away from the medical model which helped to address the long-standing problems of staffing shortages and inadequate training. For example, a Certified Nursing Assistant Task Force was formed to address the Certified Nursing Assistant shortage. The group sought to transform the work environment and to improve recruitment and retention of front-line staff. Additional initiatives included education of survey teams and creating more dialogue among regulators, providers and advocates. Administrators and owners were given the opportunity to learn first-hand from practitioners in the field of culture change at the First National Conference of Pioneers in Culture Change which was held in August of 1999 with assistance from staff of the Nursing Home Culture Change Project (Frank, 2000).

REDESIGN OF THE DEMENTIA GRANT PROGRAM IN 2001: NEW IMPETUS FOR CULTURE CHANGE

The 1999 conference "Pioneers in Culture Change" and the results of the grants provided to the Rochester facilities that engaged in culture change provided key information that contributed substantially to the redesign of the Dementia Grant Program. After nearly three years of research to identify strategies by which to increase the effectiveness of the program in reaching its goal of improving care for persons with dementia, an RFA that differed substantially from those in the past was issued in July 2001. The research upon which the new direction was based included meetings with current grantees and other stakeholders, review of previous evaluations of the program, and research to determine strategies being used to accomplish similar goals in other states. In addition, staff and consultants to the program conducted a review of the literature on facilitators and barriers to adopting change in the practices of health care organizations. The redesign of the program reflected the results of that review and subsequent discussions with program managers, contractors and other stakeholders.

The subsequent cycle of the grant program was thus the first to specifically identify supporting culture change projects as one of its goals. While a number of the interventions that have been tested over the decade of the program's existence are consistent with the principles of culture change, the program urged applicants to implement culture change per se. In its 2001 RFA, the Department stated unambiguously that the current culture is a root cause of resident and staff dissatisfaction with today's nursing homes. Some of the Department's program managers had concerns about the readiness of New York's nursing homes to pursue culture change initiatives within the context of the grant program. While some managers would have placed the entire emphasis of the grant program on fostering and evaluating culture change, others felt this was too bold of a step. However, after consulting with staff of the statewide nursing home provider associations, managers were comfortable that enough providers were ready to begin implementing culture change to warrant a major emphasis on it in the program's priorities for funding.

A NEW ROLE FOR THE COORDINATOR TO PROVIDE TECHNICAL ASSISTANCE

The 2001 RFA provided for technical assistance including the following:

- Education and training for boards of directors, department managers, other nursing home staff, residents and family members in such areas as culture change, barriers to culture change, and approaches to overcoming the barriers; systems change, change blockers, and approaches to working with blockers; person-centered care planning; informed consent; strategic planning; team development; staff empowerment; and effective communication.

- Identification of possible surveillance and compliance issues associated with implementation of culture change, and guidance in how to avoid them, or how to anticipate and plan for them such that a compliance issue does not arise.
- Education and training for surveyors in such areas as nursing home culture change; person-centered care planning; informed consent; and possibilities for the integration of such values and goals as home-like environment, resident dignity, resident choice and resident control into current quality of life and quality of care requirements.
- Guidance and encouragement for nursing homes in continuing to work toward their project's goals in the face of staff shortages, overworked staff, and a highly stressful environment.
- Approaches to improving recruiting and retaining staff, other than wage and benefit improvements.
- Project-specific problem solving.
- Cutting edge approaches to identifying and addressing the needs of nursing home residents with dementia.

The 2001 RFA also strengthened the program's focus on sound quantitative and qualitative evaluation in order to ascertain whether: (1) individual nursing home projects produce the desired outcomes; and (2) the program as a whole is successful in achieving its objectives.

CONCLUSIONS FOR A STATE POLICY PROFESSIONAL

These conclusions are drawn from this author's state-level policy experiences and reflect a personal rather than "official" perspective.

1. Insufficient progress has been made over the past three decades of attempts to solve the vexing problems around improving quality of care in nursing homes despite considerable efforts.
2. Current regulatory models and associated enforcement approaches are insufficient to produce the improvements in nursing home quality sought by residents and advocates.
3. Improvements in the quality of nursing home care must be linked with developing solutions to the crisis in recruitment and retention of nursing home staff.
4. Advocates need to expand their focus beyond only pointing out the shortcomings of nursing homes and regulators to become part of advo-

cating for new solutions that involve partnerships between providers, regulators and consumers.

5. Culture change is a viable approach for providers to improve quality, but government needs to play a key role in supporting providers in the wide-scale implementation of culture change initiatives.

6. Evaluation of the process of implementing culture change and its many outcomes is critical and government should play a role in supporting and conducting that evaluation.

REFERENCES

Culture Change Now. (n.d.). Bringing the Eden Alternative to Michigan (BEAM). Retrieved December 15, 2001 from http://www.culturechangenow.com/stories/beam.html.

Day, P. & Klein, R. (1987). The regulation of nursing homes: A comparative perspective. *The Milbank Quarterly, 65* (3), 303-347.

Eaton, S.C. (1997). *Pennsylvania's nursing homes: Promoting quality care and quality jobs.* Harrisburg: Keystone Research Center.

Eaton, S.C. (2000). Beyond 'Unloving Care': Linking human resource management and patient care quality in nursing homes. *Journal of Human Resources Management, 11* (3), 591-616.

Faculty Workgroup on Peopling Long-Term Care. (2001). *Peopling long-term care: Assuring an adequate long-term care workforce for Minnesota.* Minneapolis: University of Minnesota, Minnesota Chair in Long-term Care and Aging & Center on Aging.

Frank, B. (2000). *Ombudsman best practices: Supporting culture change to promote individualized care in nursing homes.* Washington: National Long Term Care Ombudsman Resource Center.

Harrington, C. (2001). Regulation nursing homes: Residential nursing facilities in the United States. *British Medical Journal, 323* (7311), 507-510.

Hawes, C., Mor, V., Phillips, C.D., Fries, B.E., Morris, J.N. et al. (1997). The OBRA '87 nursing home regulations and implementation of the resident assessment instrument: Effects on process quality. *Journal of the American Geriatrics Society, 45* (8), 977-985.

Hoffman, D.R. (1997). The role of the federal government in ensuring quality of care in long-term care facilities. *Annals of Health Law, 6,* 147-156.

Institute of Medicine, Committee on Nursing Home Regulation. (1986). *Improving the quality of care in nursing homes.* Washington, DC: National Academy Press.

Institute of Medicine, Committee on Quality Health Care in America. (2000). *Crossing the quality chasm: A new health system for the 21st Century.* Washington, DC: National Acadek my Press.

Pioneer Network, (2002). Personal communication with Rose Marie Fagan. January 4, 2002.

Reinhardt, S. & Stone, R. (2001). *Promoting quality in nursing homes: The Wellspring model.* Retrieved December 15, 2001 from www.cmwf.org/programs/elders/reinhard_wellspring_432.pdf.

Senge, P.M. (1990). *The fifth discipline: The art and practice of the learning organization.* New York: Currency Doubleday.

State of New Jersey, Department of Health and Senior Services. (1999). *News Release: $200,000 awarded to help nursing homes become Eden Alternative homes.* Retrieved December 14, 2001 from http://www.state.nj.us/health/news/p91203a.htm .

State of South Carolina, Department of Health and Human Services. (n.d.). *FY 1999-2000 Accountability Report for the Department of Health and Human Services.* Retrieved December 15, 2001, from http://www.dhhs.state.sc.us/reports/accountability_reports/f799_00.pdf.

State of South Carolina, Department of Health and Human Services. (2002). Personal communication with Anita Bowen, March 19, 2002.

State of Texas, Department of Human Services. (n.d.a). *Frequently asked questions (FAQ) on rider 26 project.* Retrieved December 15, 2001 from http://www.ltc.dhs.state.tx.us/policy/MDS/faq_26&32.htm.

State of Texas, Department of Human Services. (n.d.b). *Sharing the vision: 2000 Annual report Texas Department of Human Services.* Retrieved December 15, 2001 from http://www.dhs.state.tx.us/publications/AnnualReport/2000/AR%20_LTC_p46_55.pdf.

U.S. General Accounting Office. (1998). *California nursing homes: Care problems persist despite federal and state oversight: Report to the Special Committee on Aging, U.S. Senate.* GAO/HEHS-98-202, Washington, D.C., 1998.

U.S. General Accounting Office. (1999). *Nursing homes: Additional steps needed to strengthen enforcement of federal quality standards: Report to the Special Committee on Aging, U.S. Senate.* GAO/HEHS-99-46, Washington, D.C., 1999.

U.S. General Accounting Office. (2000). *Nursing homes: Enhanced HCFA oversight of state programs would better ensure quality of care: Report to the Special Committee on Aging, U.S. Senate.* GAO/HEHS-00-27, Washington, D.C., 2000.

United States Department of Health and Human Services, Health Care Financing Administration. (n.d.). *Study of private accreditation (deeming) of nursing homes, regulatory incentives and non-regulatory initiatives, and effectiveness of the survey and certification system.* Retrieved December 12, 2001 from http://www.hcfa.gov/medicaid/exectv2.htm.

Warner, J.L. (1998). *Nursing home care is improving.* Retrieved December 15, 2001 from http://www.elderlaw-sc.com/articles/12.asp.

Willging, P.R. (n.d.) The Eden Alternative to nursing home care: More than just birds. Retrieved December 15, 2001 from http://www.asaging.org/at/at-214/eden.html.

Selecting a Model
or Choosing Your Own Culture

Robyn I. Stone

SUMMARY. In this article the author reviews the practical issues related to implementing culture change in nursing homes. The merits of model replication are discussed and the barriers to creating and sustaining culture change in nursing homes are highlighted. This is followed by a description of the various dimensions of culture that must be changed including the approach to clinical training and practice, the nature of management and job design, the approach to caring, and the characteristics of the residential environment. The article then identifies the major elements required to maximize the potential for nursing homes to create and sustain culture change. *[Article copies available for a fee from The Haworth Document Delivery Service: 1-800-HAWORTH. E-mail address: <docdelivery@haworthpress.com> Website: <http://www.HaworthPress.com> © 2003 by The Haworth Press, Inc. All rights reserved.]*

Robyn I. Stone, PhD, is Executive Director for the Institute for the Future of Aging Services, Washington, DC.

Address correspondence to: Robyn I. Stone, PhD, Executive Director, Institute for the Future of Aging Services, 2519 Connecticut Avenue, NW, Washington, DC 20008 (E-mail: rstone@aahsa.org).

The information presented in this article was drawn, in part, from technical expert panels and a literature review supported by funds from the U.S. Department of Health and Human Services, Office for Disability, Aging and Long-Term Care Policy in Washington, D.C. The materials on the Wellspring model are taken from an evaluation of the program funded by the Commonwealth Fund in New York City.

[Haworth co-indexing entry note]: "Selecting a Model or Choosing Your Own Culture." Stone, Robyn I. Co-published simultaneously in *Journal of Social Work in Long-Term Care* (The Haworth Social Work Practice Press, an imprint of The Haworth Press, Inc.) Vol. 2, No. 3/4, 2003, pp. 411-422; and: *Culture Change in Long-Term Care* (ed: Audrey S. Weiner, and Judah L. Ronch) The Haworth Social Work Practice Press, an imprint of The Haworth Press, Inc., 2003, pp. 411-422. Single or multiple copies of this article are available for a fee from The Haworth Document Delivery Service [1-800-HAWORTH, 9:00 a.m. - 5:00 p.m. (EST). E-mail address: docdelivery@haworthpress.com].

KEYWORDS. Culture change, nursing homes, template

INTRODUCTION

Culture change has become a buzzword for the 21st century. It has been identified as an essential element of quality assurance and is seen as a major contributor to the successful recruitment and retention of frontline, as well as clinical, management and administrative staff. Earlier in this publication Gibson and Barsade outlined a useful framework for understanding the dimensions of organizational and cultural change in a nursing home. The case studies described in Section 3 of this volume provide an overview of the range and interventions as well as the issues related to implementing a model program. The challenge for providers, workers, consumers and policymakers, however, is to ensure that culture change becomes a normative and ongoing process in all nursing homes and that exemplary practices become a reality, rather than simply a model program, in the day-to-day operations of these organizations.

The insights and perspectives presented in this article result from this author's research and policy analysis in the area of workforce development over the past 15 years (Stone, 2001; Stone and Wiener, 2001). This includes a review of the empirical literature on culture change and other recruitment and retention strategies across long-term care settings, informal discussions and focus groups with administrators, directors of nursing and frontline workers in several states, findings from an expert panel focused on this issue, and the results of a recent evaluation of the Wellspring model of quality improvement in Wisconsin (Stone et al., 2002).

The purpose of this article is to review the issues related to creating an organizational culture in nursing homes that optimize staff recruitment and retention potential and that enhance quality of care and quality of life. The article begins with a generic discussion of the merits of model replication and the barriers to successful implementation. This is followed by a discussion of the dimensions of successful culture change, regardless of the model or models emulated. The article concludes with a summary of the major elements required to ensure the initial and ongoing success of culture change efforts in nursing homes.

SELECTING A MODEL

A review of the literature, anecdotal evidence from nursing home administrators, management staff and workers, and empirical evaluation activity underscore the fact that there is no recipe for organizational culture change. Despite this observation, however, policymakers, providers, workers and consumers are searching for the "magic bullet," a cookie-cutter approach to creating an organizational culture and work environment that fosters good intra-staff communication and staff-resident relationships, that empowers frontline workers and that creates positive links with families and the surrounding community. The nurse and nursing assistant shortages have accelerated policymaker and provider interest in developing the "culture change primer"; regulators see this as a panacea for quality of care problems and insurers are experimenting with discounting liability insurance premiums for providers who adopt a particular model (e.g., Wellspring, the Eden Alternative).

There is, however, no perfect model of organizational and culture change. As the case studies in this volume underscore, there are a range of models being tested and implemented in the field. While they may have key elements in common, the approaches to culture change–including the tools and protocols used and the change agents employed to implement the models–vary greatly. Nursing homes also vary significantly on a number of dimensions including size and auspice, resident characteristics, staff characteristics (particularly the level of ethnic and racial diversity), geography, and funding sources. As was learned in the Wellspring evaluation, for example, there is significant intra-facility variation within chains and alliances, and even more variation across units within a particular facility.

Despite the absence of the perfect model and the variation across and within facilities, the replication literature suggests that organizations interested in real, sustained culture change begin with a living template, not just a theoretical model (Szulanski and Winter, 2002). Researchers who have examined model development and dissemination in a number of industries argue that model adoption fails because the replicators place too much trust in experts and documents, and start to improve on the model before the initial replication is completed. This includes selectively choosing only those aspects of the model that seem appropriate to the particular organization's needs or interests, tinkering with the model process, and customizing the model prematurely. Individuals trying to replicate a model frequently overestimate how much they know and tend to be overly optimistic about the potential for success.

Although perfect replication is not possible, closely copying the living template should be the goal (Szulanski and Winter, 2002). This includes duplicating key physical and environmental characteristics as well as the skill sets of staff, the tools used and the practices followed. Adaptations of the model should only occur after the organization has achieved acceptable results. Adding elements from different models or implementing a new approach before the living template is adopted is likely to sabotage the effort, add confusion to an already complex activity and usually result in failure. The advantage of the living template is that it becomes a major source of ongoing technical assistance, the functioning laboratory. (Homes that have been "Edenized," members of the Wellspring charter group and other Pioneer homes are examples of natural laboratories that can help other organizations interested in various aspects of culture change.) As others attempt to replicate the model, they must keep the template in mind and use the experiences of the innovator to stay on course.

BARRIERS TO SUCCESSFUL MODEL REPLICATION

Complex models designed to change organizational arrangements and behavior are inherently difficult to replicate. The barriers identified in the following section are particularly challenging and warrant special attention by those committed to a replication process.

First-Try Failure

Most attempts to replicate a model do not succeed the first time around. Individuals become demoralized because of overoptimistic expectations and a perception that the time and resources invested have been lost. CEOs, boards and other stakeholders become disenchanted with an approach when it does not produce quick results. Several years ago, for example, an alliance of nursing homes in Texas received a state grant to help replicate the Wellspring model. Although a number of issues precipitated the termination of the replication process, one of the major reasons was the fact that the state was expecting significant positive outcomes within one year. When the model replication failed to produce such results, the disillusioned alliance discontinued the initiative.

The Model Is Not Worth Replicating

Model programs come and go. Many are developed as research projects or as the whim of a particular administrator or management consultant. The literature is replete with examples of model interventions that produced short-term success only to have the original behaviors and processes resume once the research team completed its work (Feldman et al., 1990; Schnelle et al., 1993). It is essential that organizations interested in replicating an approach to culture change have evidence that (1) the model has been implemented systematically, (2) that the elements have been codified in some way, including tools/protocols available to assist implementation, (3) that success has been measured with reliable and valid performance indicators, and (4) that the program has a track record of sustainability.

These criteria eliminate many initiatives that have strong face value and anecdotal support, but that have not demonstrated the potential for a more systematic adoption by multiple organizations. Such activities require a more rigorous and evaluative approach to model development and dissemination but are necessary if we are going to develop and sustain a quality long-term care workforce and better quality of care and quality of life for nursing home residents.

Resistance to Change

Perhaps the most serious impediment to successful and sustained model replication is staff resistance to change. Culture change in nursing homes, for example, is a radical departure from the status quo and can be threatening to staff members who do not believe that "the system is broken." Many individuals, particularly those who have had a long tenure with the organization or who have been in a position of authority that is challenged by the new approach, will resist adoption of the model. These employees are the loudest "Nay sayers" and many will also attempt (often successfully) to sabotage the process. The qualitative interviews with Wellspring management and nursing staff indicated that the directors of nurses in several facilities were the strongest opponents of model development and implementation. In most cases these individuals were "let go" rather than jeopardize the potential for success in their organizations (Stone et al., 2002).

Culture Change Interventions Take a Long Time

Changing the nature of the work environment and interpersonal relationships takes time and is an evolving process. The charter Wellspring group, for example, has been involved in this program for seven years and the evaluation found that there is still significant variation in the extent to which the model has been implemented, particularly at the unit level. Respondents to our interviews suggested that culture change is like "brushing your teeth" or "losing weight"–the process must become normative, integrated into the fabric of the organization and constantly evolving. Most nursing homes–fighting a persistent negative image and closely scrutinized by regulators, litigators, advocacy groups and the media–do not necessarily have the patience or the time to allow culture change to take hold.

THE DIMENSIONS OF CREATING A NEW CULTURE

The nursing home workplace is very labor intensive. While technological advances have helped increase efficiency and reduce staff burden, it is the "high touch" and personal care of residents that distinguishes this setting from hospitals and other acute care settings. The nursing facility is also home to the long-stay residents, those who are not receiving post-acute services for a time-limited period. Consequently, the nature of the work culture and the social and physical environments are important contributors to quality of care and quality of life for the individuals receiving care (and their families, where applicable) as well as those providing care. No single model of culture change contains all of the elements highlighted in the following section. It is useful, however, for providers, nursing and non-nursing staff, residents and their families and the public at large, to recognize and begin to address these dimensions if we are to develop and sustain a quality long-term care workforce.

Changing the Clinical Culture

The nursing home resident population has changed dramatically over the past 15 years. Nursing staff is caring for a much sicker group of people–higher acuity levels, multiple co-morbidities, greater levels of cognitive impairment, and the need for multiple medications (Spillman et al., 1997). Nursing facilities are responsible for quality outcomes, and the federal government requires all nursing homes to collect and report resident status information related to a variety of clinical indicators through implementation of the Minimum Data Set. A recent quality initiative introduced by the U.S. Department of Health and Human Services was scheduled to provide to consumers in October 2002 national comparative information on select quality indicators to help them make better decisions about nursing home placement and to enhance quality of care monitoring.

Nursing homes, therefore, must place greater emphasis on the development and fostering of clinical knowledge and skills across all levels of nursing staff and among non-nursing staff (e.g., activity staff, dietary workers, maintenance staff). This includes the implementation of state of the art clinical protocols, ongoing in-service training related to specific clinical areas (e.g., incontinence, pressure ulcers, pain management), training in assessment and data collection, and use of data for continuous quality improvement.

The Wellspring evaluation underscored the importance of the clinical culture and the need to include all levels of staff in this process. Interviews with both nursing and non-nursing personnel indicated that the staff working in Wellspring facilities had developed new knowledge of and insights into specific clinical areas, the interaction of interventions on resident health and functional status and how their activities improved clinical outcomes. While observing formal clinical module training sessions and through informal discussions with frontline workers, the research team discovered that many certified nursing assistants had become amateur epidemiologists. They understood the importance of prevalence and incidence of specific conditions and recognized the connections between their work and clinical outcomes. The clinical training, combined with an emphasis on use of data, strengthened the critical thinking and analytical skills of the direct care staff (Stone et al., 2002).

Changing the Work Culture

Teaching and fostering clinical best practices are not sufficient to produce the level of culture change that is required to retain the workforce and to improve quality of care and life in nursing homes. In fact, as the Wellspring research team learned in its evaluation, these interventions will not be effective without changing the fundamental facility culture. Organizational change involves transforming the work environment into one that (1) nurtures staff at all levels; (2) fosters empowerment of the frontline workers and non-nursing staff; (3) promotes a collaborative approach across disciplines, units and shifts as well as up and down the organizational hierarchy; (4) provides opportunities and tools to improve communication between and across staff levels, and (5) enhances and strengthens the potential for improving interpersonal relationships between staff and residents and their families (Stone et al., 2002).

Anecdotes and empirical research have underscored the importance of the supervisor/frontline staff relationship in impeding or enhancing worker retention and the development of a quality workforce in long-term care (Banaszak-Holl and Hines, 1996; Burgio and Seilley, 1994). Consequently, nursing homes committed to meaningful and lasting culture change must begin by ensuring that staff at all levels are treated with dignity and respect and that all are given the opportunity to learn, expand their skills and expertise, exercise their authority in decision making and be accountable to themselves, their peers and the organization. While the models of job redesign and worker recognition may vary, the basic principles remain the same.

Changing the Caring Culture

Long-term care is very personal and intimate. Caregivers, particularly the direct care workers, are the "eyes and ears" of the care system in the nursing home and other settings. The nature of the interpersonal relationship between caregiver and resident is a barometer of the quality of care and quality of life provided in a facility. Clinical training and skills are not sufficient to create a caring environment. Staff at all levels must learn how to communicate with residents and their families, how to treat residents as unique individuals (not just patients) with special needs and desires, and how to use touch as an emotional as well as a physical therapeutic intervention. Caring takes time and is not possible when facilities are understaffed, when workers are constantly assigned to new residents, floors and wings, and when caregivers are not rewarded for this aspect of their job. The challenges are greater for those responsible for people with serious cognitive impairment and are further heightened where racial and cultural differences exist between staff and residents. As several articles within this volume have noted, models have been developed to address the resident/staff interactions; successful elements of these approaches should be included in efforts to implement radical culture change in nursing homes.

Changing the Residential Culture

For many individuals receiving care in a nursing home, the facility is their residence. While an increasing proportion of nursing home residents are there for a relatively short period, a significant number will remain in the facility permanently. The quality of the physical and social environment, therefore, is an essential dimension of the nursing home culture.

Some Pioneer homes (e.g., Evergreen in Wisconsin, Fairport Baptist Home in Rochester, NY, Mount St. Vincent Nursing Home in Seattle) have focused special attention on innovative environmental design as well as management transformation. These organizations have reconfigured the facility wings as "neighborhoods" using a pod design that creates a homelike feel and facilitates better interaction between residents and between residents and staff. The traditional nursing home design with the hospital-like nursing stations and institutional hallways has been replaced with completely renovated or newly built structures that emulate one's private home or apartment. These facilities also include smaller communal dining areas and lots of open space for integrating families and the larger community into the nursing home.

As described in the articles on the Eden Alternative in this volume by Thomas and Monkhouse, many organizations have enhanced the living environment with plants and animals, and support intergenerational relationships with formal programs, including co-location of day care on the nursing home property. Other organizations have been successful in transforming the institutional environment by wall-papering in bright colors, disguising the nurses stations, and adding other homelike touches. All environmentally sensitive facilities pay special attention to good lighting and acoustics for residents, particularly those with Alzheimer's disease and related dementias.

CREATING YOUR OWN CULTURE CHANGE

Given the tremendous variation in the characteristics of nursing homes, it is likely that each organization will have to adapt the features of model programs to meet its own unique needs. There are, however, a series of elements that should be in place to ensure that culture change not only occurs but also continues to evolve. These are outlined briefly below.

1. *Top leadership must be committed emotionally and financially to culture change.*

It is essential that the board, chief executive officers (CEOs) and other top-level administrative officials support the concept and understand the details involved in implementation and ongoing development. Leaders may become enamored with the fad, but only those who recognize the time and burden, including the initial psychic and financial costs, associated with implementing and sustaining culture change will be successful.

2. *Commitment must exist at all levels of the organization.*

The models that have demonstrated success in executing meaningful and sustainable culture change have been those where the staff at all levels, as well as residents and their families, have understood the need for change and have supported the necessary interventions to create a new work and living environment. Mid-level managers, in particular, often create barriers to successful implementation. Directors of nursing and charge nurses must either be "bought in" to the process or be replaced by individuals who understand and support the development of an empowering, nurturing work environment.

3. *Systems of accountability must be built-in at all organizational levels.*

Findings from the Wellspring evaluation indicate that even when the culture change process has strong support throughout the organization and the various steps in the process have been systematized and codified, foci of accountability must be established at all levels to ensure successful and sustained implementation. In the case of Wellspring, accountability was essential at the alliance level, the facility level, the care resource team level and the unit level. Much of the failure to systematically implement the Wellspring approach was attributable to lack of accountability or accountability break down at one or more levels. The problem was particularly acute at the unit level. Despite the best intentions of facility leadership, supervisors and direct care staff, a number of the facilities experienced a lack of follow-through on individual units, where the day-to-day work and caregiving actually occurs.

4. *The clinical and work culture dimensions must be integrated.*

Many nursing homes have experimented with new ways to enhance the clinical skills and expertise of staff, and to build these changes into a program of internal quality improvement. Others have focused primarily on changing the work culture, including the introduction of management practices that foster worker empowerment, the development of better channels of communication across and between categories of staff, job redesign (e.g., self-managed work teams, career ladders), and other mechanisms for creating a nurturing environment for employees and residents. The interface between the clinical culture and the work culture, however, is as important as the two separate dimensions.

In the Wellspring model, the clinical module trainings, the development of the care resource teams (CRTs), the dissemination of new knowledge and skills through the CRTs and the use of data by all staff (including the frontline workers) to compare outcomes are tools for implementing organizational change and job redesign. CNAs, dietary workers and other line staff are empowered by these new responsibilities and the authority they have to make care decisions. Wellspring, therefore, provides a living example of how clinical interventions and organizational redesign intersect to foster fundamental culture change in nursing homes.

5. *The dimensions of culture change must be codified and applied systematically.*

Many nursing homes struggle with the concept of culture change because it is viewed as "touchy feely" and without structure. In fact, culture change requires a rigorous approach that recognizes the complexity of systems change and the difficulties in transforming individual and organizational behavior. Nursing homes need a template to help them create and sustain new clinical and management structures and processes. While there is no recipe for success, organizations need a guide that provides them with a set of principles, a blueprint for how to operationalize change and the protocols and other tools to facilitate the process. They also need access to targeted technical assistance from individuals who have successfully implemented certain aspects of culture change.

6. Sustained culture change requires ongoing feedback about failures as well as successes.

Organizations must develop formal information systems and feedback loops for tracking how well the nursing home is implementing culture change. This requires systematic data collection that goes beyond the current MDS activity. As new clinical practices are introduced, nursing and non-nursing staff at all levels should receive periodic feedback on how their interventions have affected the quality of care and life of their residents. Facilities also must conduct an initial organizational assessment to ascertain their readiness for culture change and then periodically reassess their organizational status and share that information with staff so that all stakeholders recognize concretely their successes and remaining weaknesses. Special attention should be paid to worker outcomes including changes in job satisfaction and turnover.

CONCLUSION

There is no single model that will address all the aspects of culture change in nursing homes. At the same time, an organization that simply believes it can change its culture in an ad hoc way is doomed for failure. As was highlighted in this article, organizations interested in radically transforming their care, work and residential environments should begin with a living template that has successfully implemented and sustained one or more dimensions of culture change. Adaptations to that model and innovation should occur once the replication is completed and evaluated. This process requires commitment at all levels, formal mechanisms of accountability and a systematic approach to changing the culture that involves all levels of the organization. This process is also never-ending. Just as an individual must change one's fundamental eating habits to sustain weight loss, so too must organizations embrace culture change as the norm and recognize its evolutionary nature.

REFERENCES

Banaszak-Holl, J., and M.A. Hines. 1996. "Factors Associated With Nursing Home Staff Turnover." *The Gerontologist* 36 (4): 512-17.

Burgio, L.D., and K. Seilley. 1994. "Caregiver Performance in the Nursing Home: The Use of Staff Training and Management Procedures." *Seminars in Speech and Language* 15 (1): 313-22.

Feldman, R.H., A. Sapienza, and N. Kane. 1990. Who Cares for Them? Workers in the Home Care Industry. Westport, CT: Greenwood Press.

Schnelle, J.F., D. Neuman, M. White, J. Abbey, K.A. Wallstrom, T. Fogarty, and M. Ory. 1993. "Maintaining Continence in Nursing Home Residents Through the Application of Industrial Quality Control." *The Gerontologist* 33: 114-21.

Spillman, B., N. Krauss, and B. Altman. 1997. "A Comparison of Nursing Home Resident Characteristics: 1987-1996." Unpublished Paper. Rockville, MD: Agency for Health Care Research and Quality.

Stone, R.I. 2001. "Frontline Workers in Long-Term Care: Research Challenges and Opportunities." *Generations* 25 (1): 49-57.

Stone, R.I., and J.M. Wiener. 2001. Who Will Care for Us? Addressing the Long-Term Care Workforce Crisis. Monograph prepared under contract with the Office of Disability, Aging and Long-Term Care Policy, U.S. Department of Health and Human Services and support from the Robert Wood Johnson Foundation, Washington, D.C.: Urban Institute and the American Association of Homes and Services for the Aging.

Stone, R.I., S. Reinhard, B. Bowers, D. Zimmerman, C. Hawes, C. Phillips, N. Jacobson, P. Beutel, and J. Fielding. 2002. Promoting Quality in Nursing Homes: Evaluating the Wellspring Model. Final report submitted to the Commonwealth Fund, Washington, D.C.: Institute for the Future of Aging Services/American Association of Homes and Services for the Aging.

Szulanski, G., and S. Winter. 2002. "Getting It Right the Second Time." *Harvard Business Review*. January: 62-69.

Successfully Surviving Culture Change

Diane L. Dixon

SUMMARY. Successfully surviving culture change is a multifaceted process. It requires leaders to have a good understanding of "self" which helps build resilience needed during challenging times. Exploring old assumptions and beliefs about the field is groundwork for adopting new mindsets that can transform long-term care. Managing the personal side of change includes being able to let go of old behaviors and mindsets, face resistance, manage stress, and maintain balance during the unsteady times of transition. Continuous learning throughout the change process is essential. Working towards alignment of key aspects of the internal and external environment enables the whole system to change effectively. *[Article copies available for a fee from The Haworth Document Delivery Service: 1-800-HAWORTH. E-mail address: <docdelivery@haworthpress.com> Website: <http://www.HaworthPress.com> © 2003 by The Haworth Press, Inc. All rights reserved.]*

KEYWORDS. Culture change, personal change management, new mindsets, leadership

---

Diane L. Dixon, EdD, is Managing Principal of D. Dixon & Associates, LLC and Faculty Associate at University of Maryland, Office of Continuing and Extended Education and Faculty Associate, Johns Hopkins University, Business of Medicine Program.

Address correspondence to: Diane L. Dixon, D. Dixon & Associates, LLC (E-mail: didixon@erols.com).

[Haworth co-indexing entry note]: "Successfully Surviving Culture Change." Dixon, Diane L. Co-published simultaneously in *Journal of Social Work in Long-Term Care* (The Haworth Social Work Practice Press, an imprint of The Haworth Press, Inc.) Vol. 2, No. 3/4, 2003, pp. 423-438; and: *Culture Change in Long-Term Care* (ed: Audrey S. Weiner, and Judah L. Ronch) The Haworth Social Work Practice Press, an imprint of The Haworth Press, Inc., 2003, pp. 423-438. Single or multiple copies of this article are available for a fee from The Haworth Document Delivery Service [1-800-HAWORTH, 9:00 a.m. - 5:00 p.m. (EST). E-mail address: docdelivery@haworthpress.com].

10.1300/J181v2n03_16

INTRODUCTION

This publication, and indeed long-term care literature, have addressed culture change models such as the Eden Alternative, the Wellspring Model, and models related to the Pioneer Movement (Stone, 2001; Lustbader, 2000; Thomas, 1994). The focus is usually on descriptions of key components of the models and their implementation. In unusual fashion, this volume has also provided the reader with an understanding of the language of culture change. However, little is written about what leaders need to do to survive leading and managing culture change. Culture change is a major organization development intervention that requires capabilities in effective change management. Culture change is particularly difficult because it requires changing shared assumptions, beliefs, and values that have been deeply held for a long time. Every aspect of the facility, such as strategy, structure, systems, staff, organizational processes, and procedures must be aligned with the new culture. Positive relationships and communication become even more important. Changing culture is a whole system intervention. Leaders and staff must have a shared vision of the future and commitment to achieving it. Hence, these are complex undertakings that occur in the midst of environmental complexity. Time, energy, and stamina are needed for a change of this magnitude. Improved quality of life for residents, patients, their families, and staff make the effort worthwhile. The issue, though, of what can leaders do to more effectively survive and lead culture change, remains a clear challenge. This chapter will focus on several simple guides and ideas intended to be helpful during this time of transformation.

FINDING STRENGTH FROM WITHIN

Leader survival starts inside the leader. Leading culture change requires inner resiliency and strength. This is only possible if long-term care leaders are willing to engage in introspection; *"Know Thyself."* Asking themselves serious questions that assists with exploring the essence of who they are is a beginning. Sample questions may include–Who am I as a person? What do I stand for? What do I believe in? What are my values? Why am I resisting change? What are my blockages? What are my hidden inner beliefs that keep me from being a better person and leader? Why do I choose to be a leader in long-term care? Continuous inquiry and self-exploration aid in building a strong inner core. This is the foundation for resilience and strength as well as authenticity.

There are several ways to engage in this type of self-inquiry. A solitary approach requires taking time for reflective thinking, asking and answering the tough introspective questions. Writing thoughts in a journal helps to organize ideas and creates a visual pattern for review and further reflection. Another alternative is to work with a trained personal coach who can facilitate a guided inquiry and development process in a safe environment. A professional colleague or friend can also play this role if they have the ability to coach and mentor effectively and maintain confidentiality.

This work helps to excavate the roots of authenticity that are centered deep within the person. Authenticity means leaders are being true to who they "really" are and their beliefs. An authentic leader is stronger and more centered because of this. They are less likely to lose focus and be swept away by the swirl of complexity so inherent in the health care environment. It is essential for effective change management to be authentic. Unfortunately, there are many examples in which members of the long-term care community–residents, families, and staff–have become disillusioned because leaders send mixed messages about starting a new way of providing care but continue doing things the old way. For example, an administrator announces to staff that the facility is moving to a decentralized model of care, yet care continues to be delivered in a centralized manner. A nurse manager establishes care teams and talks about participative decision-making but continues to make authoritarian decisions. Or the social work director who talks about the need for interdisciplinary teamwork continues to isolate his/her staff from interdisciplinary meetings. When leaders say one thing and do another, they are not authentic. These confusing signals create mistrust and heighten resistance in the environment. Leaders such as those cited in the examples often have not faced their own resistance to change. To create conditions for effective change, leaders on all levels must face how they themselves may be blocking organizational progress (Varney, 2001).

The *Tao of Leadership: Leadership Strategies for a New Age* (Heider, 1985, p. 51) highlights the importance of knowing self:

> The leader who is centered and grounded can work with erratic people and critical group situations without harm. Being centered means having the ability to recover one's balance, even in the midst of action. A centered person is not subject to passing whims or sudden excitements. The centered and grounded leader has stability and a sense of self. One who is not stable can easily get carried away by the intensity of leadership and make mistakes of judgment or even become ill.

Leaders are enabled to be more focused and maintain inner strength which helps them keep their balance in the midst of culture change. Shifting paradigms and mindsets becomes a little easier from a grounded center.

SHIFTING PARADIGMS AND MINDSETS

> The real voyage of discovery consists not in seeking new landscapes but in having new eyes. (Proust, 1982)

The culture change movement in long-term care challenges the long-held assumptions about how care should be delivered. It really is a paradigm shift in that the whole pattern of beliefs, values, techniques, and models shared by the long-term care community are moving in a different direction (Kuhn, 1970). A new worldview about what the nature of nursing home and post-acute care should be in the 21st century and beyond is emerging. Real paradigm shifts are most difficult as they require a common framework and belief set by the entire industry about the field. There is always a push and pull between old and new among multiple constituencies. Gaining consensus on the common ground is rarely easy.

As the new paradigm is evolving, so too are leaders' mindsets. For instance, an administrator's mindset is that individual's fundamental beliefs about how to lead and manage a facility. It includes the administrator's thoughts, attitudes, values, and choices about long-term care in general and specifically about how to provide care for residents and/or patients. How one sees the world is filtered through their mindset. Anderson and Anderson (2001) suggest that there is a "seamless connection between mindset and reality." Stemming from the mindset is what we perceive in reality, and our reality is our experience of what we perceive. Hence, mindsets have a powerful influence on how leaders see themselves and their roles.

UNDERSTANDING MINDSETS

Before leaders can move to a new mindset, they must first understand their current one. Chart 1 illustrates differences between traditional views of long-term care organizations and new viewpoints.

Characteristics of the new mindset, are indicative of culture change in long-term care. This is a major shift in how leaders have been trained and conditioned by the industry to think and act. Viewing nursing homes and other post-acute organizations as complex adaptive systems means seeing them as living, complex systems that adapt to a changing environment (Zimmerman, Lindberg, and Plsek, 1998). They have the ability to self-organize in high turbulence and disequilibrium characteristic of health care. This uncertainty and unpredictability requires leaders and staff to think and act differently. To be able to adapt quickly to change makes it necessary for facilities to have flat and

CHART 1

Traditional Mindset	New Mindset
• Organizations as Machines	• Organizations Adaptive Systems
• Tight Hierarchy	• Flat and Fluid Hierarchy
• Functional/Silo Thinking	• Cross-Functional Teams/Across Boundaries
• Centralized Decision-Making	• Decentralized Decision-Making
• Command and Control	• Participative Management/Empowering
• Certainty and Predictability	• Uncertainty and Unpredictability
• Order	• Complexity/Radical Change
• Linear, Stepwise Thinking	• Non-Linear, Cyclical Thinking

fluid hierarchies. If, as all of the models suggest, nursing homes are to be more resident-centered, decision-making must be decentralized and participative. This creates staff and resident empowerment. They need to work across boundaries in teams to develop innovative methods for delivering care in budget strained environments. Step-wise linear thinking is not as effective because change occurs in cycles and processes need to be ongoing. Hence, shifting mindsets is a deliberate process that requires letting go of aspects of old viewpoints that are outmoded.

LETTING GO

Moving to different worldviews is difficult because it requires letting go of portions of the old that do not work in the new context. It means taking a serious look at the behaviors associated with the old ways of thinking and determining what has to be changed and how. Letting go means that the sense of security associated with old identities and commitments is shaken. Dr. William Bridges (1991) suggests four possible reactions to "letting go":

- Disengagement—Old cues which reinforce roles and patterns of behavior are broken up. In culture change initiatives leaders and staff must change patterns of behavior to become resident-centered. Residents and families must also adjust to the resident-centered approach. *Personal Inquiry: What are the behavioral cues associated with the institutional model? What are the behavioral cues associated with the resident-centered model? What do I need to do to shift my behavior to become more resident-centered?*

- Disidentification–In breaking up former roles and patterns of behavior, leaders, residents, families, and staff lose their old identities. This means that they must develop new identities associated with culture change. For example, residents who have become so accustomed to not being involved in decisions that affect their living arrangements may be initially uncomfortable when asked for their ideas about change in the facility. They need to shift from a passive identity to an active and engaged identity that enables them to be full participants in their living environment. Leaders who have adopted a traditional command and control identity now must change to a leader that is a teacher, facilitator, change agent, listener, empowerer in the new culture. *Personal Inquiry: What was the old identity? Why am I experiencing difficulty in letting go of the old identity? What is the new identity? What aspects of the new identity are difficult for me? Why? What will help me adapt to the new identity?*
- Disenchantment–Some people become disenchanted when they recognize that the old view of long-term care was sufficient at one point in time but is not now. It means hard work to change to new ways of living and doing for residents, families, leaders, and staff. They also become upset when they feel that the past is being disrespected. *Personal Inquiry: What old views are hard to let go of and why? Was I a "bad" administrator a decade ago? What can I do to manage my feelings about change more effectively? What can I do to cope with my feelings of loss? What can I still hold to while embracing the new?*
- Disorientation–Changing strategies, structures, systems, processes, and procedures is complex and can be confusing as well as overwhelming. *Personal Inquiry: What is the source of confusion? Am I moving too fast? What action plan can be developed to help organize my thoughts and learning needs? Do I have a personal change management strategy and action plan?*

The personal inquiry process involves becoming more self-aware by taking time to reflect on the questions and answers. Investigating feelings in this manner can be enlightening. As mentioned previously, the process can either be solitary or facilitated by a coach. Engaging in personal inquiry enhances the process of comprehending why certain feelings are being experienced during different stages of letting go. With this understanding leaders, staff, residents, and families are better able to manage relinquishing long-held traditions that are no longer viable.

ADOPTING NEW MINDSETS

Adopting new mindsets begins with looking at mind habits. This means becoming aware of what one thinks on a regular basis and developing new routines of thought as appropriate. Costa and Kallick (2000) suggest that there are sixteen "Habits of Mind" that move people to enhanced effectiveness. They are: persisting; thinking and communicating with clarity and precision; managing impulsivity; gathering data through all senses; listening with understanding and empathy; creating, imagining, innovating; thinking flexibly; responding with wonderment and awe; thinking about thinking; taking responsible risks; striving for accuracy; finding humor; questioning and posing problems; thinking interdependently; applying past knowledge to new situations; and remaining open to continuous learning. Embracing this positive approach can help leaders to manage dilemmas and uncertainties more constructively. Mind conditioning supports efforts to develop new mindsets.

Practical approaches begin with "mindfulness" exercises (Kabat-Zinn, 1994). Thinking about what you think is the practice of developing an acute awareness of thoughts. There are two ways to accomplish this. One is to reflect in action on current thoughts and the other is to reflect on action about past thoughts. A daily practice of reflection tones the mind. Another exercise is personal introspection and self-assessment. For example, long-term care professionals using the traditional mindset characteristics discussed above as criteria, can assess how closely their thinking aligns to them. One question might be–*How often do I think that I am the only one who can make the best decisions?* This question is linked to command and control as well as centralized decision-making mindsets. Once an understanding is gained of how one thinks then another exercise is to determine what needs to change. That is, what new mind habits need to be acquired. A written plan with reasonable and attainable behavior change objectives can lead to concrete actions for change. Periodic monitoring of the plan assists with ongoing conditioning of the mind and thinking. Hence, adopting new mindsets is a conscious effort that requires self-discipline.

The business case for doing this work is summarized by this premise from Leebov and Scott (1990) in *Health Care Managers in Transition*. The premise states, "Your belief system and the way you conceptualize your management role, that is, your 'mindset,' powerfully influence your managerial behavior and effectiveness." These authors further suggest that thoughts, actions and results affect each other and thereby create a dynamic process that individuals have the power to influence and change. Hence, leaders and staff in long-term care must examine their mindsets before they can affect real change in the industry and in their facilities.

THE PERSONAL SIDE OF CHANGE MANAGEMENT

Surviving culture change also means managing the personal side of change. Effective change management must balance both organizational system and personal journeys. The system and business journey includes the shared vision, mission and values; redesign of facility structures, systems, and processes; and staff changes. We tend to spend the majority of our time focusing on steps for creating a restraint-free environment, for example, and not on the human impact of doing this on residents, families, staff, and leaders. Each culture change intervention brings with it a new set of responsibilities and ways of working that have personal consequences that left unmanaged can cause problems for both individuals and the collective. Managing the personal consequences involves individuals reviewing their purpose and vision and determining whether they are aligned with the culture change initiative. It means adjusting to new assumptions, beliefs, and values associated with resident-centered care which is hard work and takes time. In addition, new knowledge and skills must be attained for implementing the various resident-centered models. This requires unlearning and relearning which can be difficult for some individuals. Associated with all of this are the inner obstacles, fear, and anxiety that individuals often experience when adapting to culture change, or indeed, any change. Hence, managing the human impact of change demands equal attention and is imperative.

MANAGING RESISTANCE TO CHANGE

The typical response to resistance to change is to resist it. That is, to avoid dealing with it either as an individual or as a leader dealing with staff reactions to change. A more effective response is to embrace resistance and manage it. In this way, a window of understanding opens that allows resistance to become a source of information about what about obstacles need to be overcome. If you run away from it then you can not comprehend what is blocking movement towards culture change. Rick Maurer (2000) in the *Building Capacity for Change Sourcebook* suggests that "resistance is a natural part of change." Exploring resistance begins with leaders. They need to understand the roots of their own resistance before they can work effectively with other members of the long-term care facility's community. On the other hand, leaders must grasp the staff's perspective on culture change and listen compassionately. To explore reasons for resistance there are key areas of inquiry that might be helpful. Leaders can engage staff in meaningful dialogue and ask these questions: *Did you get the information that you needed? Do you disagree with the information or ideas? Are you confused about information or ideas? Are you afraid that you will lose control or status? Do you feel that you do not have the skills and knowledge? Are your reactions based on prior events that have nothing to do with this current change?* (Maurer, 2000). This level of inquiry can help to uncover the deep reasons for resistance and smooth the transition for moving forward.

There are several tips for embracing resistance to enhance acceptance. Active listening expands understanding of the staff's feelings about change. Clear reasons for change and articulation of the future direction helps staff to gain commitment. Open, honest, and factual communication throughout the culture change process limits resistance. Staff empowerment through participation is an esteem booster and utilizes their full potential. A demonstration of caring and compassionate behavior lets staff know that they are important. Finally, honoring the past because it has many lessons from which all can learn validates the important work and care that has come before.

MAINTAINING BALANCE AND MANAGING STRESS

Maintaining balance and managing stress during major culture change in facilities can be a real challenge. But it is also an opportunity to enhance life/work balance by engaging in positive life practices. Focusing on how to keep spirit, mind, emotions and body healthy is key to the balancing act. Loehr and Schwartz (2001) indicate that building capacity in these areas helps leaders understand the importance of recovering energy. In change of this magnitude, a great deal of energy is expended. This is why there are frequent discussions about being tired or exhausted in facilities. It is essential to balance expending energy with energy recovery. Taking time to stop, breathe, and meditate for a few minutes can have a restorative effect that is re-energizing. Slowing down to reflect for just a couple of minutes can shift a collision course of ideas in the mind to being able to refocus again. Resting the mind is as important as resting the body. Building mental capability is more than just intellectual development. It is about conditioning the mind to achieve its fullest capacity.

There is a mind-spirit connection. What we think is directly linked to the spirit. Some might say that there is no room for "spirit" at work. But to the contrary, caring for the elderly is all about the spirit. Spirit is that inner vitality. It is the light that shines deep within that fuels energy and life. The very essence of every long-term caregiver's ability to provide compassionate care is rooted in his/her spirit. Therefore, it must be nurtured as a key part of the balancing process. Regular spiritual check-ins may involve taking private time for self-inquiry by asking and answering basic questions such as–*What keeps my inner light burning? What motivates me to live and work? What can I do to maintain my spirit?* A nurtured spirit is determined, motivated, and resilient. Reflection is an important component of this spiritual awakening process.

Emotional balance is also an essential component of life/work management. Cooper and Sawaf (1998), in *Executive EQ: Emotional Intelligence in Leadership and Organizations*, state:

> It is emotional intelligence that motivates us to pursue our unique potential and purpose, and activates our innermost values and aspirations, transforming them from things we think about to what we live.

Being able to balance emotions is a vital source of positive direction and energy that moves people to a higher level of purpose. Long-term caregivers whose work is so directly linked to values of service and caring more than ever can benefit from exploring their own core values. As the industry continues to transform, the impact of transition really tests emotions. There is a direct connection between emotional wellness and the ability of leaders to be fair, build trust, and act with integrity. These can be trying times, but if professionals are emotionally sound, they can weather the storms of change.

Avoiding the "Stressed-Out Leader Syndrome" means managing stress appropriately (Dixon, 1999). Adequate physical activity and exercise helps minimize stress. Breathing effectively, body alignment, stretching, strengthening, and aerobic exercise are all part of building a physical capacity regimen. Balance is also achieved through proper nutrition and diet. Getting enough sleep is important too. Chronic sleep deprivation adds to the stressed-out syndrome and throws the human system out of balance. The physical component of balance requires ongoing attention.

Maintaining balance and managing stress means viewing life and work as a series of circles in rotation seeking symmetry. The inner circle comprised of spirit, mind, emotions, and body act as the center of gravity. The outer circle includes the forces of life and work–home, family, work, co-workers, community, and friends, etc. The ideal is to embark on the journey to becoming a whole person which requires reflection, inquiry, and positive action to continuously seek balance. One might question what this has to do with culture change in long-term care. The reality is that this is the heart and soul of the transformation. If long-term care leaders and staff are to be able to actively re-create facilities into more compassionate, caring, and resident-focused environments, then they must be taking care of themselves.

CREATING BALANCED ENVIRONMENTS

Surviving culture change is not only an individual endeavor but a collective effort shared by everyone in the facility. The environment must be conducive for residents and staff to adapt and cope with the multiple facets of facility transformation. Balanced leaders are more likely to be able to create environments that promote holistic wellness. Leaders create the milieu and set the cultural tone through their actions. They must role model the behaviors that they expect. The balanced leader provides support for residents, families, and staff. This can be accomplished in several ways. Providing education about spiritual, emotional, and physical wellness teaches important skills and expands knowledge in these areas. Educational options include traditional teacher led classroom experiences or self-directed learning aided by books, posters, videos, and computer-assisted programs. Leaders can also provide individual coaching and mentoring as needs are identified on any aspect of wellness. Bringing in specialists, such as massage therapists, yoga teachers, meditation instructors, nutritionists, fitness experts, etc., to facilitate sessions with residents, families, and staff not only furnishes vital support but helps boost morale. These actions demonstrate that leaders really care. Finally, when internal resources are not sufficient or available, employee assistance programs can provide counseling and other related assistance. In sum, positive results from culture change are more likely in healthy, balanced environments in which holistic wellness is practiced.

CONTINUOUS LEARNING

Continuous learning is the transparent currency of personal change management. It paves the way for achieving culture change. Learning is a key to surviving change. Leaders and staff can benefit from making a personal commitment to acquire new knowledge, skills and competencies needed to work in the new long-term care paradigm. Learning can be in several forms. For example, the formal leadership and staff development that takes place in workshops or seminars, whether offered in-house or by local and regional long-term care associations, can provide opportunities for education about new models of care delivery.

Informal learning abounds if individuals are open to it. For instance, in staff meetings learning occurs when a problem is discussed about difficulties with making the transition to the neighborhood model of care. In this scenario, the administrator or department head can take time for dialogue about the reasons for the difficulties, then ask a simple question—*What are the lessons learned from our experience?* In this way, learning is embedded in the normal facility routine. Learning in action is an important component of managing change. It is a method that helps continuous adaptation throughout the process. Recognizing that learning can take place anytime, anywhere, whether in hallways, conversations, or in the heat of a crisis, is key. Mistakes and failure also offer tremendous learning opportunities. The ongoing inquiry into what is being learned is a gateway to gaining new insights. As learners in the moment, leaders and staff are growing in ways that assist them in becoming not only better at their jobs but also as effective people.

As mentioned previously, reflection is a method for tapping into insights, intuition, and experience that can promote learning. The ability to pause and think about what has happened, the implications, and the inferences has tremendous learning value. Reflection is a portal for self-knowledge and also knowledge acquisition about the culture change. It does not mean going away but rather taking a few minutes during the course of the day to think about what is being or has been experienced. Active participation in the ongoing cycle of engaging in action, reflecting, and learning helps ensure ongoing openness to new ideas.

MANAGING THE "IN-BETWEEN" TIMES

Don't be swayed by external circumstances. (Chodron, 2001)

The "in-between" times are not easy to manage during culture change. This is the phase during which traditional mindsets and attendant behaviors related to long-term care culture have not been completely relinquished and new mindsets and behaviors have not been adopted. It is a zone of ambiguity and uncertainty. There is misalignment during "in-between" times because all components of the change don't quite fit together. Conflict and inconsistency are higher. There is both internal and external misalignment. From the internal perspective, strategy, staff, skills, structure, systems, and procedures may be incongruent with a social model of care. The board of directors may not fully understand their governance role during the culture change process. Regulations and a survey process that mirror the traditional institutional model of long-term care create external misalignment.

MANAGING INTERNAL MISALIGNMENT

Staff who are unable or not committed to the new assumptions, beliefs, and values in a transforming facility are misaligned. For example, department heads may be having trouble giving up command and control behaviors so characteristic of hierarchical structures in nursing homes. Staff empowerment is likely to be threatening to a nurse manager who is not accustomed to sharing power with nursing assistants. On the other hand, nursing assistants may have difficulty accepting power and knowing how to manage it in a decentralized environment. They may not trust the nursing director or administrator and resist being asked to make decisions. Staff misalignment can impede progress towards the new culture and create unrest in the facility.

Leaders have several options for managing staff misalignment. It begins with making sure that staff fully understand the reasons for change and the benefits for them—*What is in it for them?* Their involvement early in the change process helps ensure a higher level of commitment. It is important to remember that the people doing the job know best how to change it to fit the new environment. Clear expectations about new roles and responsibilities are important. Often staff resist change because either they do not understand what is expected of them or they are insecure about their ability to do work differently. Education and training are essential for supporting staff and helping them to gain confidence needed to meet new expectations. Periodic performance feedback along with adequate mentoring and coaching helps staff to adjust to different roles. Teambuilding further aids staff with the adjustment to new relationships in a more interdisciplinary, cross-functional care delivery structure. These are just a few actions leaders can take to manage staff misalignment in the culture transition process.

However, there will be some staff who will not be able to adjust. In these cases, a combination of supportive, specific performance feedback and counseling that will help these individuals move out of the facility may be the best alternative. It is critical to note that how the leader manages these situations is being observed by other staff and sends cultural cues to them. Therefore, leaders are role models for the change that they expect and must act accordingly.

MANAGING EXTERNAL MISALIGNMENT

External misalignment is one of the key challenges facing long-term care leaders on all levels. The board of directors play a key role in facilities that are transforming their cultures. Collaboration between the facility board and leadership is critical for articulating the vision, mission, and core values that guide the organization toward a new model of care. It is critical that they understand the implications of culture change for the facility. The board also needs to comprehend and embrace a potentially different governance role. They will need to be more visionary, systems thinkers, team players, and action-oriented

(Goodspeed, 1998). The board and leaders of facilities are partners in culture change. Senior leaders enhance this relationship with effective communication and education.

Other external alignment issues are regulations and the survey process. They are still aligned with the traditional views of long-term care. Sometimes regulations and surveyors who monitor their implementation have unrealistic expectations (Levenson and Crecelius, 2001). This disconnect between old and new creates a tremendous amount of stress for both leaders and staff as they work hard to move toward more enlightened resident-centered environments. Managing external misalignment is very difficult because the ability to change the issues is out of the sphere of direct control. However, leaders and staff can control the manner in which they look at the situation. That is, if they choose to look through a more positive lens, long-term care staff will likely develop creative approaches that are realistic for facilities. The focus becomes *"How can we do this in a realistic manner within the realm of the facility's capabilities?"* rather than *"We can not do this."* The other option is advocacy which means getting involved with state, regional, and/or national associations that lobby legislators for more adequate and realistic regulations and reimbursement. The challenge and opportunity is to be tenacious with culture change and not be swayed by the external forces that have the potential to throw it off course.

PACING CHANGE

The "in-between" times can be paradoxically fast and slow. They are fast times because so much must be accomplished in a short timeframe. Leaders and staff often struggle with adapting to the internal demands of transitioning to a new environment while simultaneously keeping up with the external changes that impact facilities. These can be slow times when the different components of the facility and staff do not move quickly enough to adopt the new way. Also, facility cultures do not change overnight. It takes time to transition to a new organizational culture. Hence, pacing change management becomes very important. The speed of change must be balanced between fast and slow. Finding the appropriate speed is a continuous process. Moving too fast to change strategy, systems, structures, and procedures can create havoc in facilities. Leaders, staff, residents, and families can only manage so much change at a time and can become overwhelmed. Culture change is a process that affects every aspect of facility life and must be paced appropriately. It requires a pacing discipline that allows adequate time for adapting, reflecting, learning, measuring and evaluating results. In addition, the ability to readjust when unexpected events occur that put the facility in an unstable state is essential.

While it is difficult to generalize a specific timeframe for total culture change because of variances between different facilities and the dynamic internal and external environment, leaders should expect to invest several years in this effort. Time pacing considerations for the culture change cycle include a readiness assessment, review of readiness assessment outcomes, strategy development, implementation, measurement and evaluation, and feedback about results achieved. Within each of these phases are multiple actions that require buy-in and commitment. Full participation and active involvement from all levels of the facility and community is another time factor but essential for success.

CLOSING REFLECTIONS

Surviving culture change is a multifaceted process. It requires the discipline of self-management. The keys to managing self are positive thinking, practicing self-responsibility, being purposeful, communicating effectively, building positive relationships, living a balanced life, and demonstrating personal integrity. A continuous process of inquiry, reflection, and learning are tools for ongoing resilience and focus. The obstacles faced are teachers and lessons for how to move forward. Remaining focused in unsteady times requires being centered and grounded as the *Tao of Leadership* described. Personal and professional alignment are ingredients of integrity and authenticity. Perseverance, passion, and energy are needed to make a difference in the field. This is meaningful because contributing to the transformation of long-term care provides a vital service to the frail elderly, families, and the community.

REFERENCES

Anderson, D. & Anderson, L.A. (2001). *Beyond change management.* San Francisco, CA: Jossey-Bass/Pfeiffer.

Bridges, W. (1991). *Managing transitions.* Reading, MA: Addison-Wesley Publishing Company.

Chodron, P. (2001). *The places that scare you: A guide to fearlessness in difficult times.* Boston, MA: Shambhala Publications, Inc.

Cooper, R.K. & Sawarf. (1998). *Executive EQ emotional intelligence in leadership and organizations.* New York: Perigee Book.

Costa, A.L. & Kallick, B. (2000). Describing 16 habits of mind. Retrieved from *http://wwwhabits-of-mind.net.*

Dixon, D.L. (1999). Leadership and the human touch. *Subacute Care Today.* 2(5), p. 39.

Goodspeed, S.W. (1998). *Community stewardship: Applying the five principles of contemporary governance.* Chicago: AHA Press.

Heider, J. (1985). *Tao of leadership: Leadership strategies for a new age.* New York: Bantam Books, p. 51.

Kabat-Zinn, J. (1994). *Wherever you go there you are.* New York: Hyperion, p. 3.

Kuhn, T.S. (1970). *The structure of scientific revolutions.* Chicago: The University of Chicago.

Leebov, W. & Scott, G. (1990). *Health care managers in transition.* San Francisco, CA: Jossey-Bass Publishers, p. 18.

Levenson, S. & Crecelius. (2001). SOM shortcomings: Why the heart of the survey is missing some beats. *Caring for the Ages.* 2(11), p. 36.

Loehr, J. & Schwartz T. (2001). The making of the corporate athlete. *Harvard Business Review.* 79(1), p. 120-128.

Lustbader, W. (2000). The pioneer challenge: A radical change in the culture of nursing homes. In Noelker, L.S. & Harel, Z. (Eds.) *Linking quality of long-term care and quality of life.* (pp. 185-203). New York: Springer Publishing Company, Inc.

Maurer, R. (2000). *Building capacity for change sourcebook.* Arlington, VA: Maurer & Associates, p. 2.2.

Proust, M. (1982). *Remembrances of things past: Cities of the plain.* New York: Random House/Knopf.

Stone, R. & Reinhard, S. (2001). Evaluating the Wellspring Program as a Model for Promoting Quality of Care in Nursing Homes, Research Executive Summary. Washington, DC: *Institute for the Future of Aging Services.*

Thomas, W. (1994). *The eden alternative: Nature, hope and nursing homes.* Columbia, Missouri: University of Missouri.

Varney, D. (2001). Personal reflections on leadership: Achieving sustained superior performance. *Vital Speeches of the Day, 67 (10), 313-317.*

Zimmerman, B., Lindberg, C. & Plsek, P. (1998). *Edgeware: Insights from complexity science for health care leaders.* Irving, Texas: VHA Inc.

Index